Image-guided Laser Ablation

Claudio Maurizio Pacella
Tian'an Jiang · Giovanni Mauri
Editors

Image-guided Laser Ablation

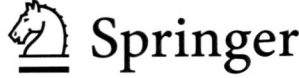

Editors
Claudio Maurizio Pacella
Department of Interventional Radiology
Ospedale Regina Apostolorum
Albano Laziale
Rome
Italy

Tian'an Jiang
Department of Ultrasound
Zhejiang University
Hangzhou
China

Giovanni Mauri
Division of Interventional Radiology
European Institute of Oncology
IRCCS
Milan
Italy

ISBN 978-3-030-21747-1   ISBN 978-3-030-21748-8   (eBook)
https://doi.org/10.1007/978-3-030-21748-8

This Springer imprint is published by the registered company Springer Nature Switzerland AG
The registered company address is: Gewerbestrasse 11, 6330 Cham, Switzerland

Foreword

My initial introduction to Claudio Pacella and his team was in 2005 when I visited his hospital near Rome to get a better understanding of the work that he was doing. As an associate editor of the *Journal of Vascular and Interventional Radiology* (*JVIR*), I had the pleasure of reviewing and commenting on his hepatic ablation article in the journal and was so impressed by his results in treating liver lesions that I booked a trip to Italy that year. Claudio's team of physicians are incredibly talented and devoted, most importantly to patient care but also to the highly technical future of laser medical therapy, which remains a largely unrecognized alternative for the obliteration of various tumors at low risk and high success. I was able to experience several ablation procedures and, afterward, sat among Claudio's team, listening to their stories and dreams. Amazingly, they asked me to discuss my experience with laser therapies, which I did (totally unrehearsed). It was a fulfilling afternoon of observing and engaging with an incredible team of clinicians. After leaving Italy, my team successfully initiated a laser ablation program for a variety of tumors culminating in local and national recognition on US television and news reports. With mentoring from Dr. Pacella and team, our Texas program is now robust with over 300 procedures performed to date. My team owes much of its success and drive to Dr. Pacella and his associates, and we continue to consult them frequently.

Dr. Pacella's book, like laser itself, is coherent in both time and location—he provides us with current information regarding laser ablation of tissue while dividing his chapters into anatomic regions. This organization allows the reader to focus on the diseases relevant to them and obtain the latest information as to the technique and follow-up required for the treatments applied. While laser ablation (LA) for some circumstances is well-established (liver, lung, thyroid, brain), some newer indications are quite promising. LA with MRI guidance and MR thermometry is progressing rapidly in the United States as the initial treatment for low- to intermediate-risk prostate cancer and LA for pancreatic lesions, locally metastatic lymph nodes, and arteriovenous malformations seems to have a bright future. Endoscopic or endovascular laser procedures are ripe for development aided by non-traumatic delivery of a small-diameter fiber. Spinal cord tumors are particularly suited for the precise MRI-guided ablations as well as paraspinal nerve ablations for long-term pain reduction. I, like Claudio, believe that the possibilities are endless for such minimally invasive laser procedures.

I am confident that the reader will find this book highly informative as they begin or continue a path down the road of laser ablative procedures. The beginning chapters are especially important in providing the physician with a bedrock of basic knowledge regarding the physics of laser and the biology of energy-guided heat transfer in human tissue. Subsequent chapters provide specific information optimizing results for LA in a variety of locations.

As an interventional radiologist (IR), it is important to have a variety of ablative techniques in one's "toolbox" (microwave, radiofrequency, cryoablation, electroporation, focused ultrasound, and others). However, laser ablation is a particular technique with numerous advantages including MRI compatibility with real-time ablation monitoring, small probe diameter reducing complications of percutaneous insertion, and a poorly understood but real reduction in pain post-procedure.

As Claudio would surely agree, the addition of laser to the IR toolbox is a valuable one.

Galveston, TX, USA   John Sealy
                                                                                              Eric Walser

Preface

From the last decade of the last century to our days, we have witnessed an impetuous flowering of clinical applications supported by so-called minimally invasive therapies (MIT). Among the techniques that use heat to kill neoplastic cells, the technique based on laser light appears fast, precise, and relatively insensitive to tissues and, even if less diffused than other techniques, has been successfully applied for several different clinical applications. Particularly, laser ablation, due to its physical characteristics, allows achieving very precise and reproducible ablations and is extremely versatile in its possible applications. Thanks to the use of very thin applicators, with laser ablation, it is possible to tackle with great success and safety several lesions that are difficult to reach and/or close to vital structures in the various organs. Also, in cases where the clinical condition of the patient to be treated is compromised, laser ablation represents a very safe and effective treatment modality. On the other hand, with the possibility of applying multiple fibers simultaneously, it is possible to obtain large and shaped ablative areas.

To date, there is no ablative technique which has been proven to be better than the others and none that can be used effectively in all applications. For some applications, one or the other technique can be more effective or safe. Furthermore, each technique has specific technical characteristics, advantages, and limits. Similarly, patients may have some contraindications to some ablation techniques, and indication can differ according to tumors number, size, and site. It follows that, in our opinion, the choice should be based on the characteristics of the patient, tumor, and ablation techniques. Ideally, each center should have all the techniques available to move toward a tailored approach to thermal ablation, and operators should be familiar with all the available techniques.

In the present book, the technical characteristics of laser ablation are described, and all the different clinical applications are illustrated, with high focus on the evidence present in the literature on the topic. Also, an overview on the potential of the technique and on its future possible development is provided. The book is divided into 16 chapters which, after the initials on history and technique, are dedicated to the different applications developed in these past three decades. Some applications are well established, while others are more recent and in the process of being perfected. The reader does not necessarily have to read the entire book but can read the chapter or chapters of his interest.

Rome, Italy   Claudio Maurizio Pacella
Hangzhou, China   Tian'an Jiang
Milano, Italy   Giovanni Mauri

Contents

Contributors

Daria Bottacci Elesta Srl, Florence, Italy

Luca Breschi Elesta Srl, Florence, Italy

Weilu Chai Department of Ultrasound, The First Affiliated Hospital, College of Medicine, Zhejiang University, Hangzhou, China

Giovan Giuseppe Di Costanzo Liver Unit, Department of Transplantation, Cardarelli Hospital, Naples, Italy

Francesca Di Vece Section of Interventional Ultrasound, St. Anna Hospital, Ferrara, Italy

Marco Guarracino Liver Unit, Department of Transplantation, Cardarelli Hospital, Naples, Italy

Rinaldo Guglielmi Department of Endocrinology and Metabolism, Regina Apostolorum Hospital, Albano Laziale, Rome, Italy

Tian'an Jiang Department of Ultrasound, First Affiliated Hospital, College of Medicine, Zhejiang University, Hangzhou, China

Ping Liang Department of Interventional Ultrasound, Chinese PLA General Hospital, Beijing, China

Guglielmo Manenti Department of Diagnostic Imaging and Interventional Radiology, Tor Vergata University, Rome, Italy

Leonardo Masotti Scientific Committee, El.En. S.p.A., Florence, Italy

Maria Mattera Liver Unit, Department of Transplantation, Cardarelli Hospital, Naples, Italy

Giovanni Mauri Division of Interventional Radiology, European Institute of Oncology, IRCCS, Milan, Italy

Rosaria Meucci Department of Diagnostic Imaging and Interventional Radiology, Tor Vergata University, Rome, Italy

Claudio Maurizio Pacella Department of Diagnostic Imaging and Interventional Radiology, Regina Apostolorum Hospital, Albano Laziale, Rome, Italy

Enrico Papini Department of Endocrinology and Metabolism, Regina Apostolorum Hospital, Albano Laziale, Rome, Italy

Gianluigi Patelli Department of Diagnostic and Interventional Radiology, Pesenti-Fenaroli Hospital-ASST Bergamoest, Alzano Lombardo, Italy

Tommaso Perretta Department of Diagnostic Imaging and Interventional Radiology, Tor Vergata University, Rome, Italy

Agnese Persichetti Department of Endocrinology and Metabolism, Regina Apostolorum Hospital, Albano Laziale, Rome, Italy

Paola Saccomandi Department of Mechanical Engineering, Politecnico di Milano, Milan, Italy

Sergio Sartori Section of Interventional Ultrasound, St. Anna Hospital, Ferrara, Italy

Emiliano Schena Department of Measurements and Biomedical Instrumentation, Università Campus Bio-Medico di Roma, Rome, Italy

Luigi Solbiati Department of Biomedical Sciences, Humanitas University, Milan, Italy

Paola Tombesi Section of Interventional Ultrasound, St. Anna Hospital, Ferrara, Italy

Raffaella Tortora Liver Unit, Department of Transplantation, Cardarelli Hospital, Naples, Italy

Jie Yu Department of Interventional Ultrasound, Chinese PLA General Hospital, Beijing, China

Weiwei Zhan Department of Ultrasound, Rui Jin Hospital, School of Medicine, Shanghai Jiao Tong University, Ruijin, China

Qiyu Zhao Department of Ultrasound, The First Affiliated Hospital, College of Medicine, Zhejiang University, Hangzhou, China

Claudio Maurizio Pacella and Giovanni Mauri

1.1 Introduction

Developing the theory of Albert Einstein on the stimulated emission of radiation, the American physicist Maiman first realized in May 1960 at the laboratories of Hughes Research in Malibu (California, USA) an artisan laser with a ruby crystal [1, 2]. Since then the invention has given life to all subsequent laser applications in the most disparate fields. Already in 1962 the laser found its first practical application for microsoldering during retinal surgery. Thus, historically, lasers were initially applied in ophthalmology because the eye and its interior belong to the most accessible organs thanks to their transparency. Following Meyer-Schwickerath's data on retinal-tissue-induced coagulation using xenon flash lamps [3], and the first experimental studies published by Zaret et al. [4], patients with retinal detachment were successfully treated by Campbell et al. [5] and Zweng [6]. Almost simultaneously, the first applications in dentistry started [7, 8]. At the beginning, laser treatment was limited to the application of ruby lasers. Then other types of lasers followed. To date, due to the variety of existing laser systems and the diversity of their physical parameters, each branch of surgery and medicine has been involved [9, 10]. And today, a large variety of laser procedures are performed all over the world [11–13]. Most of them belong to the family of *minimally invasive surgery* (MIS), a novel term that describes noncontact and blood-less surgical procedures. These two characteristics have mainly promoted the laser as a universal scalpel and an indispensable aid for the treatment of the most varied pathologies. Some patients and even some surgeons mistakenly considered the laser to be a sort of miraculous instrument and aroused excessive hope. This attitude led to erroneous indications and aroused unjustified hopes. In fact, laser technology has multiple effects that must always be evaluated with accurate evidence-based studies but cannot be considered valid and useful in all circumstances and in all types of pathology. For example, the heating of cancerous tissue can mean the death of the cancer cells but by using the same parameters in retinal coagulation we can burn the retina with consequent irreversible blindness. So the same effects can be good in some treatments but disastrous in other cases.

C. M. Pacella (✉)
Department of Diagnostic Imaging and Interventional Radiology, Regina Apostolorum Hospital, Albano Laziale, Rome, Italy

G. Mauri
Division of Interventional Radiology, European Institute of Oncology, IRCCS, Milan, Italy

1.2 Early Medical Applications of Lasers

In light of the fact that the ruby laser was able to produce holes in razor blades, it was natural that the very first studies focused on the vaporizing

© Springer Nature Switzerland AG 2020
C. M. Pacella et al. (eds.), *Image-guided Laser Ablation*,
https://doi.org/10.1007/978-3-030-21748-8_1

effects of this type of pulsed laser on small experimental tumors in animals [14]. Soon after, in 1964, Goldman and Wilson used the ruby laser to destroy a basal cell epithelioma in humans [15]. In the same year Minton reported his results on the use of a very powerful pulsed neodymium laser in two experimental tumor systems [16, 17]. The CO_2 laser was the first laser to be used in a gastroenterological application to treat rectal cancer using a rigid rectoscope [18]. The CO_2 laser was the first to be used in the treatment of bleeding erosions in the stomach by means of a cystoscopic control in laparotomy [19]. Nath in 1973 demonstrated the potential of argon and Nd-YAG lasers transmitted through fiberoptic waveguides within flexible endoscope to stop gastrointestinal bleeding [20], while Kiefhaber, in 1977 reported on the efficacy of the Nd-YAG laser as a means of stopping bleeding and obtain hemostasis in a large series of patients [21]. In the early 1980s, bronchoscopists published data on the efficiency and effectiveness of the Nd-YAG laser in recanalizing obstructed bronchi or the trachea blocked by tumors [22]. Finally, data on the use of flexible endoscopes to recanalize the esophagus obstructed by tumor masses have been reported [23].

Many of the clinical applications of lasers in gastroenterology require output powers varying from a few hundreds of joules as for hemorrhages to some thousands as happens in the palliation of an esophageal or rectal tumor (it is typically about 5000 J). Immediately below the beam, if the powers and energies are sufficient, some parts of the tissue will vaporize while the adjacent ones will undergo necrosis. The depth of the vaporized tissue will depend on the amount of total energy applied while the extent of the damage in the remaining tissue will depend much more on the wavelength of the laser light used. These clinical applications are not the object of this book and therefore refer our readers to books or dedicated works. Here we discuss the important advances achieved by reducing the 50–80 W Nd-YAG laser powers used to stopping bleeding or debulking advanced and obstructive tumors at only 1–2 W. This methodology is known as interstitial hyperthermia, and its use

with the Nd-YAG laser was reported for the first time in 1983 by Bown [11]. Interstitial therapy has opened a completely new range of lesions to laser treatment. The idea is very simple. Instead of dispensing light from a contactless fiber or a tip in contact with the tissue surface, the fiber is inserted directly into the target organ. In this way, the maximum response can be achieved within the organ with little surface effect apart from the small hole required for fiber insertion. This can be extremely valuable, even if it means that it is impossible to evaluate the results of the treatment visually and immediately. In order for this to happen safely, it is essential to be able to accurately predict or monitor the nature, extent and healing of tissue damage caused by the parameters planned for treatment. This approach is more suitable for tumors of solid organs such as the liver or other organs although it could also be useful for solid wall lesions of hollow organs, such as sessile villous adenomas in the colon. When the tip of the fiber is inside the tissue, the response takes place in a very small space. If the energy is delivered at high power, the result can be drastic, because if the water is vaporized, there is no space for its exit, and this can lead to the "breaking" of the lesion due to the local increase of the pressure. Furthermore, the tip can be damaged if it gets too hot while it is in contact with biological material. Therefore, interstitial therapy can be performed with laser powers so low as to avoid vaporization while other thermal effects such as coagulative necrosis with subsequent healing by cicatrization or regeneration occur as with the high-power laser. However, since the exposure time used is long (usually a few minutes), there is the possibility that the heat delivered by the laser further expands into the tissue, causing necrosis up to 8–9 mm from the tip of the fiber. Thus, a necrotic area of 16–18 mm of diameter can be obtained inside the target organ. This can be further increased by using multiple activated fibers simultaneously by treating overlapping regions [24]. Contrary to what was reported in the literature about the low values above the recommended, we used higher laser parameters up to 3–5 W with exposure times comparable to those reported above with effects, in our opinion, that were valid and interesting, which will be possible to read in Chap. 3 of this book.

1.3   Laser Ablation

The first coagulation zone was obtained in 1983 from Bown at the National Medical Laser Centre in London in cutaneous metastasis in a patient with lung carcinoma using Nd-YAG laser light with an output power of 20 W for a time of 10 min [11]. Bown obtained an area of coagulation necrosis around the fiber inserted in the context of the tumor with a peripheral ring of tissue still vital (partial ablation). This data represents the first example of the use of laser energy as an ablation technique. The heat generated by the energy-tissue interaction (in this case the Nd-YAG laser light) around the fiber (applicator) inserted in the lesion induces irreversible damage to the tumor cells (in situ destruction). In essence, Bown with this initial in vivo experiment has done nothing but confirm what has been known since ancient times [25] on the ability to apply local heat to a specific tumor in order to kill the malignant cells that are more sensitive to heat than normal cells [26–28]. In the same way Asher in Graz (Austria), as reported personally to Heisterkamp (Department of Surgery, Erasmus University and University Hospital, Rotterdam, Dijkzigt), obtained the coagulation of an inoperable menigeal tumor, positioning a laser scalpel in the tumor mass after craniotomy using a lower output power than that normally used for cutting. The patient quickly showed an improvement in his clinical condition after an initial paralysis due to the edematous swelling of the tumor after ablative treatment [29].

Laser technology is one of the three ablation techniques that uses heat to kill cancer cells. In fact, thermal ablation therapies, such as radiofrequency, microwaves and lasers, use the energy-tissue interaction generated around an inserted applicator to adequately heat target cells to induce irreversible lesions (50–54 °C for 4–6 min is a commonly used endpoint). So, as I have already mentioned in the introductory paragraph, it belongs fully to the group of minimally invasive therapies (MIT). These techniques uses thermal (or chemical) technologies to induce cell death within the focal target tumor, ideally including an additional margin of 0.5–1.0 cm of ablation of the contiguous normal-appearing parenchyma to target while limiting damage to large amounts of normal tissue [30].

It may be appropriate here in this specific chapter to mention the different synonyms that the various authors have used over time to define this type of technique. Bown, as a pioneer, baptized the technique calling it interstitial laser hyperthermia (ILH) [31]. Amin called it interstitial laser phototherapy (ILP) to distinguish it from hyperthermia at low temperatures [32]. Interstitial laser ablation (ILA) [33], laser-induced thermotherapy (LITT) [34], interstitial laser thermotherapy (ILT) [35], interstitial laser coagulation (ILC) [29], and interstitial laser thermal ablation (ILTA) or laser thermal ablation (LTA) [36, 37] have been adopted over time by Nolsoe in 1989, from Vogl in 1995, from Tramberg in 1996, from Heisterkamp in 1999, and from Pacella in 1993 and in 2000, respectively. Each of these acronyms underlines an element of the technique as the anatomical site (interstitial), the means used (laser), the effects of treatment (coagulation) or, more properly, the destruction of substance (ablation). But following the efforts of a committee of experts who have worked for years on the standardization of terminology in order to provide an appropriate vehicle for reporting the various aspects of image-guided ablation therapy, the technique must simply be called laser ablation (LA) [38]. In fact, the committee expresses itself as follows: "The term *laser ablation* should replace terms as "laser induced interstitial tumor therapy", "laser coagulation therapy," and "laser interstitial photocoagulation." This term should be used for all types of ablation using light energy. Given multiple laser technologies and application methods, including superficial therapy (contact/noncontact mode) or transcutaneous ablation, the term "interstitial" or "direct" can be reported to clarify that the laser is applied with fibers directly inserted into the tissue" [38–40].

1.4 Historical Notes on the Use of Heat to Stop Bleeding and Destroy Tumors

Cauterization, clearly described for the first time in the ancient medical literature in Edwin Smith's Papyrus dating to 1700 BC, has been used in the treatment of breast cancers. The verb is "to burn", and the instrument used as the burning tip was a piece of wood used by the Egyptians to light fire [25]. Cautery was widely used in ancient Greek and Roman medicine and we know a considerable amount of instruments designed in different forms for different applications. The ancient cautery instruments were usually made of iron, which despite being a more perishable material than bronze was harder than the softer bronze. Cauterization was used in a wide variety of medical purposes for example, as a hemostatic or to disrupt benign and malignant tumors. The writings of Hippocrates (c. 400 BC) refer to cauterization tools as "the irons." With specific ovoid shapes they were used to destroy nasal polyps or in tubular forms protected by tubular sheaths to block bleeding from hemorrhoids in the anus. Celsius (first century AD) says that this tube must be a calamus or a ceramic tube. Ezio's descriptions in the fourth century AD on the use of cautery as a means of destroying tumors are known. Cautery remained the most used medium as a hemostatic until the sixteenth century when Ambroise Parè in 1951 popularized ligation as a method of hemostasis for large vessels after amputation. Cautery was first used in 1880 to treat bleeding from gastric ulcers in man by Mikulicz and Kuster during early operative attempts to control gastrointestinal bleeding as reported by Dieulafoy, G in Krasner, N [10].

References

1. Maiman TH. Optical and microwave-optical experiments in ruby. Phys Rev Lett. 1960;4:564–6.
2. Maiman TH. Biomedical lasers evolve toward clinical applications. Hosp Manage. 1966;101(4):39–41.
3. Meyer-Schwickerath G. [Experiments with light-coagulation of the retina and iris]. Doc Ophthalmol. 1956;10:91–118; discussion 9–31.
4. Zaret MM, Breinin GM, Schmidt H, Ripps H, Siegel IM, Solon LR. Ocular lesions produced by an optical maser (laser). Science. 1961;134(3489):1525–6.
5. Campbell CJ, Rittler MC, Koester CJ. The optical maser as a retinal coagulator: an evaluation. Trans Am Acad Ophthalmol Otolaryngol. 1963;67:58–67.
6. Zweng HC. Retinal laser photocoagulation. Trans Pac Coast Otoophthalmol Soc Annu Meet. 1964;45:423–39.
7. Goldman L, Hornby P, Meyer R, Goldman B. Impact of the laser on dental caries. Nature. 1964;203:417.
8. Stern RH, Sognnaes RF. Laser beam effect on dental hard tissue. J Dent Res. 1964;43:873.
9. Muller GJ, Roggan A. Laser-induced interstitial thermotherapy. Bellingham, WA: SPIE-The International Society for Optical Engineering; 1995.
10. Krasner N. Lasers in gastroenterology, Lasers in medicine and surgery series. London: Chapman & Hall Medical; 1991.
11. Bown SG. Phototherapy in tumors. World J Surg. 1983;7(6):700–9.
12. Muschter R, Hofstetter A. Technique and results of interstitial laser coagulation. World J Urol. 1995;13(2):109–14.
13. Schena E, Saccomandi P, Fong Y. Laser ablation for cancer: past, present and future. J Funct Biomater. 2017;8(2):E19.
14. McGuff PE, Bushnell D, Soroff HS, Deterling RA Jr. Studies of the surgical applications of laser (light amplification by stimulated emission of radiation). Surg Forum. 1963;14:143–5.
15. Goldman L, Wilson RG. Treatment of basal cell epithelioma by laser radiation. JAMA. 1964;189:773–5.
16. Minton JP, Ketcham AS, Dearman JR, McKnight WB. The effect of neodymium laser radiation on two experimental malignant tumor systems. Surg Gynecol Obstet. 1965;120:481–7.
17. Minton JP, Ketcham AS, Dearman JR, McKnight WB. The application of pulsed, high-energy laser radiation to multiple intra-abdominal tumor implants in experimental animals. Surgery. 1965;58:12–21.
18. Versheuren RSC. Technical problems of carbon dioxide laser surgery in the rectum. In: Goldman L, editor. The biomedical laser. New York: Springer; 1981. p. 163–74.
19. Youmans CR Jr, Patterson M, McDonald DF, Derrick JR. Cystoscopic control of gastric hemorrhage. Arch Surg. 1970;100(6):721–3.
20. Nath G, Gorisch W, Kiefhaber P. First laser endoscopy via a fibreoptic transmission system. Endoscopy. 1973;5:208–13.
21. Kiefhaber P, Nath G, Moritz K. Endoscopical control of massive gastrointestinal hemorrhage by irradiation with a high-power Neodymium-YAG laser. Prog Surg. 1977;15:140–55.
22. Toty L, Personne C, Colchen A, Vourc'h G. Bronchoscopic management of tracheal lesions using the neodynium yttrium aluminium garnet laser. Thorax. 1981;36(3):175–8.

23. Fleischer D, Kessler F, Haye O. Endoscopic Nd:YAG laser therapy for carcinoma of the esophagus: a new palliative approach. Am J Surg. 1982;143(3):280–3.
24. Steger AC, Lees WR, Shorvon P, Walmsley K, Bown SG. Multiple-fibre low-power interstitial laser hyperthermia: studies in the normal liver. Br J Surg. 1992;79(2):139–45.
25. Breasted J. The Edwin Smith surgical papyrus. Chicago, IL: University of Chicago; 1930.
26. Jacques SL. Laser-tissue interactions. Photochemical, photothermal, and photomechanical. Surg Clin North Am. 1992;72(3):531–58.
27. Castren-Persons M, Schroder T, Lehtonen E. Sensitivity to Nd:YAG induced laserthermia is a cell-type-specific feature not directly related to tumorigenic potential or proliferation rate. Lasers Surg Med. 1996;18(4):420–8.
28. Bhuyan BK, Day KJ, Edgerton CE, Ogunbase O. Sensitivity of different cell lines and of different phases in the cell cycle to hyperthermia. Cancer Res. 1977;37(10):3780–4.
29. Heisterkamp J, van Hillegersberg R, Ijzermans JN. Interstitial laser coagulation for hepatic tumours. Br J Surg. 1999;86(3):293–304.
30. Ahmed M, Brace CL, Lee FT Jr, Goldberg SN. Principles of and advances in percutaneous ablation. Radiology. 2011;258(2):351–69.
31. Masters A, Bown SG. Interstitial laser hyperthermia in tumour therapy. Ann Chir Gynaecol. 1990;79(4):244–51.
32. Amin Z, Bown SG, Lees WR. Local treatment of colorectal liver metastases: a comparison of interstitial laser photocoagulation (ILP) and percutaneous alcohol injection (PAI). Clin Radiol. 1993;48(3):166–71.
33. Nolsoe CP, Torp-Pedersen S, Burcharth F, Horn T, Pedersen S, Christensen NE, et al. Interstitial hyperthermia of colorectal liver metastases with a US-guided Nd-YAG laser with a diffuser tip: a pilot clinical study. Radiology. 1993;187(2):333–7.
34. Vogl TJ, Muller PK, Hammerstingl R, Weinhold N, Mack MG, Philipp C, et al. Malignant liver tumors treated with MR imaging-guided laser-induced thermotherapy: technique and prospective results. Radiology. 1995;196(1):257–65.
35. Tranberg KG, Moller PH, Hannesson P, Stenram U. Interstitial laser treatment of malignant tumours: initial experience. Eur J Surg Oncol. 1996;22(1):47–54.
36. Pacella CM, Rossi Z, Bizzarri G, Papini E, Marinozzi V, Paliotta D, et al. Ultrasound-guided percutaneous laser ablation of liver tissue in a rabbit model. Eur Radiol. 1993;3:26–32.
37. Pacella CM, Bizzarri G, Magnolfi F, Cecconi P, Caspani B, Anelli V, et al. Laser thermal ablation in the treatment of small hepatocellular carcinoma: results in 74 patients. Radiology. 2001;221(3):712–20.
38. Ahmed M, Solbiati L, Brace CL, Breen DJ, Callstrom MR, Charboneau JW, et al. Image-guided tumor ablation: standardization of terminology and reporting criteria—a 10-year update. Radiology. 2014;273(1):241–60.
39. Rosenberg C, Puls R, Hegenscheid K, Kuehn J, Bollman T, Westerholt A, et al. Laser ablation of metastatic lesions of the lung: long-term outcome. AJR Am J Roentgenol. 2009;192(3):785–92.
40. Vogl TJ, Dommermuth A, Heinle B, Nour-Eldin NE, Lehnert T, Eichler K, et al. Colorectal cancer liver metastases: long-term survival and progression-free survival after thermal ablation using magnetic resonance-guided laser-induced interstitial thermotherapy in 594 patients: analysis of prognostic factors. Investig Radiol. 2014;49(1):48–56.

Claudio Maurizio Pacella, Luca Breschi,
Daria Bottacci, and Leonardo Masotti

2.1 Introduction

In the early 1960s, after the first positive results in the development of a new generator of special light in the visible and almost-visible regions of the electromagnetic spectrum [1], several research laboratories and some industrial organizations have made available valid devices for the continuation of researches for possible practical applications [2]. Such generators go under the designation of "lasers" or optical masers; the first term is an acronym for the "amplification of light by stimulated emission of radiation." These lasers were quickly used in communication technologies and in physics experiments. The researchers soon realized that since the laser was an emitter of light with a wide range of controllable optical properties and very high intensity, it can be a new source of energy with which one can explore its effects in ophthalmology and other organs in view of biomedical applications.

From the point of view of medical interest, there are two important properties of laser light beam, the extremely collimated behaviour,

i.e., coherence in space, and its high degree of monochromaticity, i.e., coherence in time. The collimation property implies the possibility of obtaining large energy densities in narrow beams [3] for cutting and precisely ablating soft tissue. The monochromaticity permits to utilize selective interaction with tissue both for diagnostic applications and for therapeutic ones. Thanks to the fact that the laser light is coherent and monochromatic, it can be propagated in a very thin flexible optical fiber (200 μm in diameter or less) and can be used to reach every part of the body and deliver substantial amount of energy even over long distances without significant losses. So, lasers are sophisticated light sources capable of yielding large amounts of energy to vital tissues with great precision [4].

The laser is based, among other involved phenomena, on the spontaneous emission of photons characteristic of excited atoms or molecules. Each of the emitted photon can stimulate the emission of a couple of identical and coherent photons mainly from nearby excited atoms or molecules. In this way a cascade effect is activated that could amplify the number of coherent photons. But the non-excited atoms or molecules tend to absorb the emitted characteristic photons, so that to activate the amplification of photons effect most of the atoms must be in the excited state. According to the thermodynamic statistics laws, equilibrium in an isolated medium implies that the number of nonexcited particle population

C. M. Pacella (✉)
Department of Diagnostic Imaging and Interventional Radiology, Regina Apostolorum Hospital, Albano Laziale, Rome, Italy

L. Breschi · D. Bottacci
Elesta Srl, Florence, Italy

L. Masotti
Scientific Committee, El.En. S.p.A., Florence, Italy

© Springer Nature Switzerland AG 2020
C. M. Pacella et al. (eds.), *Image-guided Laser Ablation*,
https://doi.org/10.1007/978-3-030-21748-8_2

is higher than that of the excited population. The required "inversion of the population" is obtained by pumping energy into the system in various forms, including electrical sources, radiation of photons of appropriate energy and the energy generated by chemical reactions. The pumped energy allows the system to sustain the amplification, and the energy that is extracted from this kind of sources is used for different applications. In this simplified and synthetic explanation it is worthwhile to mention that the directivity of the laser beam is obtained because the phenomena of the light amplification is realized into a resonant cavity equipped with two parallel mirrors at the extremities. The photons inside the cavity move, according to thermal agitation, in a random way; only the photons having the direction of movement parallel to the axis of the cavity, i.e., normal to the mirror surface, moving forward and backward, reflected each time by the mirrors, contribute to the amplification phenomenon. In fact only in this direction the stimulated emission becomes a cascade effect. This is the direction of propagation of the beam of photons which are extracted from the cavity through one of the two mirrors. The mirror from which the output energy is transmitted is made only partially reflecting for this purpose, so that only a fixed percentage of the impinging photons are reflected back inside the cavity; the others come out of the resonant cavity.

2.2   Laser-Tissue Interactions

The nature of the effects of the interaction of the laser light with the tissues depends on many factors: mainly the laser wavelength, the laser power, the exposure time, the pulse duration and repetition frequency (when pulsed emission is used), the beam characteristics, the physical properties of the tissue and the optical applicator features [5]. In living tissue the final biological effect depends not only on what happens to each particular portion of tissue exposed to the light beam, but also on what happens in the surrounding areas, as these will determine the type of response to local thermal insult and how it will evolve towards necrosis or healing. Therefore, it is essential to observe the entire volume of the affected tissue from the beginning of exposure to the end of the treatment and then to the subsequent evolution of the tissue. It is relatively easy to evaluate the effects of a laser like a CO_2 laser, whose beam is absorbed into a very thin layer of water (0.1 mm), since the most evident and interesting effect for surgical applications is tissue vaporization to obtain cutting or ablation or hemostatic effects precisely. With deeper penetrating beams, like those of the Nd:YAG laser, the situation is more complex [4].

The range of laser-tissue interaction effects that can be produced is very wide. We limit mentioning only three important effects utilized for medical applications: (1) thermal effects: (a) vaporization, (b) necrosis, (c) coagulation; (2) photochemical effects: photodynamic therapy; (3) mechanical effects: lithotripsy [4, 6]. In this chapter and in the remaining chapters of the book, we will not deal with photochemical or mechanical effects but only with the thermal effects that underline the mechanisms of tumor destruction. The thermal effect is the main laser-tissue interaction. The light is emitted at a specific wavelength that determines the property of the laser when it is interacting with the biological tissue. The laser acts as a means of delivering light energy into tissue where it is transformed into heat. Within tissue, light can be reflected, transmitted, scattered or absorbed. Only absorbed energy can produce biological effects; reflection, transmission and scattering determine where the light goes, and, consequently, the areas in which it can be absorbed. All factors that influence the ablative effect resulting from temperature increase due to heat generation must be taken into account during treatment in order to ablate the tumor with no risks of damaging healthy surrounding tissue. Among these, the penetration depth, defined as the tissue depth needed to absorb 63% of the incident light intensity, is the most important parameter. The penetration depth is typical of each laser type because it depends on the light wavelength and on the characteristics of the tumor and of the surrounding healthy tissue [7]. As we said before laser lights which are strongly absorbed by biological soft tissue are used for superficial treat-

Fig. 2.1 The drawing shows that a high depth of optical penetration is required to treat deep tumors (Courtesy of Elesta Srl, Calenzano, Florence, Italy)

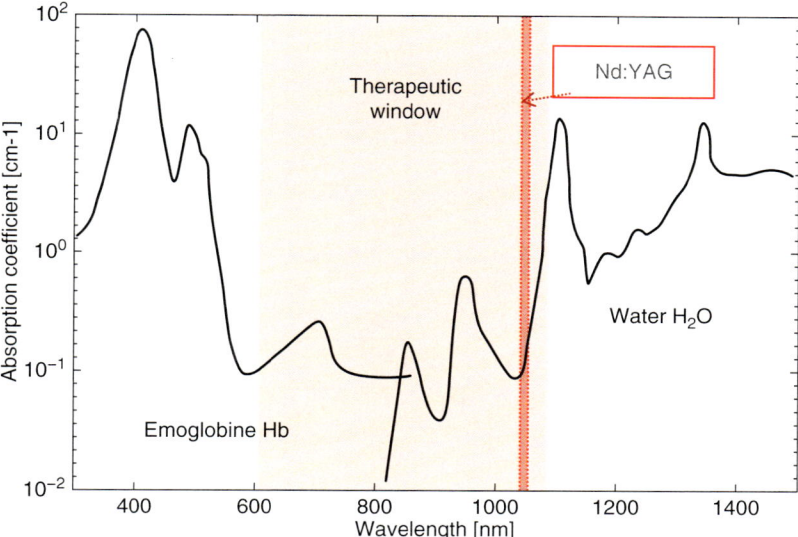

ment. Conversely, in order to treat deep tumors, a high optical penetration depth is required (Fig. 2.1). This is the reason why, in clinical practice, different lasers are used to obtain different effects. The operator must choose the laser (wavelength) and its setting most suitable for the purposes that he or she wants to obtain during the procedure [8].

LA can be performed by using the laser emission in continuous wave (CW) or pulsed mode (PW). In continuous wave, the laser power level is ranging from 2 to 3 W up to 30 W (and the treatment time range is from a few minutes to more than 20 min) [9]. In pulsed mode the laser energy is intermittently released in a series of pulses, the pick power, i.e., the power level of each pulse, is higher in comparison with the CW emitting laser but the average power has a level comparable with that of the CW laser.

2.2.1 Tissue Alterations Due to the Temperature Increase: Thermal Dosimetry

It should be noted that increasing the tissue temperature by setting the laser at a higher level and/or longer treatment time the dimensions of the ablated tumor does not increase proportionally

[10]. This nonlinear relationship between laser settings and the amount of ablation is due to the mechanism by which the ablation is obtained. For most applications involving temperatures where tissue coagulation necrosis is achievable within an exposure time from seconds to minutes, generally the NIR light part of the spectrum is used. One of first mathematical models that takes into account the various elements involved in the process of biological heat transfer (biotransfer) is the Pennes model. This model also takes into account the role that the flow of blood circulating in vascular networks in the context of the tissue plays as a source of heating or sink (cooling effect)[1] [11]. This model can be further

---

[1]The Pennes equation was developed around 1948 [11] and, in the years to follow, it has been deeply analyzed and reinterpreted also at the mathematical level. Pennes conducted a study on a mathematical model based on the energy balance of an arbitrary volume of tissue. In this model the energy transfer is due to the phenomenon of conduction, metabolism and movement of blood or convection. In more detail, it takes into account many parameters including the thermal conductivity of the tissue—the capacity of the tissue to conduct heat, the rate of perfusion and the specific heat capacity of the blood, the specific heat and the mass density of the tissue, the density of the absorbed power—the external heat input to the tissue or the energy released from the outside, and again the heat generated by tissue metabolism (generally negligible compared to other heat inputs), the tissue and arterial

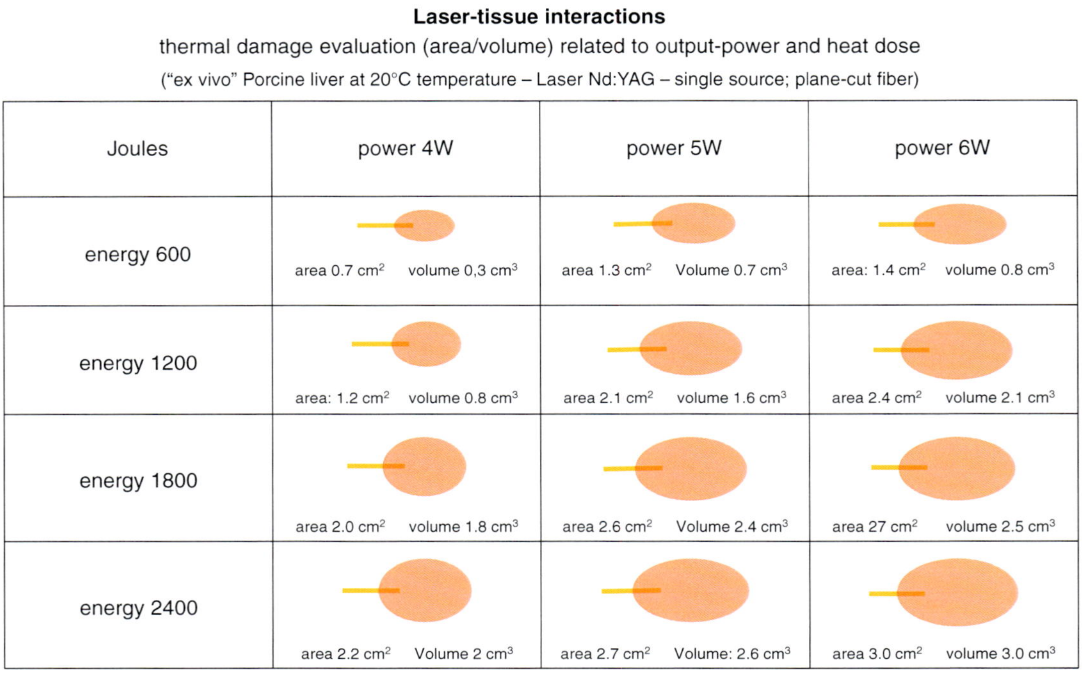

Laser-tissue interactions
thermal damage evaluation (area/volume) related to output-power and heat dose
("ex vivo" Porcine liver at 20°C temperature – Laser Nd:YAG – single source; plane-cut fiber)

Joules	power 4W	power 5W	power 6W
energy 600	area 0.7 cm² | volume 0,3 cm³	area 1.3 cm² | Volume 0.7 cm³	area: 1.4 cm² | volume 0.8 cm³
energy 1200	area: 1.2 cm² | volume 0.8 cm³	area 2.1 cm² | volume 1.6 cm³	area 2.4 cm² | volume 2.1 cm³
energy 1800	area 2.0 cm² | volume 1.8 cm³	area 2.6 cm² | Volume 2.4 cm³	area 27 cm² | volume 2.5 cm³
energy 2400	area 2.2 cm² | Volume 2 cm³	area 2.7 cm² | Volume: 2.6 cm³	area 3.0 cm² | volume 3.0 cm³

Fig. 2.2 Correlation between energy transferred (heat dose) outpower and volume of thermal damage induced with single fiber in ex vivo porcine liver (Courtesy of Elesta Srl, Calenzano, Florence, Italy)

exploited for treatment planning and to develop a model for real-time monitoring and controlling of procedures of LA guided by magnetic resonance (MR-g LA) [12].

The complex mathematical description based on Arrhenius rate analysis allows us to estimate cell death as a function of both temperature and exposure time [13–15] (Fig. 2.2). Assuming a body temperature of 37 °C, no measurable effects are observed for the next 5 °C above this. The first mechanism by which tissue is thermally affected can be attributed to conformational changes of molecules. These effects,

blood temperatures over time—the kinetics of heat transfer caused, respectively, by thermal conduction (fats and proteins) and convection (blood flow). Alternative theoretical models have been studied to describe the characteristics of heat transfer of tumors more accurately, considering the "thermally significant" blood vessels, but the bioheat transfer (BHTE) serves as a good starting point. The balance equations are linear and, therefore, the tissue studies can be solved by various methods. For this last reason, the Pennes equation is universally recognized as the equation of human warmth ("bioheat equation").

accompanied by bond destruction and membrane alterations, are commonly classified with the term hyperthermia for the temperature interval ranging from approximately (42–50 °C). If such a status is maintained for several minutes, a significant percentage of the tissue will undergo necrosis. Beyond 50 °C, a measurable reduction in enzyme activity is observed, resulting in reduced energy transfer within the cell and immobility of the cell. Consequently, certain repair mechanisms of the cell are also disabled. Thereby, the fraction of surviving cells is further reduced. At 60 °C, denaturation of proteins and collagen occurs which leads to coagulation of tissue and necrosis of cells (Fig. 2.3). At even higher temperatures (>80 °C), the membrane permeability is drastically increased, thereby destroying the otherwise maintained equilibrium of chemical concentrations. At 100 °C, the intra- and intercellular water molecules begin to vaporize. The great heat of water vaporization is advantageous since the generated steam takes away the heat and helps prevent any fur-

Fig. 2.3 The drawing shows the critical temperature for cellular death (Courtesy of Elesta Srl, Calenzano, Florence, Italy)

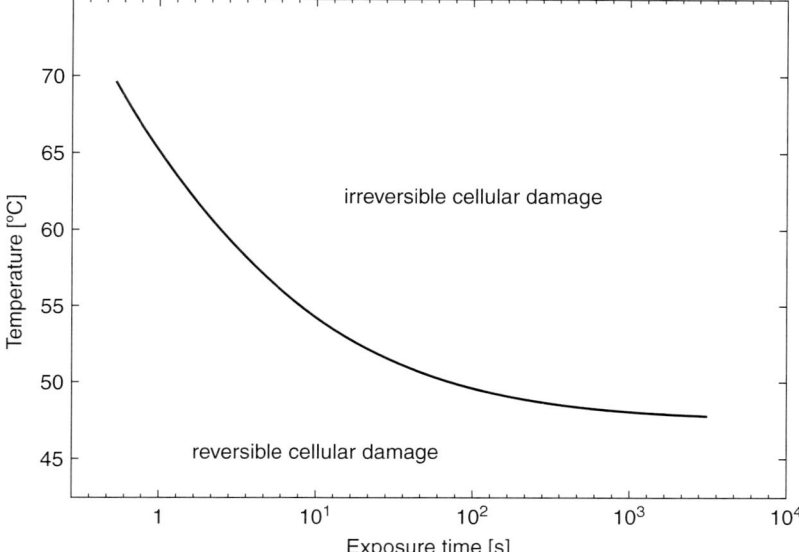

ther increase in the temperature of the adjacent tissue. Due to the strong increase in volume during this phase transition, gas bubbles are formed which induce sudden mechanical breakage and thermal decomposition of tissue fragments. Once all the water molecules have been vaporized and the laser exposure continues, the temperature continues to increase. At temperatures above 100 °C, carbonization occurs which is observable by the black appearance of a thin superficial layer of the adjacent tissue and by smoke escape. Over 300 °C sublimation or fusion may occur depending on the target material. Sublimation occurs when the target material is a soft biological tissue. This phase transition from solid to gas generates a cavity around the applicator at the expense of a portion of the energy supplied by the laser light. In other words, when the tissue is completely dehydrated, further heating produces a very thin film of carbonized tissue on the surface of this cavity (Fig. 2.4). The carbonized film with the further increase in temperature, due to continuous exposure to laser light, sublimates and enlarges the cavity. The inner cavity continues to increase until the intensity of light (photons per unitary surface) decreases to a level that is no longer capable of giving rise to sublimation. The energy of light continues to heat the internal surface which, in turn, by conduction mechanism, transmits heat to the surrounding tissue which is cooled by contact with healthy tissue perfused by blood. After a certain exposure time, the energy supplied to the tissue no longer has the effect of enlarging the volume of the ablated area; so the amount of ablated tissue increases with a nonlinear and less efficient behavior.

2.2.2 Equipment for LA

2.2.2.1 Laser Source
Superficial treatments, as previously said, require CO_2 lasers, thulium lasers or holmium lasers (Ho:YAG) with wavelengths of 10,600, 2016 and 2100 nm, respectively, with lower penetration (from about 0.1 mm to almost 1 mm). Neodymium:YAG lasers (1064 nm) have been the most widely used for decades due to the excellent penetration (millimeters) of its light into deep tissues and, therefore, very suitable for successfully treating internal tumors (Fig. 2.1). During the 1980s, advances in solid-state lasers allowed the creation of portable water-cooled devices, but with the semiconductors diodes of the 1990s, lasers became even smaller and more compact. Such systems weigh less than 20 lb.

Fig. 2.4 The surgical postoperative specimen shows the area of coagulation necrosis that surrounds the central elliptical area of carbonization (Courtesy of Elesta Srl, Calenzano, Florence, Italy)

Laser-tissue interactions
heat-dose and treated volume with a single fiber

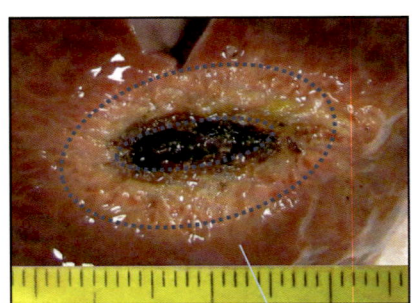

Experimental Set-Up (ex vivo):
Tissue: porcine liver
Basal Tissue Temperature: 20°C
Power:5W
Energy: 600÷4,800J
Plane-cut fiber: 300μm
1 plane-cut fiber used

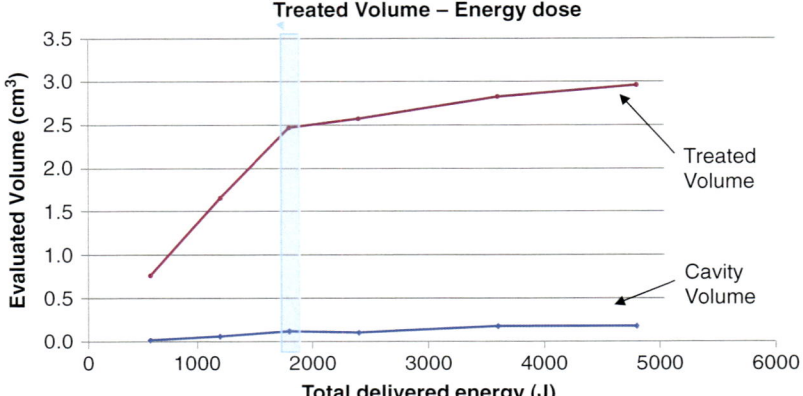

Currently, most LA procedures use Nd:YAG (λ = 1064 nm) or semiconductor diode lasers (λ = 800–980 nm) operating in the range of 2–40 W and use a standard 110/220 V socket and are air cooled. These lasers do not require water cooling, do not require pump lamps, and they, hence, are also more cheap and easier to maintain than the first lasers.

2.2.2.2 Laser Transmission and Cooling
The laser applicator must be inserted into the tumor in a minimally invasive way; it must be stable and allow maximum light transmission. Optical fibers are used to deliver the laser light with high efficiency; they are very small in diameter (few tenths of a millimeter) and are flexible, allowing to reach every part of the body via natural apertures or by very small diameter needles. An efficient device is the one that is able to obtain maximum volume of ablated tis-

sue for a given amount of laser energy. For this purpose an accurate design of the applicator is very important. The emission characteristics of the optical applicator play an important role in the geometry of the damaged tissue. Laser energy is delivered to the site of interest interstitially and percutaneously. Images obtained with real-time ultrasound imaging, computed tomography (CT), fluoroscopy or magnetic resonance imaging are used to guide the applicator through the tissue to the context of the lesion to be treated.

In some laser applications a diffusing tip fiber is used, which is designed to radiate light radially over a length of 0.5–2.5 cm in order to heat simultaneously and symmetrically large isotropic volumes of tissue. Diffusing tip fibers often incorporate small, dispersed particles, such as gold or titanium dioxide, into a mixture of elastomers such as a silicone epoxy resin. Both the diffusive material and the epoxy resin must be able to withstand high temperatures. The distribution of the light emitted along the entire length of the diffusing fiber can be modulated by varying the diffusion properties, i.e., via varying the particle concentration or size along the whole diffuser according to Beer's law; for example, a region with a high concentration of particles followed by a region of lower concentration can be used to obtain a fairly constant emission along the length of the diffuser.

The optical fiber for delivering the laser light consists of a silica-based core with a thin surrounding coating also made of silica or a hard polymeric material. The fiber is enclosed in a jacket, often made of fluoropolymer or polyamide-type materials, whose purpose is to provide a nonstick surface for the coagulated tissue and provide strength and flexibility. The optical fibers used for ablation have a diameter of 400–600 μm and can transmit large amounts of energy over a long distance with minimal losses (for MR imaging–guided procedures the fiber can be 10 m long). Bare fibers with the distal surface emittent are used for LA applications. Appropriate design and production of the applicator's emitting surface allows to reduce the power density and the temperature on their surface and of the tissue that is in contact with it as well as to increase the possibility to check the geometry of the damaged tissue [16]. These fibers operating at powers of the order of 2–4 W for 15 min slowly heat large volumes of tissue with minimal vaporization and carbonization of

the irradiated area [17, 18]. Experimental study in rat tumor found that the maximum lesion diameter produced with this fiber was 1.6 cm [19]. Others have confirmed that the maximum achievable lesion size by a bare fiber is approximately 2 cm [20]. Of course the lesion size is also dependent on the type of tissue and tumor. These fibers are ideal for treating small lesions in a suitable anatomical location using a fine-bore (21- to 23-gauge) cannula/needle for access. We ourselves used this type of fiber in the 1990s and in the first 5 years of 2000 and successfully treated tumors at risk-sites and in locations difficult to approach because of close proximity to vital structures. Using a power setting of 3–5 W with exposure times of 6–10 min with four 21-gauge introducers and fibers of 300 μm, appropriately positioned to create a square configuration in the context of the tumor nodule, spaced 1.5–1.8 cm, we have effectively ablated hundreds of tumors with sizes up to 4 cm [21–23] (Fig. 2.5) (see also Chap. 3).

In the same period, other researchers used quartz diffusing laser fibers with cylindrical shaped applicators with larger diameters. The light is emitted on the whole diffusing surface usually at a power setting of between 4 and 10 W [24–26]. Laser energy is distributed with minimal intralesion variation, producing a large volume of coagulative zone, with minimal carbonization [27–30]. Subsequently, other applicators have been designed and validated, such as zebra applicators [8, 31], or sapphire-tipped applicators in order to

Fig. 2.5 Introducer sheath and optical fiber: the drawing and the image show the introducer needle and the flat-tipped bare fiber. A schematic drawing indicates the laser beam. The caliber of the introducer and of the fiber are shown in the drawing (Courtesy of Elesta Srl, Calenzano, Florence, Italy)

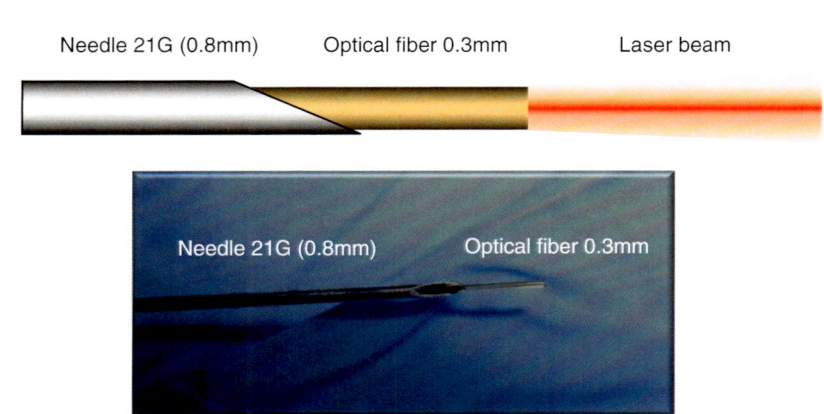

Needle 21G (0.8mm)   Optical fiber 0.3mm   Laser beam

Needle 21G (0.8mm)   Optical fiber 0.3mm

Fig. 2.6 The figure shows how the water-cooled device is constructed. It consists of two concentric tubes that create a cavity where a cooling fluid (saline) flows. The innermost tube houses the optical fiber with a distal diffusing tip of 10 mm. Note how the ablated area in a live pig liver does not show the central carbonization zone (Courtesy of Elesta Srl, Calenzano, Florence, Italy)

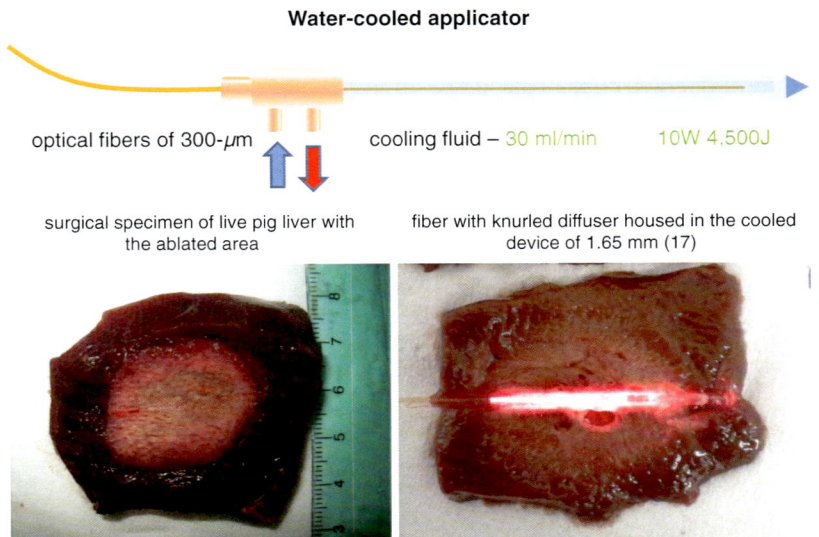

limit the carbonization around the tip of the fiber [32, 33] and to penetrate with the ablation more deeply into the tissue [28, 30, 34]. Finally, various solutions based on the development of cooled applicators have been proposed [29, 35–40]. To obtain large areas of coagulation both with flat-tipped fibers and with cooled devices, multiple applicators were simultaneously used [22, 23, 35, 41].

Since high light intensities increase the risk of producing the carbonization of the tissue nearest to the applicator and of damaging itself, the cooling of the laser fiber was introduced with the dual purpose of reducing these limitations and at the same time with purpose of obtaining larger coagulation areas. The cooled tip fibers are now a promising technology for an approach of the ablative technique even if being more expensive [42]. Most of solutions of this new technology are based on the adoption of a dual-lumen design to circulate the cooling liquid (often a physiological solution at room temperature) around the fiber during the procedure (Fig. 2.6). These systems allow

control of the temperature of the tissue nearer to the applicator, avoiding early generation of a highly dehydrated area and obtaining in this way a larger volume of ablation. In the case that the laser light source that impinges the tissue is too intense, the temperatire reaching the surface layer will be so high that the tissue will lose by evaporation all the water intra- and intercellular and it becomes very poorly transparent to the laser light and poorly heat conducting, so that very soon the heat produces carbonization followed by sublimation of the soft tissue. If we use a lower level of laser light intensity, we make the dehydration take place more slowly because the water abandons the tissue gradually and it is partially replaced by water coming from the farthest layers of the tissue. The longer the transparency time of light and heat conduction, the more the phenomenon approaches the "reduced heat cooking mode" as we know from the barbecue hobby that a violent fire give you a carbonized superficial layer but not total cooking of the internal parts. On the contrary when putting the meat more far from the fire (i.e., lower intensity heat source) one obtains completely cooked meat also on the inside. The current cooled applicators operating at 980 nm are able to obtain lesions up to 3 cm with an appropriate combination of power, exposure times and type of irradiated tissue. The cooled applicator implies that a negligible part of the energy coming from the laser source is lost because the cooling liquid draws away part of the heat from the system. During the same treatment session, multiple ablations are possible so that larger areas of ablation can be achieved by simply pulling the applicator back or advancing it forward; this is possible with bare fiber applicators. To generate even larger lesions safely and to reliably deliver the greatest energy needed, when the apparatus used is equipped with several independent laser sources, various applicators can be positioned and activated in a selectable sequence separately or simultaneously. Power settings of 25–30 W can achieve tissue coagulation zones of 4–6 cm as maximum diameters [43, 44]. A large diameter (3 mm) of the cooled fiber necessitates wide bore cannula (9- to 11-gauge) for percutaneous insertion and positioning.

Because this is not the place to discuss widely the RMN guidance system, however, a mention on this topic deserves to be made to the reader. Since the technique that uses laser fibers does not require metal applicators, it becomes compatible with MR even with higher field strengths (>1.5 T). Despite the costs and complexities inherent in working in the MR environment, magnetic resonance imaging has many advantages for performing thermal therapy procedures such as LA. Magnetic resonance imaging gives us an extraordinary contrast between soft tissues and it is able to give us functional images and information on tissue metabolism. Furthermore, the optical fiber does not affect or degrade the quality of the images acquired during the procedure. MR images can be acquired in almost real time on any arbitrarily chosen plane. This has advantages in the optimal planning of the procedure with more precise monitoring and controlling of the treatment area and of nearby critical structures. After therapy delivery, in addition to the routine relaxation mechanisms (T1 and T2 weighing), it is possible to use changes in many parameters, such as tissue perfusion or diffusion, to visualize the actual extent of therapy. One of the most useful advantages of performing LA in the MR environment is the availability of periprocedural multiplanar temperature-sensitive imaging. Because modern LA delivery aims to generate lesions in tissues that have many convective heat sinks and critical structures (such as brain and prostate), the ability to visualize and to quantify tissue temperature changes can be crucial feedback for safety, efficacy and overall outcomes of these procedures. So, MR temperature imaging (MRTI) is a noninvasive method for qualitatively and/or quantitatively characterizing changes in tissue temperature [12, 45–47]. In simpler words, complete destruction of the target tumor with or without safety margin can be guided by magnetic resonance imaging. In practice, after having performed the correct positioning of the devices in the lesion to be treated (targeting) under US guidance or preferably under CT guidance, as reported by the Frankfurt group, which uses and has used this imaging technique most of all, we can perform monitoring and assessment in real time and the entire operation is concluded as soon as it is established that the target has been achieved. It will be possible to clearly observe that during the heating process the tissue adjacent to the catheter containing the fiber rapidly undergoes coagulative necrosis while the contiguous vessels are occluded and the water near the coagulated area is expelled. The heat expands into the surrounding tissue by conduction as the temperature increases (Fig. 2.7).

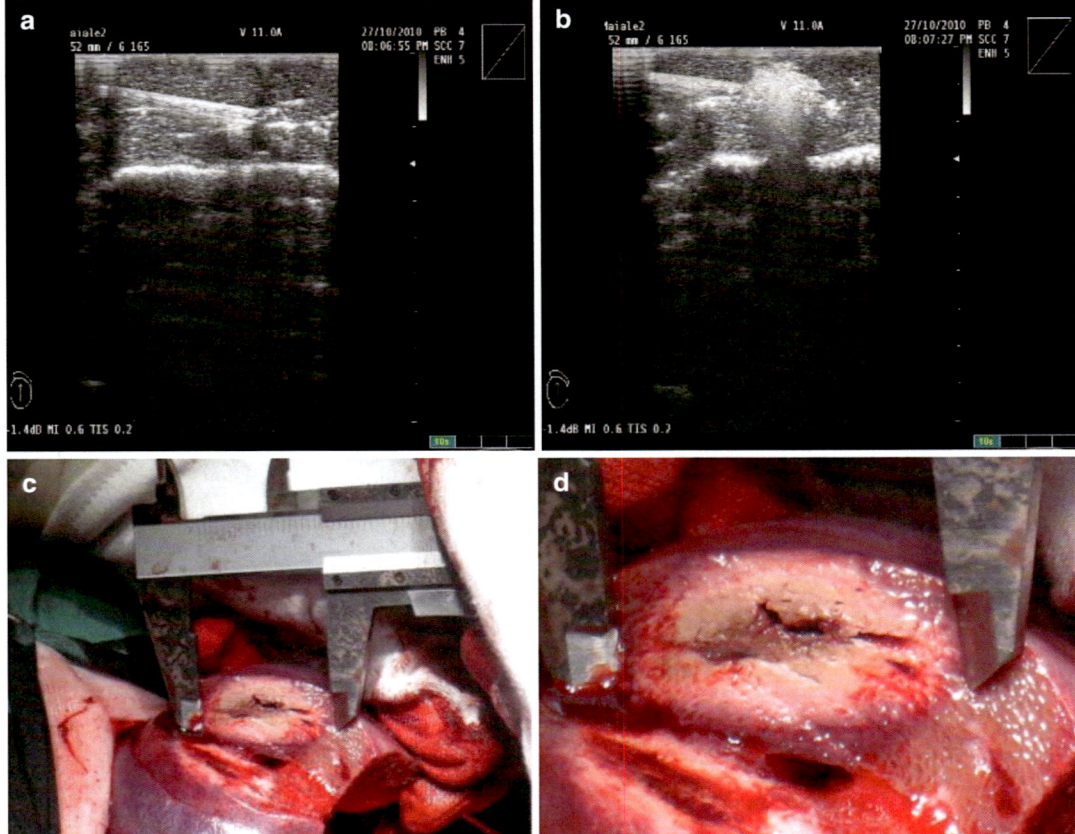

Fig. 2.7 In vivo experimentation on a healthy pig liver for the macroscopic and histological evaluation of a thermal lesion induced by LA treatment performed by a 17-gauge cooled device positioned laparoscopically and under ultrasound guidance in the liver tissue of the right lobe. (**a**) The longitudinal ultrasound scan shows a good position of the needle cannula in the hepatic tissue before starting the delivery of the thermal energy. (**b**) The ultrasound image documents the appearance of an ill-defined hyperechogenic zone in the treated area due to the vaporization of the tissue fluid and the formation of gas microbubbles. (**c, d**) The treatment has led to a thermal damage lesion around 35 × 20 mm. It should be noted that the thermal lesion has reached the surface of the parenchyma. Note the thin peripheral ring of hyperemia at the edge of the coagulated zone and the sharp boundaries between thermally coagulated tissue and normal tissue. There are no signs of carbonization. We used a one laser source with semiconductors diodes with a wavelength of 1064 nm and a 300 μm optical fiber (Echolaser, Elesta, Srl, Florence, Italy). We have delivered a total amount of 5400 J in 6 min with an output power of 15 W, taking in account a pullback added ablation. The peristaltic pump circulated the cooling fluid (water at room temperature) at a rate of 10 mL/min (Courtesy of Elesta Srl, Calenzano, Florence, Italy)

References

1. Townes CH. Optical masers and their possible applications to biology. Biophys J. 1962;2(2 Pt 2):325–9.
2. Maiman TH. Biomedical lasers evolve toward clinical applications. Hosp Manage. 1966;101(4):39–41.
3. Solon LR, Aronson R, Gould G. Physiological implications of laser beams. Science. 1961;134(3489):1506–8.
4. Bown SG. Phototherapy in tumors. World J Surg. 1983;7(6):700–9.
5. Muller GJ, Roggan A. Laser-induced interstitial thermotherapy. Bellingham, WA: SPIE-The International Society for Optical Engineering; 1995.
6. Jacques SL. Laser-tissue interactions. Photochemical, photothermal, and photomechanical. Surg Clin North Am. 1992;72(3):531–58.
7. Jacques SL. Optical properties of biological tissues: a review. Phys Med Biol. 2013;58(11):R37–61.

8. Schena E, Saccomandi P, Fong Y. Laser ablation for cancer: past, present and future. J Funct Biomater. 2017;8(2):E19.
9. Nikfarjam M, Christophi C. Interstitial laser thermotherapy for liver tumours. Br J Surg. 2003;90(9):1033–47.
10. Saccomandi P, Schena E, Caponero MA, Di Matteo FM, Martino M, Pandolfi M, et al. Theoretical analysis and experimental evaluation of laser-induced interstitial thermotherapy in ex vivo porcine pancreas. IEEE Trans Biomed Eng. 2012;59(10):2958–64.
11. Pennes HH. Analysis of tissue and arterial blood temperatures in the resting human forearm. J Appl Physiol. 1948;1(2):93–122.
12. Stafford RJ, Shetty A, Elliott AM, Klumpp SA, McNichols RJ, Gowda A, et al. Magnetic resonance guided, focal laser induced interstitial thermal therapy in a canine prostate model. J Urol. 2010;184(4):1514–20.
13. Dewhirst MW, Viglianti BL, Lora-Michiels M, Hanson M, Hoopes PJ. Basic principles of thermal dosimetry and thermal thresholds for tissue damage from hyperthermia. Int J Hyperth. 2003;19(3):267–94.
14. Dewey WC. Arrhenius relationships from the molecule and cell to the clinic. Int J Hyperth. 2009;25(1):3–20.
15. Stafford RJ, Fuentes D, Elliott AA, Weinberg JS, Ahrar K. Laser-induced thermal therapy for tumor ablation. Crit Rev Biomed Eng. 2010;38(1):79–100.
16. Schwarzmaier H-J, Goldbach T, Ulrich F, Schober R, Kahn T, Kaufmann R, et al. Improved laser applicators for interstitial thermotherapy of brain structures. In: Cerullo LJ, Heiferman KS, Liu H, Podbielska H, Wist AO, Zamorano LJ, editors. Proceedings of the clinical applications of modern imaging technology II, Los Angeles, CA, USA, 23 Jan 1994. Orlando, FL: International Society for Optics and Photonics; 1994. p. 4–12.
17. Amin Z, Donald JJ, Masters A, Kant R, Steger AC, Bown SG, et al. Hepatic metastases: interstitial laser photocoagulation with real-time US monitoring and dynamic CT evaluation of treatment. Radiology. 1993;187(2):339–47.
18. Schroder T, Castren-Persons M, Lehtinen A, Taavitsainen M. Percutaneous interstitial laser hyperthermia in clinical use. Ann Chir Gynaecol. 1994;83(4):286–90.
19. Matthewson K, Coleridge-Smith P, O'Sullivan JP, Northfield TC, Bown SG. Biological effects of intrahepatic neodymium:yttrium-aluminum-garnet laser photocoagulation in rats. Gastroenterology. 1987;93(3):550–7.
20. Matsumoto R, Selig AM, Colucci VM, Jolesz FA. Interstitial Nd:YAG laser ablation in normal rabbit liver: trial to maximize the size of laser-induced lesions. Lasers Surg Med. 1992;12(6):650–8.
21. Pacella CM, Bizzarri G, Ferrari FS, Anelli V, Valle D, Bianchini A, et al. [Interstitial photocoagulation with laser in the treatment of liver metastasis]. Radiol Med. 1996;92(4):438–47.
22. Pacella CM, Bizzarri G, Francica G, Bianchini A, De Nuntis S, Pacella S, et al. Percutaneous laser ablation in the treatment of hepatocellular carcinoma with small tumors: analysis of factors affecting the achievement of tumor necrosis. J Vasc Interv Radiol. 2005;16(11):1447–57.
23. Pacella CM, Francica G, Di Lascio FM, Arienti V, Antico E, Caspani B, et al. Long-term outcome of cirrhotic patients with early hepatocellular carcinoma treated with ultrasound-guided percutaneous laser ablation: a retrospective analysis. J Clin Oncol. 2009;27(16):2615–21.
24. Huang GT, Wang TH, Sheu JC, Daikuzono N, Sung JL, Wu MZ, et al. Low-power laserthermia for the treatment of small hepatocellular carcinoma. Eur J Cancer. 1991;27(12):1622–7.
25. Nolsoe CP, Torp-Pedersen S, Burcharth F, Horn T, Pedersen S, Christensen NE, et al. Interstitial hyperthermia of colorectal liver metastases with a US-guided Nd-YAG laser with a diffuser tip: a pilot clinical study. Radiology. 1993;187(2):333–7.
26. Vogl TJ, Mack MG, Straub R, Roggan A, Felix R. Magnetic resonance imaging-guided abdominal interventional radiology: laser-induced thermotherapy of liver metastases. Endoscopy. 1997;29(6):577–83.
27. van Hillegersberg R, van Staveren HJ, Kort WJ, Zondervan PE, Terpstra OT. Interstitial Nd:YAG laser coagulation with a cylindrical diffusing fiber tip in experimental liver metastases. Lasers Surg Med. 1994;14(2):124–38.
28. Moller PH, Lindberg L, Henriksson PH, Persson BR, Tranberg KG. Temperature control and light penetration in a feedback interstitial laser thermotherapy system. Int J Hyperth. 1996;12(1):49–63.
29. Heisterkamp J, van Hillegersberg R, Sinofsky E, Ijzermans JN. Heat-resistant cylindrical diffuser for interstitial laser coagulation: comparison with the bare-tip fiber in a porcine liver model. Lasers Surg Med. 1997;20(3):304–9.
30. Sturesson C. Interstitial laser-induced thermotherapy: influence of carbonization on lesion size. Lasers Surg Med. 1998;22(1):51–7.
31. Mensel B, Weigel C, Hosten N. Laser-induced thermotherapy. Recent Results Cancer Res. 2006;167:69–75.
32. Möller PH, Lindberg L, Henriksson PH, Persson BRR, Tranberg K-G. Interstitial laser thermotherapy: comparison between bare fibre and sapphire probe. Lasers Med Sci. 1995;10:193–200.
33. Heisterkamp J, van Hillegersberg R, Ijzermans JN. Critical temperature and heating time for coagulation damage: implications for interstitial laser coagulation (ILC) of tumors. Lasers Surg Med. 1999;25(3):257–62.
34. Muralidharan V, Christophi C. Interstitial laser thermotherapy in the treatment of colorectal liver metastases. J Surg Oncol. 2001;76(1):73–81.
35. Steger AC, Lees WR, Shorvon P, Walmsley K, Bown SG. Multiple-fibre low-power interstitial laser hyperthermia: studies in the normal liver. Br J Surg. 1992;79(2):139–45.

36. Germer CT, Albrecht D, Roggan A, Buhr HJ. Technology for in situ ablation by laparoscopic and image-guided interstitial laser hyperthermia. Semin Laparosc Surg. 1998;5(3):195–203.

37. Germer CT, Albrecht D, Isbert C, Ritz J, Roggan A, Buhr HJ. Diffusing fibre tip for the minimally invasive treatment of liver tumours by interstitial laser coagulation (ILC): an experimental ex vivo study. Lasers Med Sci. 1999;14(1):32–9.

38. Heisterkamp J, Van Hillegersberg R, Sinofsky EL, Ijzermans JNM. Interstitial laser photocoagulation with four cylindrical diffusing fibre tips: importance of mutual fibre distance. Lasers Med Sci. 1999;14:216–20.

39. Heisterkamp J, van Hillegersberg R, Ijzermans JN. Interstitial laser coagulation for hepatic tumours. Br J Surg. 1999;86(3):293–304.

40. Saccomandi P, Schena E, Giurazza F, Del Vescovo R, Caponero MA, Mortato L, et al. Temperature monitoring and lesion volume estimation during double-applicator laser-induced thermotherapy in ex vivo swine pancreas: a preliminary study. Lasers Med Sci. 2014;29(2):607–14.

41. Vogl TJ, Muller PK, Hammerstingl R, Weinhold N, Mack MG, Philipp C, et al. Malignant liver tumors treated with MR imaging-guided laser-induced thermotherapy: technique and prospective results. Radiology. 1995;196(1):257–65.

42. Vogl TJ, Mack MG, Roggan A, Straub R, Eichler KC, Muller PK, et al. Internally cooled power laser for MR-guided interstitial laser-induced thermotherapy of liver lesions: initial clinical results. Radiology. 1998;209(2):381–5.

43. Vogl TJ, Eichler K, Straub R, Engelmann K, Zangos S, Woitaschek D, et al. Laser-induced thermotherapy of malignant liver tumors: general principals, equipment(s), procedure(s)—side effects, complications and results. Eur J Ultrasound. 2001;13(2):117–27.

44. de Jode MG, Lamb GM, Thomas HC, Taylor-Robinson SD, Gedroyc WM. MRI guidance of infrared laser liver tumour ablations, utilising an open MRI configuration system: technique and early progress. J Hepatol. 1999;31(2):347–53.

45. Rieke V, Butts Pauly K. MR thermometry. J Magn Reson Imaging. 2008;27(2):376–90.

46. Diederich CJ, Nau WH, Kinsey A, Ross T, Wootton J, Juang T, et al. Catheter-based ultrasound devices and MR thermal monitoring for conformal prostate thermal therapy. Conf Proc IEEE Eng Med Biol Soc. 2008;2008:3664–8.

47. Ahrar K, Gowda A, Javadi S, Borne A, Fox M, McNichols R, et al. Preclinical assessment of a 980-nm diode laser ablation system in a large animal tumor model. J Vasc Interv Radiol. 2010;21(4):555–61.

Experimental Data and Clinical Studies of Laser Ablation

Claudio Maurizio Pacella and Tian'an Jiang

3.1 Experimental Data and Initial Clinical Studies (1980–2000)

In the last 30 years or so, after the first studies on the tissue-laser interactions conducted by Bown in 1983 [1], a long series of experimental studies took place on healthy or diseased tissues and on animal models. Over time there have been many clinical trials that have validated laser technology as a means of treating neoplastic focal lesions in different organs with sufficient efficacy and safety.

After the first works of the 1960s [2], numerous experimental studies were conducted both in vivo and ex vivo on healthy tissues and on tumor models of various animals in the 1980s in order to establish the most suitable parameters to obtain a coagulation area as large as possible in the shortest possible time [3–12]. More precisely, while studies on induced tumors aimed to assess the toxicity of laser energy, studies on normal liver aimed to develop the best strategy to obtain large areas of coagulative necrosis. In fact, the main objective of the research was the development of a technique able to obtain large areas of coagulation safely and quickly in a single session. In his early work, Matthewson inserted into a rat liver lobe via laparotomy a 0.4 mm diameter fiber using an Nd-YAG laser light. Using an output power of 0.5–2.0 W for an exposure time of 2400 s, he was able to achieve a well-defined coagulation zone, clearly distinct from the surrounding healthy tissue. Matthewson also observed that an increase in the applied outpower meant a corresponding increase in the size of the coagulation area [3]. Subsequent experimental studies on tumor models have confirmed this relationship between the size of the lesion and the applied energy without deterioration of liver function [10]. The damaging effect was also confirmed on some tumors implanted subcutaneously in some rodents [7, 13]. Finally, to increase the volume of the coagulation zone in a single session, Steger first applied multiple light sources activated simultaneously on a normal dog liver through a device (beamplitter) able to distribute energy to four fibers equidistant 1.5 cm from each other, obtaining a coagulation necrosis area of $3.6 \times 3.1 \times 2.8$ cm equal to 15.6 mL using 1.5 W for 670 s (4020 J in total) [14].

Hashimoto [15] treated the first patients with hepatic metastases and hepatocellular carcinoma in 1985 by laparotomy using a bare-tip fiber and an Nd-YAG laser. This author has used powers of 5 W for a relatively long time obtaining a fall

C. M. Pacella (✉)
Department of Diagnostic Imaging and Interventional Radiology, Regina Apostolorum Hospital, Alabano Laziale, Rome, Italy

T. Jiang
Department of Ultrasound, First Affiliated Hospital, College of Medicine, Zhejiang University, Hangzhou, China

© Springer Nature Switzerland AG 2020
C. M. Pacella et al. (eds.), *Image-guided Laser Ablation*,
https://doi.org/10.1007/978-3-030-21748-8_3

of the carcinoembryonic antigen (CEA) and of the α-fetoprotein (AFP). Although it is not yet clear what the benefit was for patients, but the study showed that the technique was free of major complications. In subsequent studies, other authors used different combinations of power and exposure times with fibers and diffusers that were able to avoid carbonization. Hahl in 1990 [16] and Huang in 1991 [17] performed a simple hyperthermia using cooled devices able to maintain a constant temperature around 41–45 °C for 10–30 min in order to avoid a direct coagulation of the tissue. Since the air systems used to cool the devices have caused a fatal complication (gas embolism), these options have been completely abandoned. Today, cooling systems with salt solutions are used for this purpose.

In the 1990s the first works on percutaneous procedures guided by ultrasound appeared in the literature. Amin [18] in 1993 using four hollow 18-gauge needle and four flat bare-tip fibers of 600 nm activated simultaneously with 2 W for 8 min treated 55 metastases with a diameter between 1 and 15 cm in 21 patients. Metastases smaller than 4 cm in diameter were treated more effectively and required fewer treatment sessions than did those larger than 4 cm. Complications were minor and included severe pain in four cases, persistent pain for up to 10 days in 11 cases, and asymptomatic subcapsular hematoma (four cases) and pleural effusion (six cases) seen with CT. Of the 21 patients 14 remained alive, with a median survival of 7.5 months (range, 4–29 months). Nolsoe in the same year [19], with the use of a specific modification of the bare laser fiber diffuser tip, demonstrated how it was possible to produce spherical coagulations with a diameter comparable to that of liver metastases. With ultrasound (US) guidance, a 1.2 mm (18-gauge) lumbar needle was introduced via the multipuncture needle guide and positioned with its tip in the center of the metastasis (two of these were treated in laparotomy). The Nd-YAG laser was turned on, and the laser treatment continued until the temperature display read 60 °C or had stayed constant at 45 °C for 15 min. The laser output was varied between 4 and 8 W, and the activation time varied between 5 and 45 min, depending on the size and the vascularity of the metastases. This technique was used in 11 patients with 16 colorectal liver metastases with diameters of 1–4 cm, 12 of which were radically ablated. Schroder in 1994 [20] used bare-tip fibers with output powers of 2–6 W for 8–15 min on both secondary (6 cases) and primary (2 cases of hepatocellular carcinoma and 2 cases of breast cancer) lesions of 0.5–7 cm. Treatment was technically possible in all cases. The smallest metastasis disappeared totally while some larger tumors were reduced in size during a follow-up period of 6 months to 5 years. There were no serious complications. Vogl in 1995 [21] treated 33 metastases with a diameter of 1–4 cm in 20 patients using a cooled diffuser with powers of 3–8 W for 10–35 min. Under ultrasound guidance and with laparotomic access using an "icy" sapphire fiber with powers of 6–10 W for 5 min with simultaneous complete occlusion of hepatic flow, Tranberg in 1996 [22] treated 3 HCC, 18 colorectal metastases and 1 cancer of pancreas with diameters between 1 and 10 cm. Pacella in 1996 [23] under US guidance treated metastases with an average diameter of 2.9 cm (14 from colorectal cancer, 5 from breast cancer and 1 from lung cancer) in 14 patients with 21-gauge thin needles and flat bare-tip fibers of 300 μm using output powers of 5 W for 6 min. Gillams in 1997, as reported by Heisterkamp [24], treated percutaneously 148 metastases in 55 patients with a diameter between 1 and 6 cm with US and MRI approaches using bare tips simultaneously at 2 W × 7 min in multiple sessions. The authors cited above report to the control with CT and NMR a percentage of complete coagulative necrosis between 16% and 58%. All of them underline the difficulty of obtaining complete response in lesions with diameters above 2.3 cm. Finally, it should be noted that it is difficult to compare the data available for the different selection and recruitment criteria of the patients used by the different researchers.

Regarding the impact of the survival, Vogl [25] in 1997 reported the local tumor control and survival of 134 consecutive patients with a total of 383 hepatic metastases treated with magnetic resonance laser-induced thermotherapy (LITT)[1] with 1048 applications. The major groups were liver metastases from colorectal cancer (88 patients) and liver metastases from breast cancer (20 patients) as well as miscellaneous primary tumors (26 patients). All of the patients tolerated the procedure under local anesthesia well, and no severe complications or side effects were observed. During the follow-up period, 29 of the 134 patients treated died. The mean survival time was 35 months in the colorectal cancer group, 30 months in the breast cancer group, and 34 months in the group with miscellaneous primary tumors. The statistical assessment of the equality of survival distribution showed no significant differences between the three groups. These results suggest that in patients with liver metastases local tumor destruction using minimally invasive percutaneous LITT[1] under local anesthesia results in improved clinical outcomes, independently of the type of primary tumor.

3.2 Complications

As far as complications are concerned, it must be said that the major ones are really rare in this initial group of works. Pain of varying intensity is described at the point of insertion of the needles and the right shoulder as a consequence of the irritation of the diaphragm. The temperature usually rises in the days following the treatment as well as the levels of GOT and GPT as a sign of tissue coagulative necrosis and cytolysis. After a few days the temperature values return to normal and within one month the serum levels of GOT and GPT are restored. A case of biloma, two cases of subcapsular hematoma, a vasovagal reaction during treatment and a high percentage of pleural effusions that heal without sequelae and

without the need for special therapies have been described. In some cases the administration of antibiotics for a few days was needed, especially when an area of coagulation zone of discrete volume was associated. Two fatal cases have been reported. A fatal case of Budd-Chiari syndrome was reported by Bown to Heisterkamp [24] probably for the treatment of a lesion close to the suprahepatic veins and another by Tranberg [22] for acute multi-organ failure after treatment of a tumor of 8 cm. The author, in order to increase the volume of necrosis, completely excluded the blood supply to the liver during treatment. Massive necrosis probably induced a shock similar to that caused by Lee [26] after treatment of large lesions with cryosurgery without excluding the blood supply. It therefore remains to be clarified what role is played by the volume of induced necrosis and the role played by the occlusion of blood flow in multi-organ failure. Finally, as the case reported by Bown demonstrates, it is necessary to use caution and prudence when treating tumors close to vital structures. From the above it emerges that with the techniques used initially laser ablation was safe, well tolerated and effective in the local treatment of lesions with dimensions below 3 cm.

3.3 Recent Clinical Studies (2000–2018)

In 2000 Gillams and Lees [27] adopted Amin's technique to treat 69 patients with multiple liver metastases from colorectal cancer. The mean number was 2.9 (range, 1–16), the mean maximum diameter was 3.9 (range, 1–8) cm and the mean initial total liver tumor volume was 47 (range, 1–371) mL. Eighteen (26%) had undergone previous hepatic resection. Sixty-two of 67 (93%) received chemotherapy at some stage. Twenty (29%) had extrahepatic disease. Median survival time from the liver metastasis diagnosis was 27 months. Of a group of 24 patients with less than four metastases and less than 5 cm in maximum diameter, the median survival time was 33 months from first thermal ablation versus 15 months for the remainder ($P = 0.0004$). Major

---

[1] As previously explained in the first chapter and reiterated in the second chapter of this book, the term "laser ablation" (LA) is associated with several alternative acronyms in the literature, including laser-induced thermal therapy (LITT), interstitial coagulation of laser (ILC) interstitial laser therapy, interstitial laser phototherapy (ILP) and photothermal therapy, a term that has gained popularity among scientists working in the field of nanotechnology.

morbidity occurred in 3.2%, lower morbidity occurred in 12% and there was one periprocedural death. Based on these data, Gillams concluded that percutaneous therapy with laser improved survival in patients with inoperable but limited liver metastases. Thermal ablation produced an improvement in the natural history of the disease and the results of known chemotherapy.

Later, Vogl provided updated data in a more robust series of patients in 2004 [28]. In detail, MR imaging–guided LITT[1] was performed in 603 patients (mean age, 61.2 years) with 1801 liver metastases of colorectal cancer. Local tumor control and tumor volume were evaluated with nonenhanced and contrast material–enhanced MR imaging. Indications for the procedure were defined for patients with five or fewer metastases, none of which were larger than 5 cm in diameter. Local recurrence rate at 6-month follow-up was 1.9% (9 of 474) for metastases up to 2 cm in diameter, 2.4% (13 of 539) for metastases 2.1–3.0 cm in diameter, 1.2% (4 of 327) for metastases 3.1–4.0 cm in diameter and 4.4% (13 of 294) for metastases larger than 4 cm in diameter. The mean survival rate for all treated patients, with calculation started on the date of diagnosis of the metastases, was 4.4 years (95% CI: 4.0, 4.8) (3-year survival, 56%; 5-year survival, 37%). Median survival was 3.5 years (95% CI: 3.0, 3.9). Mean survival after the first LITT[1] treatment was 3.8 years (95% CI: 3.4, 4.2). So with this well-documented and detailed work, Vogl, the author, who has systematically used the laser technique for years in Frankfurt using cooled devices (9-F sheath) inserted under CT guidance in the context of metastatic lesions and monitored the entire ablation maneuver with MRI, states that MR imaging–guided LITT[1] yields high local tumor control and survival rates in well-selected patients with limited liver metastases of colorectal carcinoma.

In the same years Pacella published the results of his group on a small series of metastases from colorectal cancer treated with the technique of thin needles with low-power laser. The study included 44 individuals with 75 unresectable liver metastases and no known extrahepatic disease. The median number of metastases treated for each patient was one, with a range of 1–4. Metastases had a median diameter of 3.4 cm (range 0.5–9 cm) and a median volume of 16.8 cm^3 (range 0.4–176.4 cm^3). All patients also received systemic chemotherapy with modalities that differed according to the type of response to LA. After treatment, 61% (46/75) of the tumors were ablated completely. The likelihood of achieving a complete ablation was significantly higher when metastases had a diameter <3.0 cm ($P = 0.004$). Overall survival was 30.0 ± 12.7 months in patients with a complete ablation and 20.2 ± 10.2 months in those with a partial ablation ($P = 0.002$). There were no major complications during or after LA. These findings indicate that this LA technology can be safely used as an adjunct to chemotherapy in unresectable colorectal liver metastases and may have a positive impact on survival [29].

In the same year Gillams signaled his experience in the treatment of unresectable hepatic metastases from neuroendocrine tumors in 25 patients. Since the early 1990s Gillams has treated 189 tumors in 66 treatment sessions. Thirty of these treatment sessions were performed with a solid-state laser and 36 with radiofrequency. All treatments except one were performed percutaneously under the guidance of the image. The authors do not report significant differences between the two techniques. Sixteen patients had metastases from primary carcinoids, three from gastrinoma, two from insulinoma and four from various causes. Fourteen out of 25 had symptoms of hormone secretion. Imaging follow-up was available in 19 patients with a median of 21 months (range, 4–75 months). There was a complete response in six patients, a partial response in seven and stable disease in one. The tumor burden was controlled in 14 out of 19 patients (74%). The relief of hormone-related symptoms was achieved in nine out of 14 patients (69%). The median survival period from the diagnosis of hepatic metastases was 53 months. A patient with end-stage heart disease died after a carcinoid tumor seizure. There were eight (12%) complications, five local and three distant, four main and four minor [30]. It is not possible to draw valid considerations and conclusions from this particular experience since the data of the two techniques have not been clearly defined since the beginning of the study. For this particular type of metastasis from neuroendocrine tumors (NET) it may be useful to read the chapter dedicated to them in this book (see Chap. 14).

In 2006, the Frankfurt group published promising results of the first feasibility study to evaluate the safety and efficacy of laser-induced interstitial LITT[1] MR-thermometry) in adrenal metastases in nine patients with nine unilateral metastases (mean diameter 4.3 cm) from colorectal carcinoma (n = 5), renal cell carcinoma (n = 1), esophageal carcinoma (n = 1), carcinoid (n = 1) and hepatocellular carcinoma (n = 1). Follow-up studies were performed at 24 h at 3 months and thereafter at 6-month intervals (median 14 months). All patients tolerated the procedure under local anesthesia. No complications were reported. The average number of laser applications per tumor was 1.9 (range 1–4) with an average energy of 33 kJ (range, 15.3–94.6 kJ). A coagulation necrosis induced by the laser system with an average diameter of 4.5 cm (range, 2.5–7.5 cm) was obtained. Complete ablation was achieved in seven lesions, verified by MR imaging, while progression was observed only in two lesions [31].

This solid body of good quality studies has been the background behind further research on the use of laser technology in the treatment of focal malignant pathology in different organs and tissues. Additionally, over the same period of time it has been possible to open a new and interesting field of study for the treatment of benign focal lesions (see Chap. 7). So in the following years interesting works were done in other organs and on metastases of different nature both with cooled and noncooled devices. The experience in the treatment of hepatocellular carcinoma (HCC) with variable dimensions without or in combination with transarterial chemoembolization (TACE) belongs to this period [32–35] as well as to this period belongs the treatment of HCCs at risk sited in close contiguity (less than 5 mm) with vital structures such as the gallbladder, the biliary tract, portal vessels and the hepatic hilum [36]. As

well as studies on the role of safety margin in the study of local or remote relapses and in the survival [37] (see Chap. 4). Equally important are the combined studies with repeated embolization or those associated with antiblastic drugs (irinotecan) of metastasis from colorectal carcinoma, gastric cancer or from ovarian tumors performed by the Vogl group with cooled devices[2] [38–40]. In 2014, the same Vogl group gave us convincing data on the predictive factors of the survival of patients with metastases treated with LITT.[1] The number and size of metastases, together with the status of the initial lymph nodes, are significant prognostic factors for long-term survival [41].

Worthy of note is the work on the unresectable primary and metastatic adrenocortical carcinoma by the Pacella group. After three sessions of LA, the primary tumor of 15 cm was ablated by 75%. After 1–4 (median 1) sessions of LA, five liver metastases ranging from 2 to 5 cm were completely ablated while the sixth tumor of 12 cm was ablated by 75%. There were no major complications. Treatment resulted in an improvement of performance status and a reduction of the daily dosage of mitotane in all patients. The three patients with liver metastases presented a marked decrease of 24 h urine cortisol levels, an improved control of hypertension and a mean weight loss of 2.8 kg. After a median follow-up after LA of 27.0 months (range, 9–48 months), two patients had died of tumor progression while two other patients remained alive and free of disease [42].

3.4 Complications

Regarding the rate and type of complications in this more recent period two works have allowed to update the data. The first work reports the updated data of the experiences carried out with the cooled devices. On the basis of a total of 2132

[2]An MR-compatible cannulation needle (length, 20 cm; diameter, 1.3 mm) with a tetragonally beveled tip and stylet, a guide wire (length, 100 cm), a 9-F sheath with stylet and a 7-F double-tube thermostabile (up to 400 °C) protective catheter with a stylet that enables internal cooling with saline solution (0.9% NaCI).

LITT[1] procedures performed, complications were divided into major and minor categories and detected at clinical or imaging studies. Major complications included three deaths (0.1%) within 30 days after treatment, pleural effusion requiring thoracentesis in 16 (0.8%) cases, hepatic abscess requiring drainage in 15 (0.7%) cases, bile duct injury in four (0.2%) cases, segmental infarction in three (0.1%) cases and hemorrhage requiring transfusion in one (0.05%) case. Minor complications included postprocedural fever in 710 (33.3%), pleural effusion not requiring thoracentesis in 155 (7.3%), subcapsular hematoma in 69 (3.2%), subcutaneous hematoma in 24 (1.1%), pneumothorax in seven (0.3%) and hemorrhage in two (0.1%) cases. These data for treating 899 patients with 2520 malignant hepatic tumors over a period of 8 years document, according to the authors, that the MR-guided LITT with local anesthesia was a safe technique with an acceptably low rate of complications [43].

In a multicenter study involving 9 Italian centers, 520 patients were selected with 647 HCC nodules treated with 1004 sessions of LA. There were 15 (1.5%) major complications, including four deaths (0.8%), without any seeding, and 62 (7.2%) minor complications. Major complications were associated with higher laser energy delivered to the HCC nodule and with HCC deeply located in the liver. Minor complications were associated with higher energy deployed and in patients with low serum level of bilirubin and altered prothrombin time. Complete response was achieved in 314/387 nodules <3 cm and 94% of patients were free of local recurrence 12 months after LA. Therefore, also the thin needle technique appears safe and has low complication rates [44] (see also Chap. 4).

3.5   Conclusions

Before closing this section, it will be useful to mention some other applications that will be illustrated in the respective chapters of this book. Regarding the treatment of pulmonary metastases or primary tumor lesions during the last few years, works have been published with cooled devices [45, 46] while surprisingly few works have been published with thin noncooled devices. It is known that the laser technique is more manageable, faster and does not present the problems of conductivity of the radiofrequency and the difficulty that the microwaves have in the distribution of their energy in the tissue. We know that about 40 cases (metastases and primary tumors) have been treated in Italy and have been communicated in an international meeting [47, 48]. Chapter 12 is dedicated to this application. Finally, recent interesting applications in small renal tumors should be mentioned in patients at risk of bleeding [49] and in the benign and malignant pathology of the prostate [50] (see Chaps. 6 and 13). In light of the numerous applications in the most diverse fields of study, it is worth pointing out the recent update review of some experts who have listed them taking into account the different wavelengths of the lasers available [51].

3.6   Technique

We believe it is useful and appropriate to provide information on the characteristics of the technique used in the numerous applications described in this book. The laser technique has been described and commented in 2005 [52, 53].

Tumor ablation with the use of laser technique involves the placement of laser fibers (one or several) into a tumor via a needle or sheath, which is then retracted, exposing the laser fiber itself to the tumor. The laser sources used in the last decade of the 1990s and in the first decade of the 2000s were mainly continuous-wave Nd:YAG devices. Neodymium rods are energized to produce photons and those emitted along the long axis of the rod are deflected by a mirror, resonated in a cavity, and emitted as a 1064 nm wavelength beam, which is propagated through a 300 μm quartz-core fiberoptic (see Chap. 2). We used a laser generator with a beam-splitting device, allowing us to place four separate laser fibers in a square configuration within a tumor with the use of 21-gauge needles. The optical fibers are illuminated simultaneously. The wavelength and power of an Nd:YAG laser is well suited to medi-cal applications with tissue scatter and absorption able to create an ablation zone of approximately 1–1.5 cm, allowing finally the four fibers to achieve a tumor ablation zone of approximately 4 cm.

The laser system with which the most recent applications have been performed and is still used on an inpatient basis is a commercially available system consisting of a US device and a multisource laser unit (EchoLaser, Elesta Srl, Florence, Italy). The laser unit uses semi-conductors diodes with a wavelength of 1064 nm which carry the light beam into the tissue through the quartz-core fiberoptic of the same caliber of 300 μm used in previous historical applica-tions. The laser unit allows the use of up to four sources both simultaneously and separately from each other even at different output powers. Laser diodes are replacing the Nd:YAG laser because they are more compact and portable (weighing less than 10 kg), less expensive and have a tissue penetration similar to that obtained by Nd:YAG lasers. The system also integrates special guiding systems with software tools for the guidance of needles and advanced laser heat treatment plan-ning software.

Given that laser tumor ablation has equivalent local control, survival and complications rates as RF ablation [54], Eric Walser pointed out in his editorial the peculiar and faster mechanism of cell death from laser light than the radiofre-quency technique. He argues that "Although heat from laser light absorption is the primary mechanism of cell death, there is some evi-dence that laser ablation may cause coagulation of microvessels and progressive ischemic injury as long as 72 h after the ablation procedure [55]. Other forms of heat generation may also cause these microvascular injuries, but the laser may be more capable of "tuning" to wavelength to cause lethal endothelial injury (as in laser vein ablation procedures). Additionally, anyone performing RF ablation of large lesions will appreciate the increased efficiency afforded by laser tumor abla-tion. The illuminations performed by Pacella and colleagues [52] were done over a 6 min period as opposed to approximately 20 min for RF abla-tion." And again, "This time factor may seem inconsequential, but when multiple ablations or illuminations are being performed, the proce-dural time becomes considerably longer with the use of RF. This is of great importance in proce-dures performed in the CT area, where patient throughput and scheduling issues are extremely important" [53].

The use of thin needles reduces the size of the puncture and allows to more safely treat cirrhotic patients who often have poor coagulation param-eters. The simultaneous positioning of several needles also reduces the number of punctures and allows the four fibers to be advanced into the tumor in any geometry desired by the opera-tor. In other words, it is possible to adapt both the number and the spatial configuration of the heat sources to the size and shape of the lesion to be treated (tailored treatment). This explains the possibility of treating high-risk and/or hard-to-reach tumors effectively [36]. This technique inevitably requires skillful and experienced operators. The use of thin needles also explains the choice to treat predominantly hepatocellular carcinomas in cirrhotic patients [34] unlike what happened in Frankfurt where the number of cir-rhotic patients were considerably lower than the Italian experience [35]. Conversely, the German group has gained more experience in treating a large number of patients with liver metastases with larger devices (see previous paragraph) [28]. In fact, the method of the Vogl's group consists of a laser fiber enclosed in a cooling sheath with a diameter of 9 F. This sheath is provided with a diffusing tip, which allows the light to diffuse 12–15 mm from the point of origin. With this method, the group treated metastases and hepato-mas of up to 2 cm in diameter with a single appli-cator but also treated tumors as large as 8 cm with the use of four or five carefully positioned laser sheaths [28].

Since the fibers used in the laser tumor abla-tion are fully compatible with MR, Vogl's group uses this advantage to perform the ablation of the MR-guided liver tumor. Special RM sequences designed to evaluate thermal models (i.e., MR imaging thermometry) can monitor the actual for-mation of ablation zone. This allows theoretically to complete tumor ablation and obtain a variable safety margin in a more controlled and reproducible fashion compared to the hyperechoic focus that is formed when performing RF ablation under US guidance. Because the light generator laser is not MR compatible, it remains in the shielded MR control room. The laser energy does not decrease along the long fibers necessary to travel from the MR console to the gantry where the ablation treatment takes place. So the main advantage of MR over other imaging modalities is its sensitivity to thermal changes [56–58], which enables to monitor the heating process in near real time to ensure that the entire lesion has been treated and to reposition the applicators in case of residual tumor. Obviously, this is not possible with the Pacella group's technique, which therefore must program in advance the parameters of outpower and time to obtain both the death of the tumor and a sufficient safety margin. Clinical data have shown a correlation between the amount of energy distributed to the tumor and the volume of induced necrosis. With 3600 J (two fibers) it is possible to obtain a volume coagulation zone of 5.3 ± 1.6 (range, 5.0–8.0), with 7200 J (four fibers) a volume equal to 15.0 ± 5.1 (range, 8.0–25.0) and with 28,800 J (four fibers and two pullbacks) a volume of 30.8 ± 12.0 (range, 13.0–60.0) [52]. Knowing these parameters and the relative areas of ablation, the operator can easily plan the exposure times at fixed powers of 3–5 W to successfully ablate the tumor and thanks to the thin needles' reach with sufficient safety of nodules at risk sites and those difficult to approach.

Lastly, it should be emphasized that the introduction in the clinical practice of the contrast agent-enhanced US [(CEUS) a solution of encapsulated microbubbles stabilized by a phospholipid shell] performed 10 min from the end of the ablation maneuver by using a low mechanical index contrast specific nonlinear technique (CnTI) allows to verify the completeness of the ablation procedure. The accuracy of postprocedural CEUS in early evaluation of the ablation procedures has been reported to be comparable to CT performed at 24 h [59, 60]. So at present CEUS is recommended as a valid tool in the postprocedural assessment of the completeness of ablation [60]. Therefore, we think that postprocedural CEUS can counterbalance the advantage of MR in terms of correct evaluation of the completeness of the treatment, allowing for US-guided ablation whenever the tumor can be well visualized and confidently targeted by US with obvious cost savings and shorter duration of the procedure.

Additionally, it should be emphasized that an obvious disadvantage of the Frankfurt technique is the use of a large sheath with a cooled jacketing with consequent large size puncture in the liver during procedures, which are often repeated in as many as four or five locations. Bleeding problems are minimized by the use of fibrin sealant; however, the 9-F sheaths used by the Vogl group [43] generate hesitation between the interventional radiologists more accustomed to the smaller needles used for RF ablation. These problems are not present with the technique of the Rome group, which still achieves high rates of complete ablation and which compare favorably with the Frankfurt group, especially in the treatment of hepatocellular carcinomas, even without real-time monitoring.

Lastly but not least important is the relatively recent update of the guidance system to precisely position the needles and fibers into the tumor making the technique less operator dependent. Needles are positioned inside the target nodule easily and quickly, and correct spacing (1.5–1.8 cm) between light sources is immediately achieved. This guide allowed to obtain a high rate (92%) of complete ablation in lesions up to 5 cm [61] (Fig. 3.1).

Finally, it is worth noting that it is possible to activate the four sources simultaneously and separately to treat multiple nodules located in separate sites in the liver in a single session. In other words it is possible to treat four lesions of one centimeter in different segments distant from each other as in the miliary-shaped metastatic forms of some NETs, or two lesions of 2 cm each or a lesion from one centimeter and another 2–3 cm at various distant, etc. We consider it useful for readers and operators to draw up a list of practical points that can effectively highlight the

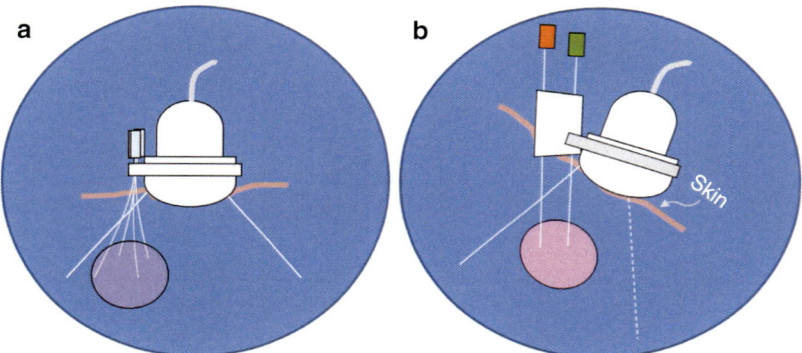

Fig. 3.1 Drawing of the two guiding systems of the multifiber technique with thin applicators: (**a**) system that allows to place the needles and the fibers one after the other from a single point of entry into central tumor mass; (**b**) novel dedicated probe that allows the precise insertion of the needles in a parallel fashion, facilitating precise positioning of the needles in geometrical configurations to maximize the ablative effect—*see also refs.* [48, 55] (Elesta Srl, Calenzano, Florence, Italy)

characteristics of this technology whose multiple applications are described and discussed in this book.

3.7 Practical Points

1. Laser energy, like RF and microwave energy, induces electromagnetic heating to raise the temperature of tissues to lethal levels. It is a fast, precise and relatively tissue-insensitive technique and can be delivered very easily and safely with simultaneous techniques to obtain large areas of coagulation.
2. The laser technique uses very thin applicators considerably smaller (<1 mm) than radiofrequency ablation electrodes and microwave ablation antenna. Up to now they represent the smallest energy applicators available in the tumor ablation field with minimally invasive approach.
3. The laser ablation shows an efficacy and safety profile with very short (up to 4–6 min) treatment time per session.
4. Usually, one to two fibers with or without a pullback technique are used to treat nodules up to 1.5–2.5 cm in diameter and four fibers arranged in a square configuration equidistant from each other of 1.2–1.8 cm to treat the nodules up to 4.0 cm. With the pullback technique it is possible to treat nodules

greater than 4 cm with excellent results. After a single session complete tumor ablation was achieved in 92% of nodules up to 5.0 cm in size.
5. Thanks to fine applicators, laser light technology is safer and more suitable for ablating lesions in high risk sites or in locations that are difficult to reach. It is possible to obtain complete ablation in a high percentage of cases (up to 93%) without using special technical devices to protect adjacent structures.
6. In addition to the possibility of obtaining an effective and safe ablation of tumors up to 4 cm due to a volume amplification mechanism, thanks to the simultaneous and separate activation of the thin devices, it is possible to treat several lesions in different segments of the liver in the same session of ablation as in the case of four tumors of 1 cm each or two tumors of 2 cm each and so on (Fig. 3.2).
7. The laser ablation technique can become the ablative technique of choice in patients with small or recurrent lesions of varying sizes ranging from 5–6 mm to 3–4 cm in diameter. Therefore, patients with disseminated hepatic metastases of varying sizes as sometimes occurs in neuroendocrine tumors can be treated at different times with the intention of reducing tumor burden and improving local or general symptoms. Furthermore,

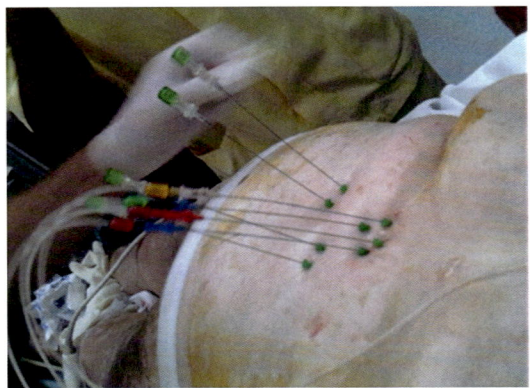

Fig. 3.2 Representative case of multiple HCCs of different sizes (two lesions of 2 cm and one of 3 cm) treated in the same session with the insertion of 8 needles through the new dedicated probe (CA431). The treatment was performed by first treating the HCC of 3 cm in 12 min placing four fibers spaced 1.5 cm apart and immediately afterward with simultaneous ablation of the remaining two lesions of 2 cm each in 6 min (Courtesy of Giovanni Giuseppe Di Costanzo, Liver Unit, Department of Transplantation, Cardarelli Hospital, Naples, Italy)

the laser technique can be repeated several times safely for a period of years.

8. LA, thanks to the recent introduction in clinical practice of a novel guide system which facilitates both the parallel insertion of multiple thin needles and their positioning in geometrical configurations to maximize the ablative effect, is more effective in achieving large volumes of coagulative necrosis and effectively treat lesions of 5–6 cm in diameter with safety at any location without using sequential combined treatment.

9. In case of pauci-lesional disease the multimodality locoregional ischemic treatment alternating catheter-based technique (i.e., radioembolization, ethiodized oil based or drug-eluting bead (DEB), bland embolization) with laser thermal ablation can be performed even with multiple sessions.

10. In the case of unresectable metastatic hepatic lesions or hepatocellular carcinomas larger than 4–5 cm in size, in which a combined treatment can be planned (laser followed by TACE), it is possible to obtain a reduction in the volume of the large lesion with the laser technique so as to allow a more effective ablative action of

TACE which, as is known, can be effective for lesions of a discrete volume around 3 cm in maximum diameter (see also Chap. 4).

References

1. Bown SG. Phototherapy in tumors. World J Surg. 1983;7(6):700–9.
2. Hoye RC, Thomas LB, Riggle GC, Ketcham A. Effects of neodymium laser on normal liver and Vx2 carcinoma transplanted into the liver of experimental animals. J Natl Cancer Inst. 1968;41(5):1071–82.
3. Matthewson K, Coleridge-Smith P, O'Sullivan JP, Northfield TC, Bown SG. Biological effects of intrahepatic neodymium:yttrium-aluminum-garnet laser photocoagulation in rats. Gastroenterology. 1987;93(3):550–7.
4. Dachman AH, McGehee JA, Beam TE, Burris JA, Powell DA. US-guided percutaneous laser ablation of liver tissue in a chronic pig model. Radiology. 1990;176(1):129–33.
5. Bosman S, Phoa SS, Bosma A, van Gemert MJ. Effect of percutaneous interstitial thermal laser on normal liver of pigs: sonographic and histopathological correlations. Br J Surg. 1991;78(5):572–5.
6. Matsumoto R, Selig AM, Colucci VM, Jolesz FA. Interstitial Nd:YAG laser ablation in normal rabbit liver: trial to maximize the size of laser-induced lesions. Lasers Surg Med. 1992;12(6):650–8.
7. Dowlatshahi K, Babich D, Bangert JD, Kluiber R. Histologic evaluation of rat mammary tumor necrosis by interstitial Nd:YAG laser hyperthermia. Lasers Surg Med. 1992;12(2):159–64.
8. Amin Z, Thurrell W, Spencer GM, Harries SA, Grant WE, Bown SG, et al. Computed tomography-pathologic assessment of laser-induced necrosis in rat liver. Investig Radiol. 1993;28(12):1148–54.
9. Pacella CM, Rossi Z, Bizzarri G, Papini E, Marinozzi V, Paliotta D, et al. Ultrasound-guided percutaneous laser ablation of liver tissue in a rabbit model. Eur Radiol. 1993;3:26–32.
10. van Hillegersberg R, van Staveren HJ, Kort WJ, Zondervan PE, Terpstra OT. Interstitial Nd:YAG laser coagulation with a cylindrical diffusing fiber tip in experimental liver metastases. Lasers Surg Med. 1994;14(2):124–38.
11. Malone DE, Wyman DR, DeNardi FG, McGrath FP, De Gara CJ, Wilson BC. Hepatic interstitial laser photocoagulation. An investigation of the relationship between acute thermal lesions and their sonographic images. Investig Radiol. 1994;29(10):915–21.
12. Germer CT, Albrecht D, Roggan A, Isbert C, Buhr HJ. Experimental study of laparoscopic laser-induced thermotherapy for liver tumours. Br J Surg. 1997;84(3):317–20.

13. Matthewson K, Barr H, Tralau C, Bown SG. Low power interstitial Nd YAG laser photocoagulation: studies in a transplantable fibrosarcoma. Br J Surg. 1989;76(4):378–81.

14. Steger AC, Lees WR, Shorvon P, Walmsley K, Bown SG. Multiple-fibre low-power interstitial laser hyperthermia: studies in the normal liver. Br J Surg. 1992;79(2):139–45.

15. Hashimoto D, Takami M, Idezuki Y. In depth radiation therapy by Nd-YAG laser for malignant tumors of the liver under ultrasound imaging. Gastroenterology. 1985;88:1663.

16. Hahl J, Haapiainen R, Ovaska J, Puolakkainen P, Schroder T. Laser-induced hyperthermia in the treatment of liver tumors. Lasers Surg Med. 1990;10(4):319–21.

17. Huang GT, Wang TH, Sheu JC, Daikuzono N, Sung JL, Wu MZ, et al. Low-power laserthermia for the treatment of small hepatocellular carcinoma. Eur J Cancer. 1991;27(12):1622–7.

18. Amin Z, Donald JJ, Masters A, Kant R, Steger AC, Bown SG, et al. Hepatic metastases: interstitial laser photocoagulation with real-time US monitoring and dynamic CT evaluation of treatment. Radiology. 1993;187(2):339–47.

19. Nolsoe CP, Torp-Pedersen S, Burcharth F, Horn T, Pedersen S, Christensen NE, et al. Interstitial hyperthermia of colorectal liver metastases with a US-guided Nd-YAG laser with a diffuser tip: a pilot clinical study. Radiology. 1993;187(2):333–7.

20. Schroder T, Castren-Persons M, Lehtinen A, Taavitsainen M. Percutaneous interstitial laser hyperthermia in clinical use. Ann Chir Gynaecol. 1994;83(4):286–90.

21. Vogl TJ, Muller PK, Hammerstingl R, Weinhold N, Mack MG, Philipp C, et al. Malignant liver tumors treated with MR imaging-guided laser-induced thermotherapy: technique and prospective results. Radiology. 1995;196(1):257–65.

22. Tranberg KG, Moller PH, Hannesson P, Stenram U. Interstitial laser treatment of malignant tumours: initial experience. Eur J Surg Oncol. 1996;22(1):47–54.

23. Pacella CM, Bizzarri G, Ferrari FS, Anelli V, Valle D, Bianchini A, et al. [Interstitial photocoagulation with laser in the treatment of liver metastasis]. Radiol Med. 1996;92(4):438–447.

24. Heisterkamp J, van Hillegersberg R, Ijzermans JN. Interstitial laser coagulation for hepatic tumours. Br J Surg. 1999;86(3):293–304.

25. Vogl TJ, Mack MG, Straub R, Roggan A, Felix R. Magnetic resonance imaging-guided abdominal interventional radiology: laser-induced thermotherapy of liver metastases. Endoscopy. 1997;29(6):577–83.

26. Lee FT Jr, Mahvi DM, Chosy SG, Onik GM, Wong WS, Littrup PJ, et al. Hepatic cryosurgery with intraoperative US guidance. Radiology. 1997;202(3):624–32.

27. Gillams AR, Lees WR. Survival after percutaneous, image-guided, thermal ablation of hepatica metastases from colorectal cancer. Dis Colon Rectum. 2000;45(5):656–61.

28. Vogl TJ, Straub R, Eichler K, Sollner O, Mack MG. Colorectal carcinoma metastases in liver: laser-induced interstitial thermotherapy—local tumor control rate and survival data. Radiology. 2004;230(2):450–8.

29. Pacella CM, Valle D, Bizzarri G, Pacella S, Brunetti M, Maritati R, et al. Percutaneous laser ablation in patients with isolated unresectable liver metastases from colorectal cancer: Results of a phase II study. Acta Oncol. 2006;45(1):77–83.

30. Gillams A, Cassoni A, Conway G, Lees W. Radiofrequency ablation of neuroendocrine liver metastases: the Middlesex experience. Abdom Imaging. 2005;30(4):435–41.

31. Vogl TJ, Lehnert T, Eichler K, Proschek D, Floter J, Mack MG. Adrenal metastases: CT-guided and MR-thermometry-controlled laser-induced interstitial thermotherapy. Eur Radiol. 2007;17(8):2020–7.

32. Pacella CM, Bizzarri G, Magnolfi F, Cecconi P, Caspani B, Anelli V, et al. Laser thermal ablation in the treatment of small hepatocellular carcinoma: results in 74 patients. Radiology. 2001;221(3):712–20.

33. Pacella CM, Bizzarri G, Cecconi P, Caspani B, Magnolfi F, Bianchini A, et al. Hepatocellular carcinoma: long-term results of combined treatment with laser thermal ablation and transcatheter arterial chemoembolization. Radiology. 2001;219(3):669–78.

34. Pacella CM, Francica G, Di Lascio FM, Arienti V, Antico E, Caspani B, et al. Long-term outcome of cirrhotic patients with early hepatocellular carcinoma treated with ultrasound-guided percutaneous laser ablation: a retrospective analysis. J Clin Oncol. 2009;27(16):2615–21.

35. Eichler K, Zangos S, Gruber-Rouh T, Vogl TJ, Mack MG. Magnetic resonance-guided laser-induced thermotherapy in patients with oligonodular hepatocellular carcinoma: long-term results over a 15-year period. J Clin Gastroenterol. 2012;46(9):796–801.

36. Francica G, Petrolati A, Di Stasio E, Pacella S, Stasi R, Pacella CM. Effectiveness, safety, and local progression after percutaneous laser ablation for hepatocellular carcinoma nodules up to 4 cm are not affected by tumor location. AJR Am J Roentgenol. 2012;199(6):1393–401.

37. Francica G, Petrolati A, Di Stasio E, Pacella S, Stasi R, Pacella CM. Influence of ablative margin on local tumor progression and survival in patients with HCC </=4 cm after laser ablation. Acta Radiol. 2012;53(4):394–400.

38. Eichler K, Zangos S, Mack MG, Hammerstingl R, Gruber-Rouh T, Gallus C, et al. First human study in treatment of unresectable liver metastases from colorectal cancer with irinotecan-loaded beads (DEBIRI). Int J Oncol. 2012;41(4):1213–20.

39. Vogl TJ, Naguib NN, Lehnert T, Nour-Eldin NE, Eichler K, Zangos S, et al. Initial experience with repetitive transarterial chemoembolization (TACE) as a third line treatment of ovarian cancer metastasis to the liver: indications, outcomes and role in patient's management. Gynecol Oncol. 2012;124(2):225–9.

40. Vogl TJ, Gruber-Rouh T, Eichler K, Nour-Eldin NE, Trojan J, Zangos S, et al. Repetitive transarterial chemoembolization (TACE) of liver metastases from gastric cancer: local control and survival results. Eur J Radiol. 2013;82(2):258–63.

41. Vogl TJ, Dommermuth A, Heinle B, Nour-Eldin NE, Lehnert T, Eichler K, et al. Colorectal cancer liver metastases: long-term survival and progression-free survival after thermal ablation using magnetic resonance-guided laser-induced interstitial thermotherapy in 594 patients: analysis of prognostic factors. Investig Radiol. 2014;49(1):48–56.

42. Pacella CM, Stasi R, Bizzarri G, Pacella S, Graziano FM, Guglielmi R, et al. Percutaneous laser ablation of unresectable primary and metastatic adrenocortical carcinoma. Eur J Radiol. 2008;66(1):88–94.

43. Vogl TJ, Straub R, Eichler K, Woitaschek D, Mack MG. Malignant liver tumors treated with MR imaging-guided laser-induced thermotherapy: experience with complications in 899 patients (2,520 lesions). Radiology. 2002;225(2):367–77.

44. Arienti V, Pretolani S, Pacella CM, Magnolfi F, Caspani B, Francica G, et al. Complications of laser ablation for hepatocellular carcinoma: a multicenter study. Radiology. 2008;246(3):947–55.

45. Vogl TJ, Fieguth HG, Eichler K, Straub R, Lehnert T, Zangos S, et al. [Laser-induced thermotherapy of lung metastases and primary lung tumors]. Radiologe. 2004;44(7):693–9.

46. Rosenberg C, Puls R, Hegenscheid K, Kuehn J, Bollman T, Westerholt A, et al. Laser ablation of metastatic lesions of the lung: long-term outcome. AJR Am J Roentgenol. 2009;192(3):785–92.

47. Sponza M, Aprile G, Gasparini D, Iaiza E, De Pauli F, Giovannoni M, et al. Percutaneous laser-induced thermoablation (LIT) of non-resectable lung metastases and primary lung tumors: a preliminary evaluation of technical aspects and local efficiency. ASCO annual meeting proceedings (post-meeting edition). J Clin Oncol. 2006;24:18S.

48. Regine R, Stavolo C, Maglione F. Laser thermoablation of small pulmonary tumors: immediate and long-term follow-up CT features. In: C 23; First world congress of thoracic imaging and diagnosis in chest disease, Pozzuoli, Italy, 2005.

49. Sartori S, Mauri G, Tombesi P, Di Vece F, Bianchi L, Pacella CM. Ultrasound-guided percutaneous laser ablation is safe and effective in the treatment of small renal tumors in patients at increased bleeding risk. Int J Hyperth. 2018;35(1):19–25.

50. Patelli G, Ranieri A, Paganelli A, Mauri G, Pacella CM. Transperineal laser ablation for percutaneous treatment of benign prostatic hyperplasia: a feasibility study. Cardiovasc Intervent Radiol. 2017;40(9):1440–6.

51. Schena E, Saccomandi P, Fong Y. Laser ablation for cancer: past, present and future. J Funct Biomater. 2017;8(2):E19.

52. Pacella CM, Bizzarri G, Francica G, Bianchini A, De Nuntis S, Pacella S, et al. Percutaneous laser ablation in the treatment of hepatocellular carcinoma with small tumors: analysis of factors affecting the achievement of tumor necrosis. J Vasc Interv Radiol. 2005;16(11):1447–57.

53. Walser EM. Percutaneous laser ablation in the treatment of hepatocellular carcinoma with a tumor size of 4 cm or smaller: analysis of factors affecting the achievement of tumor necrosis. J Vasc Interv Radiol. 2005;16(11):1427–9.

54. Di Costanzo GG, Tortora R, D'Adamo G, De Luca M, Lampasi F, Addario L, et al. Radiofrequency ablation versus laser ablation for the treatment of small hepatocellular carcinoma in cirrhosis: a randomized trial. J Gastroenterol Hepatol. 2015;30(3):559–65.

55. Nikfarjam M, Muralidharan V, Malcontenti-Wilson C, Christophi C. Progressive microvascular injury in liver and colorectal liver metastases following laser induced focal hyperthermia therapy. Lasers Surg Med. 2005;37(1):64–73.

56. Germain D, Chevallier P, Laurent A, Savart M, Wassef M, Saint-Jalmes H. MR monitoring of laser-induced lesions of the liver in vivo in a low-field open magnet: temperature mapping and lesion size prediction. J Magn Reson Imaging. 2001;13(1):42–9.

57. Vogl TJ, Eichler K, Straub R, Engelmann K, Zangos S, Woitaschek D, et al. Laser-induced thermotherapy of malignant liver tumors: general principals, equipment(s), procedure(s)—side effects, complications and results. Eur J Ultrasound. 2001;13(2):117–27.

58. Vogl TJ, Straub R, Zangos S, Mack MG, Eichler K. MR-guided laser-induced thermotherapy (LITT) of liver tumours: experimental and clinical data. Int J Hyperthermia. 2004;20(7):713–24.

59. Claudon M, Dietrich CF, Choi BI, Cosgrove DO, Kudo M, Nolsoe CP, et al. Guidelines and good clinical practice recommendations for Contrast Enhanced Ultrasound (CEUS) in the liver—update 2012: A WFUMB-EFSUMB initiative in cooperation with representatives of AFSUMB, AIUM, ASUM, FLAUS and ICUS. Ultrasound Med Biol. 2013;39(2):187–210.

60. Meloni MF, Andreano A, Zimbaro F, Lava M, Lazzaroni S, Sironi S. Contrast enhanced ultrasound: roles in immediate post-procedural and 24-h evaluation of the effectiveness of thermal ablation of liver tumors. J Ultrasound. 2012;15(4):207–14.

61. Di Costanzo GG, D'Adamo G, Tortora R, Zanfardino F, Mattera S, Francica G, et al. A novel needle guide system to perform percutaneous laser ablation of liver tumors using the multifiber technique. Acta Radiol. 2013;54(8):876–81.

Liver Tumors Laser Ablation

Giovan Giuseppe Di Costanzo, Raffaella Tortora,
Marco Guarracino, Maria Mattera, Tian'an Jiang,
and Claudio Maurizio Pacella

4.1 Introduction

Surgical resection is considered the best treatment to eradicate liver tumors. However, it is applicable only in a minority of cases due to the position of cancer nodules, comorbidities, and liver function. Furthermore, it is expensive, requires in some cases long hospital stay, and may cause significant morbidity. In patients affected by hepatocellular carcinoma (HCC), the rate of cancer recurrence is about 15% per year and 70% at 5 years; in these cases repeat resection may be often not feasible. Resection, mainly when performed with open procedure, causes the release of intracellular molecules known as alarmins or damage-associated molecular patterns which may be linked with inflammatory response and tumor proliferation [1, 2]. Due to all these factors, mini-invasive treatments of liver tumors have become more and more popular. Among these, the local

application of high temperatures through the insertion of needles inside cancer nodules is one of the most widely employed techniques. Since the first use of radiofrequency ablation (RFA) in 1990, new devices, generator machines, and energy sources have been introduced in clinical practice. Currently, there are three main types of percutaneous hyperthermic treatments for liver tumors, including RFA, microwave (MWA), and laser ablation (LA). The primary mechanism of action of these techniques is the focal increase of temperatures inside the tumor nodule in a relatively short period of time (6–12 min) with the goal of inducing irreversible cell injury [3]. Among these treatments, LA is the less-known and -employed technique. The aim of this chapter is to describe the technique and the results of LA in the treatment of liver tumors.

4.2 Technique and Devices

Quartz fibers with different sizes and designs have been used to transmit the laser light inside the liver. According to the shape of the tip, fibers may be classified as bare-tip or cylindrical diffusing fibers. The traditional bare-tip fibers have a diameter ranging between 300 and 600 µm; the light is emitted only at the tip and are introduced through fine needles (21–22 gauge). Real-time ultrasound (US), computed tomography (CT), or magnetic resonance imaging (MRI) is used to

G. G. Di Costanzo (✉) · R. Tortora · M. Guarracino
M. Mattera
Liver Unit, Department of Transplantation, Cardarelli
Hospital, Naples, Italy
e-mail: giovangiuseppe.dicostanzo@aocardarelli.it

T. Jiang
Department of Ultrasound, First Affiliated Hospital,
College of Medicine, Zhejiang University,
Hangzhou, China

C. M. Pacella
Department of Diagnostic Imaging and Interventional
Radiology, Regina Apostolorum Hospital,
Albano Laziale, Rome, Italy

guide the insertion of the needles, and the choice between them is determined mainly by the experience of the operators and their availability. LA is the only percutaneous ablative technique that may be used with MRI that is theoretically the best method for planning and monitoring ablation. In fact, MRI allows the implementation of the real-time monitoring of thermometry that is useful for adjusting power settings and treatment duration to obtain appropriate temperature elevations beyond tumor margins [4]. Furthermore, MRI with specific liver contrast media is well suited to detect residual vital tissue which should still be ablated [5]. However, MRI use is limited by machine availability and complexity of the technique with a procedural time ranging between 60 and 120 min. CT is less used because it is less effective in evaluating thermal tissue effects immediately after ablation. Many centers use US guidance to position multiple thin fibers because it is simple, fast, and widely available. The used light sources are usually neodymium-doped yttrium aluminum garnet (Nd:YAG) and solid-state diode lasers with a wavelength of 980–1064 nm, and the power settings range between 2 and 5 W. A single bare fiber, when illuminated for 4–6 min, releases 1800 J to the tissue producing an almost spherical lesion with a maximum diameter of 12–16 mm [6]. To ablate larger tumours, 2–4 fibers can be introduced with a distance of 15 mm between tips, and up to four fibers may be activated simultaneously. When four fibers are used, the tips are arranged in a square configuration with a side length of 15–18 mm. In nodules larger than 30 mm, after a first illumination the needles may be pulled back for 15 mm and further illuminations can be done according to the size of the nodule. All needles are positioned before starting LA so that any gas caused by the treatment would not prevent the correct positioning of the needles. Experimental ex vivo studies have shown that the simultaneous activation of four fibers produces an ablation zone up to 11 times larger of that obtained by using a single fiber [7]. In patients, multifiber treatment produces ablation zones ranging between 20 and 50 mm. Because the insertion of multiple needles may be challenging and

time consuming, we have designed a guide that, attached to the ultrasound probe, allows the insertion of two needles in a parallel fashion at a prefixed distance, permitting a geometrical arrangement of needles [8]. The precise disposition of needles is crucial to obtain a large volume of necrosis. In fact, using this guide in case of nodules >30 mm, we obtained an ablation rate >90%, higher than the 60% rate observed in a previous large series where the operators inserted the needle through a standard biopsy needle guide [9]. Precise disposition of applicators is crucial also when large diffusing tips or other methods are used [10]. At the end of the procedure, the still-illuminated fibers are withdrawn to induce hyperthermia along the needle tract in order to avoid neoplastic seeding and to achieve the coagulation of this tract.

Diffusing laser fibers are larger than bare-tip fibers and are introduced through wide-bore needles or cannulas with a diameter of 1.0–3.8 mm (9–17 gauge) that are mainly positioned under MRI guidance. These fibers have cylindrical diffuser endings which emit light up to a distance of 10–30 mm and are cooled by a continuous water flow that avoids tissue charring and allows the use of high power settings up to 45 W. The largest successful experience with the use of large applicators (9 gauge) under MRI guidance for the treatment of liver metastases has been reported by Vogl and Coll [11]. Also with this technique, to destroy nodules larger than 20 mm, 2–4 applicators should be simultaneously used [12]. In our opinion this technique is less applicable in cirrhotic patients that have often impaired coagulation. Recently a smaller LA applicator with a flexible diffusing fiber and 17-gauge internally cooled catheter (Visualase®, Medtronic) was introduced. When illuminated at 15 W for 3 min, one or two applicators can achieve an ablation zone of 25 or 42 mm, respectively [13]. In Europe this applicator is used in neurosurgery, and studies in liver tumors are awaited.

The use of multiple thin bare-tip fibers as compared to diffusing fibers with large-bore cannulas has the advantage of being more simpler to perform and of increasing the applicability of the procedure. In fact, nodules located in difficult areas, for example, behind large vessels, in the caudate lobe, near the hepatic hilum, or in the liver dome, may be treated more easily and safely using thin needles [14, 15] (Figs. 4.1, 4.2, 4.3, 4.4, 4.5, 4.6, and 4.7). Furthermore, these needles can be inserted through the branches of the intra-hepatic portal vein without risk so that segmental neoplastic thrombosis may be safely treated (Fig. 4.8).

As compared to the standard RFA technique, LA has some theoretical advantages when large nodules should be treated. First, LA releases the energy precisely in a well-defined area limiting the risks of damaging adjacent structures, mainly when large amounts of energy are used. Second, the simultaneous activation of laser applicators may be more effective than alternate activation of radiofrequency needles in obtaining large ablation areas.

Fig. 4.1 A 10 mm HCC nodule located near recanalized umbilical vein (arrow): (**a**) before LA and (**b**) after LA using two 300 μm fibers

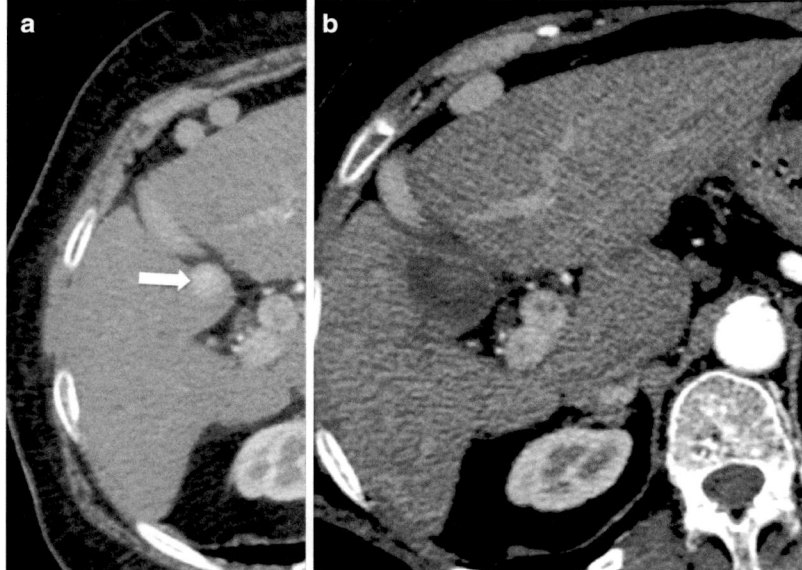

Fig. 4.2 CT scan of an exophytic 30 mm nodule, adjacent to the colon: (**a**) before LA and (**b**) after LA using four 300 μm fibers

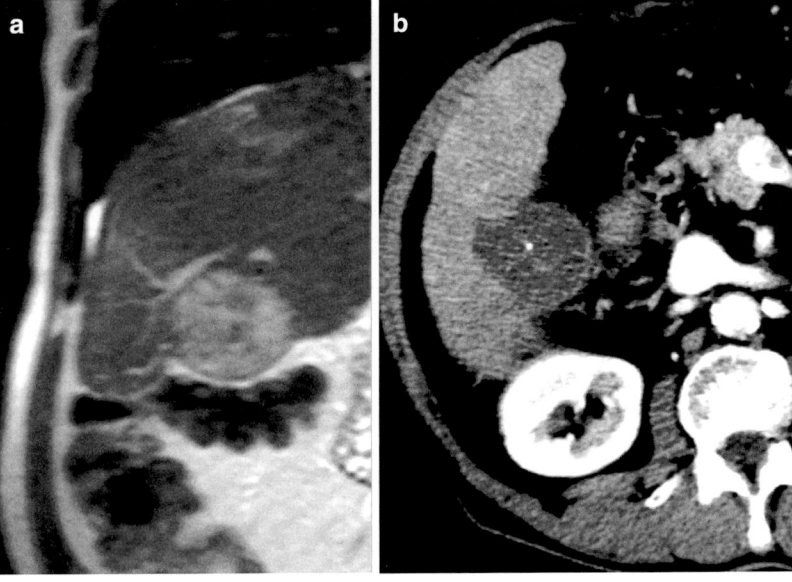

Fig. 4.3 MRI scan of an exophytic 35 mm nodule, adjacent to the right kidney: (**a**) before LA and (**b**) CT scan after LA using four 300 μm fibers

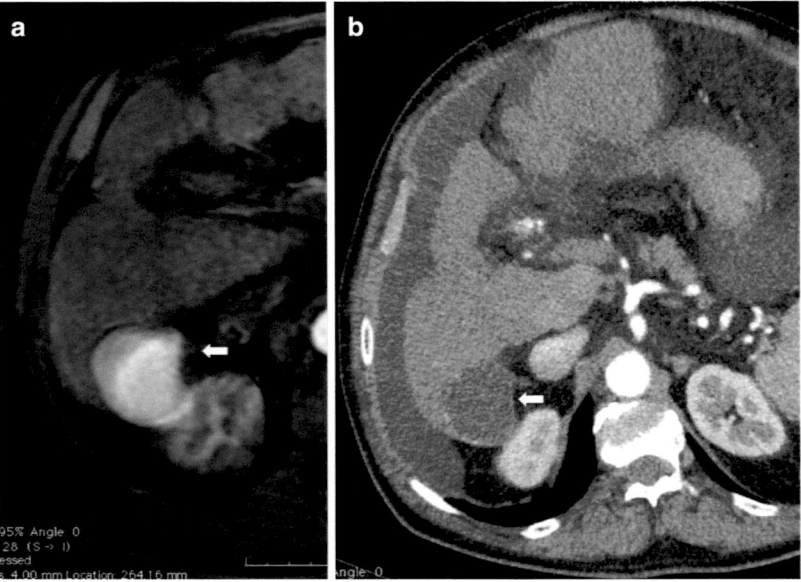

Fig. 4.4 CT scan of a 20 mm HCC nodule (arrow) located in the caudate lobe: (**a**) before LA and (**b**) after LA using two 300 μm fibers

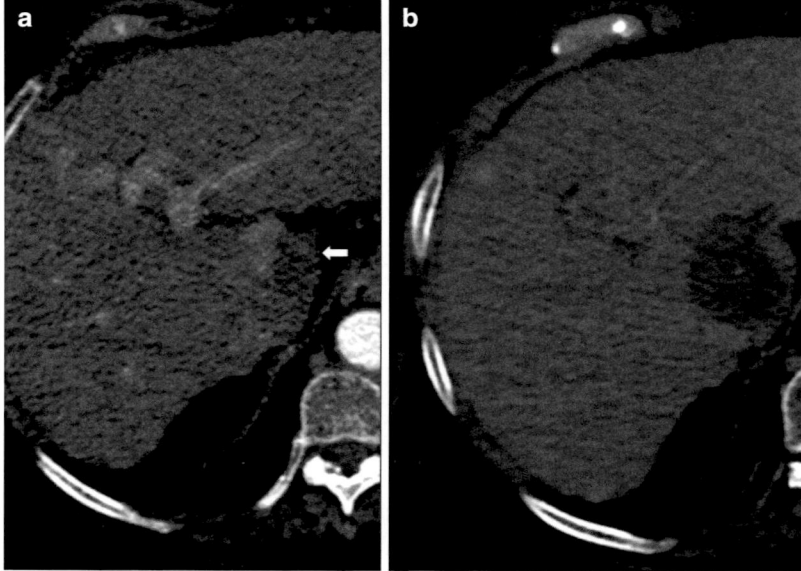

Fig. 4.5 MRI scan
showing a 30 mm HCC
nodule located near the
hepatic hilum: (**a**) before
LA and (**b**) CT scan
after LA with four
300 μm fibers

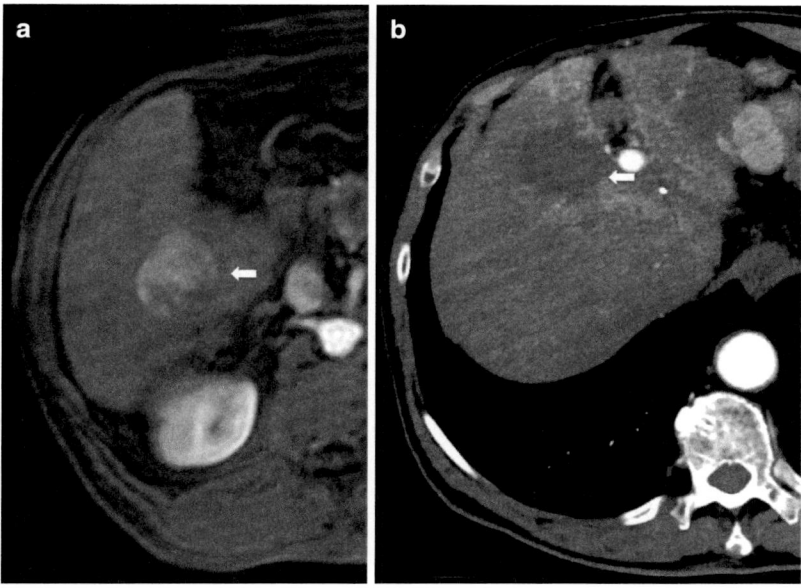

4.3   Endoscopic Approach

In very selected cases of tumors located in the left
liver, especially in the caudate lobe, inconspicu-
ous on conventional ultrasound or when there is
no perforation path and there is risk to damage
adjacent major structures, percutaneous intervention cannot be performed. The data reported by
Kazuyama et al. indicate that RFA as an effective
treatment modality for HCC in the caudate lobe
does not appear to be very convincing [16].

In the last 30 years, the development of ultrasound endoscopy (EUS) and its functional expansion have enabled its use not only in diagnostics
but also in the treatment of focal lesions. The
EUS can clearly show the relationship between
the lesion and surrounding tissue as in the case of

peri-esophageal lesions [17]. Therefore, EUS
guidance may be a good alternative to display
and treat the lesions in the left liver and caudate
lobe.

Cases of LA of left hepatic and caudate lobe
tumors have been reported. Di Matteo et al. in
2011 reported that the treatment of caudate lobe
tumors by laser ablation under EUS is effective
and safe [18]. Jiang et al. reported and discussed
10 cases of tumors located in the caudate lobe
(Fig. 4.9) and left liver treated with LA under
EUS guidance [19]. The sizes of the lesions
treated ranged from 0.9 × 0.7 to 3.4 × 2.7 cm. The
EUS-guided laser ablation (EUS-LA) of these
tumors was successfully completed without complications in all patients. However, long-term
prospective studies are still lacking.

Fig. 4.6 Images of a 54-year-old patient with a hepatic tumor located in the portal cava interval and treated with ultrasound (US)-guided laser ablation. (**a**) Pre-op (MRI) T2-weighted image depicted the tumor (*arrows*) located in the portal cava interval; (**b**) the contrast-enhanced MRI scanning described the tumor as an enhanced signal (*arrows*); (**c**) pre-op US image showed a 1.7 × 1.2 cm tumor in the portal cava interval of the liver; (**d**) the location of the guiding needle and laser fiber during the operation; (**e**, **f**) the post-operative contrast-enhanced ultrasonography (CEUS) image revealed the lesion was a well-defined perfusion defect throughout all phases; (**g**, **h**) the post-op contrast-enhanced MRI scanning revealed there was no enhanced signal during the arterial phase and portal phase, which indicated the ablation was complete

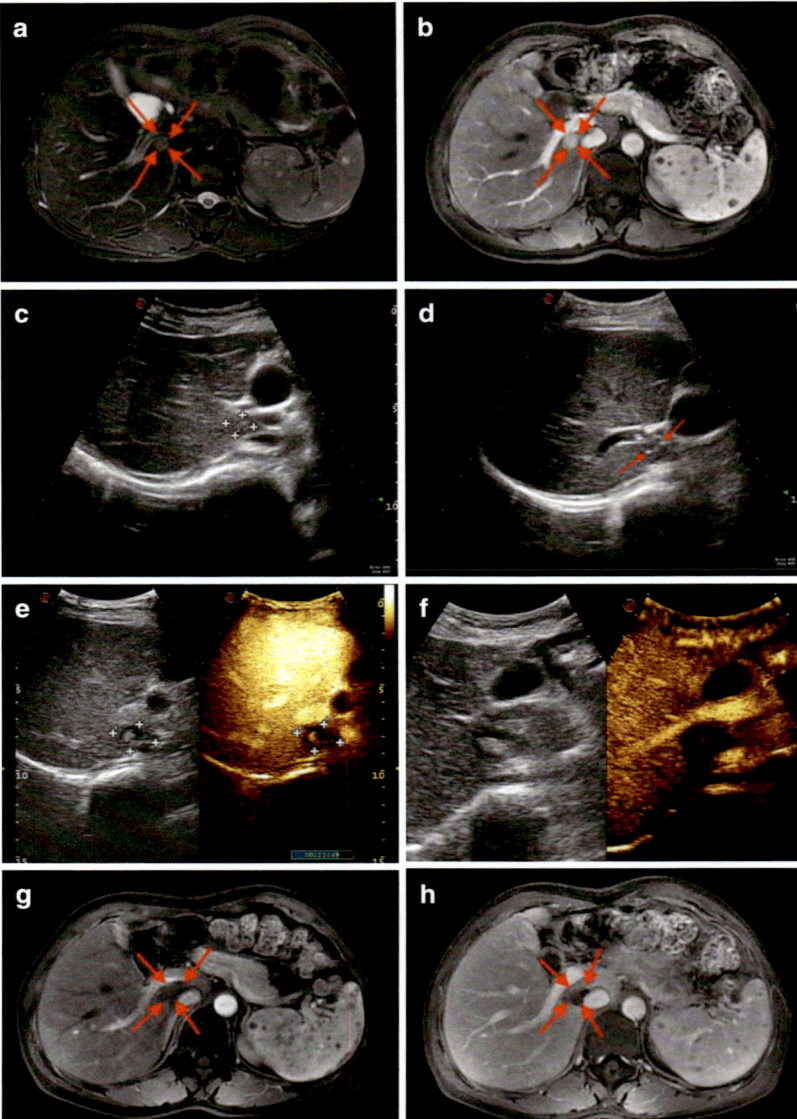

4.4 Results

4.4.1 Hepatocellular Carcinoma

HCC is a lethal disease being the fifth most common cancer worldwide and the second most common cause of death due to cancer [20]. HCC occurs in most patients affected by cirrhosis. In these patients the choice of the best available therapy may be hard, and the majority is treated with mini-invasive locoregional treatments. Several retrospective studies have shown that LA is a safe and effective treatment of HCC. Using multiple thin bare fibers a complete ablation of HCC nodules sized up to 50 mm has been achieved in 82–97% of cases [8, 9, 21–23]. Adding up the results of three studies, a complete ablation was obtained in 85–100% of 288 nod-

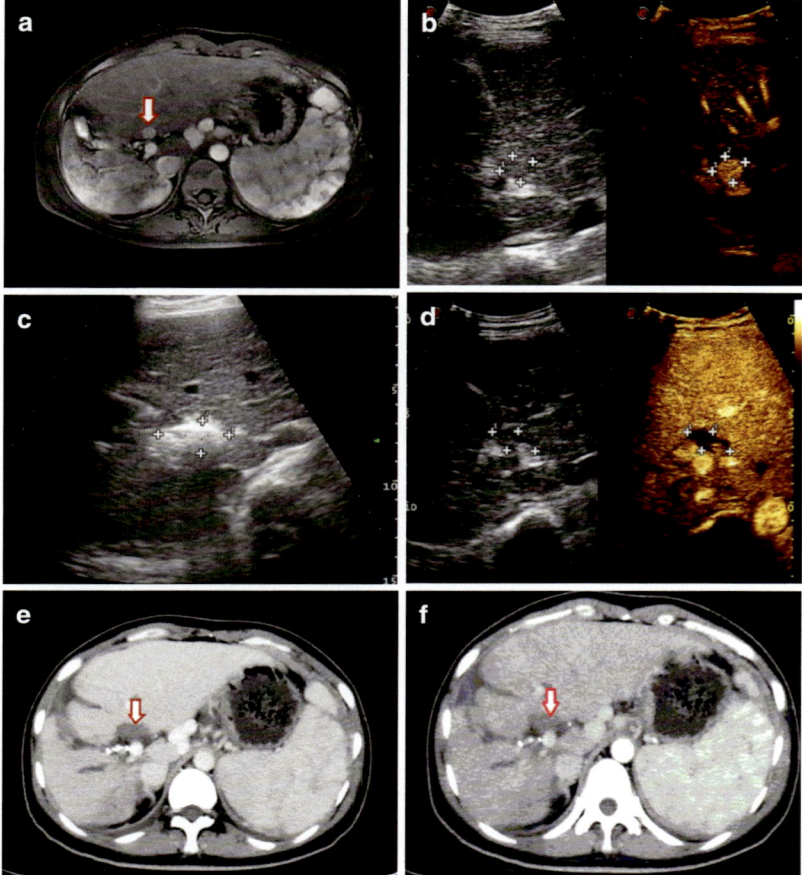

Fig. 4.7 Images of a 37-year-old patient with recurrence of hepatocellular carcinoma. Contrast-enhanced magnetic resonance imaging (MRI): (**a**) right lobe of the liver demonstrates a 1.5 × 1.0 cm tumor nodule (*arrow*) located in porta hepatic close to the right branch of the portal vein which was hardly treatable for radiofrequency ablation (RFA) or trans-arterial arterial chemoembolization (TACE). (**b**) Contrast-enhanced ultrasound (CEUS) before laser ablation (LA). (**c**) Ultrasound image during ablation shows an area of coagulative necrosis and the total energy is 1800 J. (**d**) CEUS was repeated after the LA and the lesion was not enhanced, suggesting complete ablation. (**e**, **f**) The contrast-enhanced CT after LA and the lesion (*arrow*) revealed no enhancement during the whole period

ules ≤20 mm, in 82–100% of 324 nodules between 20 and 30 mm and in 60–94% of 148 nodules between 30 and 40 mm [9, 24, 25].

The use of diffusing applicators introduced through 9-gauge (3.8 mm) cannulas (Somatex, Berlin, Germany) has been reported in 113 cirrhotic patients with 175 HCC nodules ≤50 mm. To limit the risk of peritoneal bleeding due to the use of large bore applicators, only patients with normal coagulative parameters (platelets >100,000 and prothrombin time >70%) were treated. Complete ablation rate was 98% with a

very low local recurrence of 2%. However, due to the complexity, costs and long duration of the procedure (up to 90 min), this technique is less frequently used [26].

LA for the treatment of HCC in cirrhotic patients has been validated in a randomized non-inferiority trial. One-hundred forty patients with HCC within Milan criteria were treated with RFA using a 17-gauge cooled-tip single electrode (Cool-Tip, Valleylab, Burlington, MA, USA) or LA with multiple thin fibers using a commercially available system (EchoLaser, Elesta Srl,

Fig. 4.8 Treatment of tumor thrombosis: (**a**) US showing infiltrating HCC (1) and segmental thrombosis (2); (**b**) contrast-enhanced US showing hyper-enhancement of nodule and of thrombus; (**c**) a 21G needle was inserted in the thrombus (1: tip of the needle) and a 300 μm fiber was introduced (2: tip of fiber); (**d**) contrast-enhanced US after LA showing complete ablation of nodule and thrombus

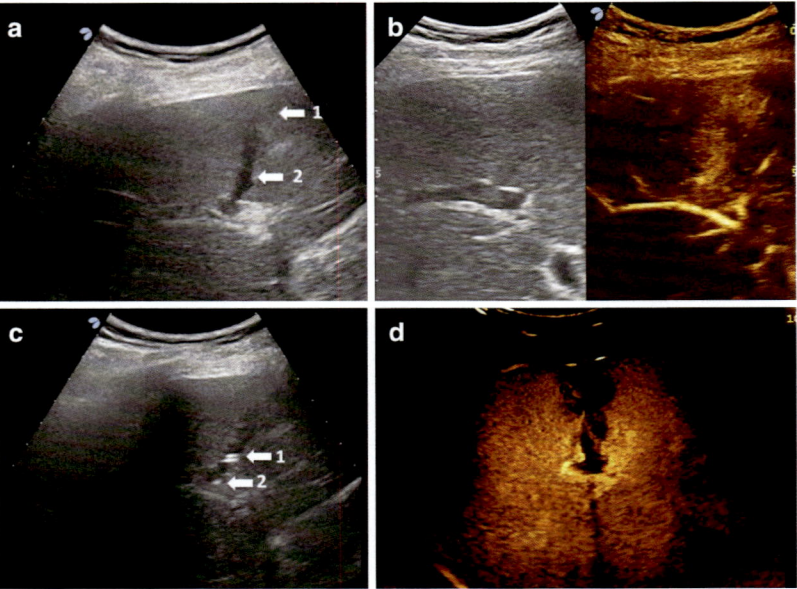

Calenzano, Florence, Italy) equipped with a diode laser. The rate of complete tumor ablation was comparable among the RFA (97%) and LA (96%) groups. Both procedures were reported safe, and the occurrence of local tumor progression and overall survival were similar in the two groups. The study also suggests that LA may be cheaper than RFA, but appropriate designed trials are needed to confirm this finding.

Local tumor progression is a relevant factor affecting the long-term results of local ablation. Among factors related to the occurrence of local progression, one of the most significant is the achievement of large safety margin to kill occult foci of cancer cells [27–29]. In a study evaluating LA, a safety margin >5 mm was observed in 82/132 nodules (62%) and >7.5 mm in 43/132 nodules (32.5%). A safety margin >7.5 mm resulted related to a lower incidence of local progression (*P* 0.020, OR 4.1 [1.1–14.7]) [30].

An advantage of LA as compared to radiofrequency and microwave ablation is the possibility of treating the majority of nodules located at high risk sites without the need of using artificial methods as artificial ascites [31]. According to the literature, nodules are defined to be in high-risk location when they are located less than 5 mm from large vessels or vital organs. In a study on 116 nodules with a diameter <40 mm in 106 patients, complete ablation was achieved in 92.2%. Major complications occurred in two patients (1.9%): one death due to liver failure and one deep jaundice due to biliary stricture [15].

Treatment of large unresectable HCCs with a diameter ≥40 mm is still a matter of debate and research; transarterial chemoembolization (TACE) is the most applied treatment. In these cases, we evaluated the efficacy of LA using eight fibers. The fibers are positioned in two-squared fashion and four fibers per time are simultaneously activated; in our experience maximum energy deposition of 55,000 J is safe. In a case-control study in patients with HCC up to 75 mm, we have compared this technique with

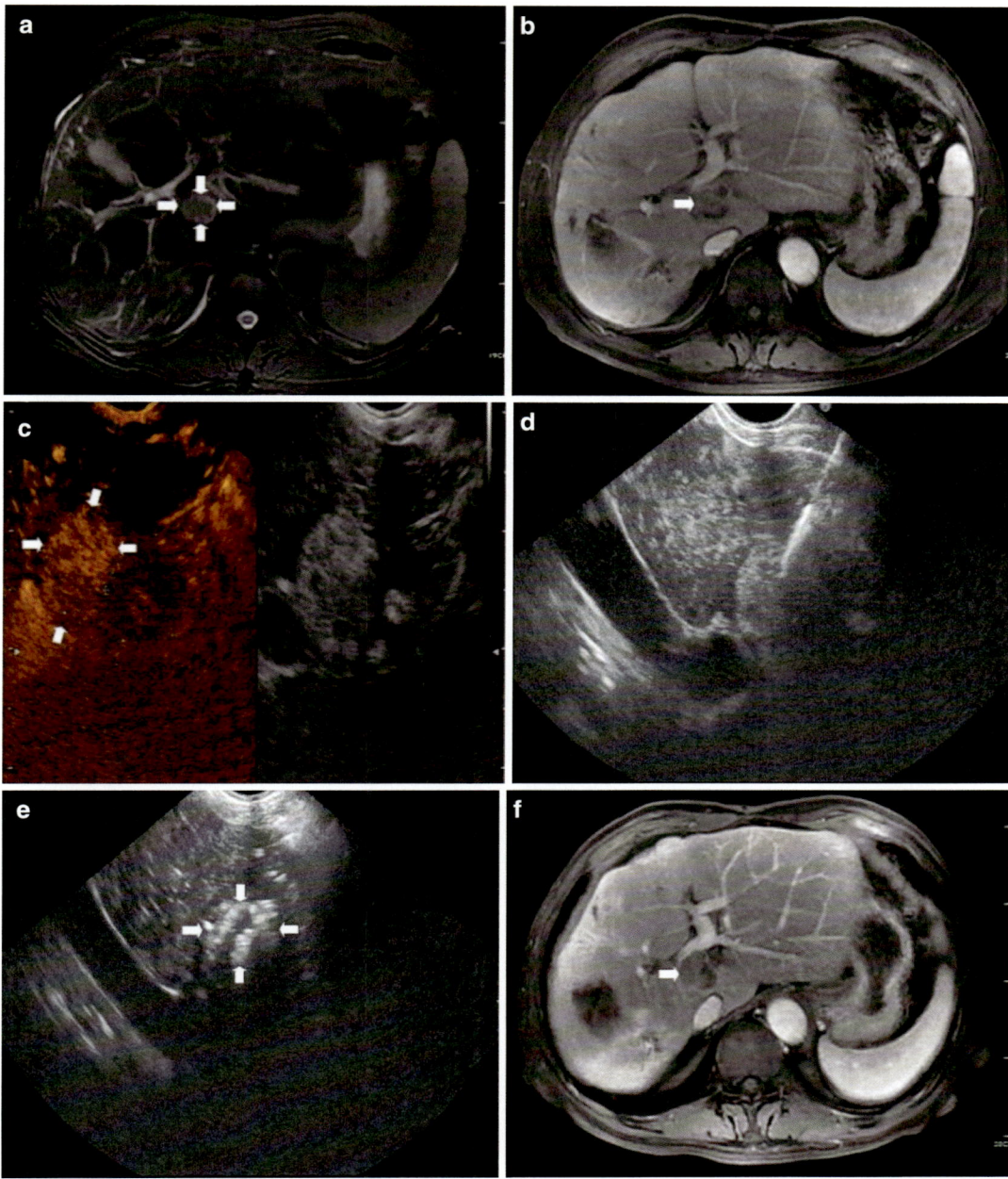

Fig. 4.9 A case of EUS-guided LA in hepatocellular carcinoma in the caudate lobe. 63-year-old man with hepatocellular carcinoma. Pre-operative MR and CEUS images showed a mass of 2.2 × 1.7 cm in size in the caudate lobe (**a–c**) (*white arrows*). EUS-guided laser fiber inserted into the tumor (**d**) and then total enhancement of the lesion (**e**) (*white arrows*). One year later, substance phase MR image showed that the mass has a complete response (**f**) (*white arrows*)

TACE in 82 patients [32]. No major complications occurred; complete ablation was obtained in 67% of cases with LA and in 19.5% with TACE ($P < 0.001$). The best response rate, up to 75%, was observed in nodules sized ≤60 mm, and we believe that LA treatment should be restricted to nodules up to this size. Combined treatment with LA and TACE whether as adjuvant or as neoadjuvant treatment seems promising and may be applied in multifocal and large HCC. In large HCC, a protocol of repeated TACE sessions before LA or TACE after LA gave excellent results, but further studies are needed [22, 33].

In a small series, LA was reported safe and effective in cirrhotic patients waiting for liver transplantation. Complete necrosis at explant was found in 8/12 nodules (67%), and no major complications occurred [34]. Further data on this topic are needed.

The rate of complications for LA is comparable to those reported for RFA and MWA. In a large multicentric Italian study, 520 patients with 647 HCC nodules treated with 1064 sessions were evaluated [35]. One hundred and eighty-one patients had poor liver function (Child-Pugh grade B–C), in 10% ascites was present and 39% of nodules had a size >30 mm. Fifteen patients (1.5%) had major complications and 4 patients deceased (0.8%). Large tumor size, poor liver function and uncontrolled ascites resulted related to these events. Seeding was not observed.

Long-term outcome of early HCC (single nodule ≤40 mm or three nodules ≤30 mm) treated with LA was investigated in a retrospective study involving 432 patients [9]. Median overall survival was 47 months and resulted independently related to age <73 years, albumin >3.5 g/dL and complete ablation. According to the results of this study, the ideal candidates for LA are younger patients with albumin >3.5 g/dL and HCC ≤20 mm in whom a 5-year survival probability of 60% was observed. The median time to recurrence was 24 months, and the median disease-free survival time was 26 months.

4.4.2 Metastases

Liver metastases account for the vast majority of hepatic malignant masses, usually carcinomas, and the most common sites of origin are colorectum, pancreas and breast. Resection of colon metastases is unfeasible in 75–90% of cases [36, 37] and prognosis of patients treated only with systemic therapy is dismal; therefore, minimally invasive techniques have been attempted in selected cases, in particular, in oligonodular and metachronous metastases. However, robust data regarding the efficacy of thermal ablation for treating liver metastases, mainly controlled randomized trials, are lacking; oncological and surgical communities are not yet totally convinced that ablation may improve patient survival. Among ablative techniques, LA alone or combined with adjuvant or neo-adjuvant treatments has been used also because it has some favorable characteristics. In an experimental model of colorectal metastasis, laser hyperthermia produced progressive microvascular and tissue injury that peaked by 72 h after starting illumination [38]. Therefore, after a first phase of direct thermal damage there is a second phase of progressive ischemic damage that causes the increase of ablation area. Laser light seems more effective than other hyperthermic treatments in inducing damage of endothelial cells as observed in the treatment of varicose veins. Furthermore, it was demonstrated both in experimental models and in patients that LA might stimulate host immune defenses against cancer-inducing local and systemic Th1 immune responses [39, 40].

Several studies using mainly large-bore diffusing tip applicators showed a positive effect of LA in unresectable colorectal metastases. The largest experience have been reported by Vogl et al. that treated patients with no more than five metastases and a size up to 50 mm. A similar cut-off was indicated by two panels of experts evaluating radiofrequency ablation: the best nodule size should be <30 mm, but ≤5 nodules <50 mm can be effectively treated depending on anatomical location

Fig. 4.10 Contrast-enhanced US of a 60 mm neuroendocrine metastasis after LA with eight thin fibers showing complete necrosis

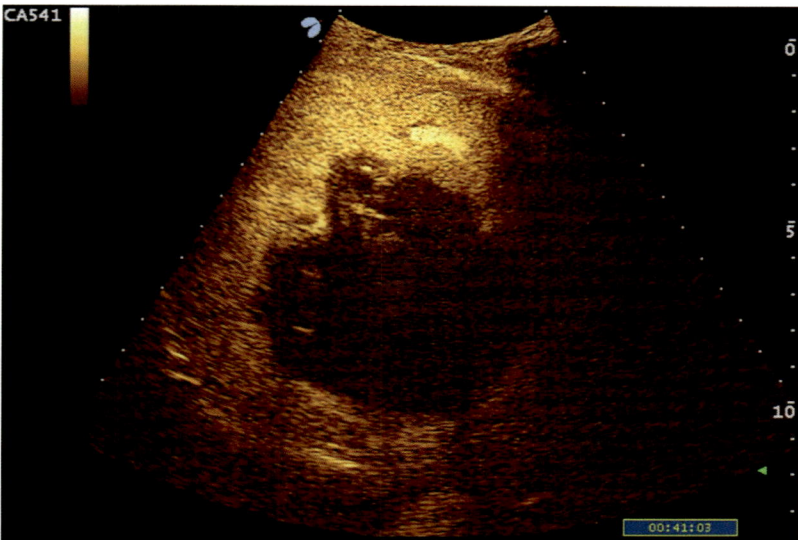

[41, 42]. Six-month local recurrence rate was <5% in patients with nodules <40 mm. The median survival was 3.5 years: 94% at 1 year, 77% at 2 years, 56% at 3 years and 37% at 5 years [43]. Comparable results were reported in another series using the same technique [44]. Concerning the complete ablation rate, it was reported to be 100% for nodules <20 mm in diameter, 71% between 20 and 30 mm, 46% between 30 and 40 mm and 30% for metastases >40 mm [45]. Pacella et al. obtained similar results using multiple thin fibers with a complete ablation rate of 87% in metastases ≤30 mm and 23% in nodules >30 mm [46].

LA may be used in patients with liver metastases from neuroendocrine tumors who are unfit for surgery. Two small series have shown that LA with multiple thin bare-tip fibers, alone or combined with TACE, is safe and allows for complete ablation in 80–100% of cases [47, 48] (Fig. 4.10). Comparable results were obtained with the use of large diffusing-tip applicators [49]. In most of patients a multimodality approach is chosen to fight neuroendocrine metastases and in the therapeutic strategy LA may be considered a very useful tool [50].

Liver metastases from breast are a controversial indication to local ablation. Good results have been reported in patients with oligonodular, non-resectable tumors, recurrent tumor after resection, bilobar tumors and those without extrahepatic involvement except for bone metastases under control [51]. In a study evaluating 232 patients with 578 metastases, an ablation area larger than the initial volume was obtained in all except two cases. The median survival was 4.3 years: 1-year survival was 96%, 3-year 63% and 5-year 41%. Comparing data from literature, the local tumor progression after RFA and LA was 13.5–58.0% and 2.9%, respectively [52].

In some cases, mainly when multiple and large metastases should be treated, combination of catheter-based treatments (transarterial embolization, chemoembolization and radioembolization) and percutaneous ablation may be used [53, 54]. Transarterial treatments may be performed in a neoadjuvant setting to reduce the tumor load and to increase tumor ischemia for increasing LA applicability and success rate. Alternatively, catheter treatments are also used in an adjuvant setting to complete the ablation performed with LA, mainly when residual tumor persists after ablation at the periphery of cancer nodules.

Prospective studies to confirm the effectiveness of LA in the treatment of liver metastases are needed.

References

1. Ramirez MF, Ai D, Bauer M, Vauthey JN, Gottumukkala V, Kee S, et al. Innate immune function after breast, lung, and colorectal cancer surgery. J Surg Res. 2015;194:185–93.
2. Fretland AA, Sokolov A, Postriganova N, Kazaryan AM, Pischke SE, Nilsson PH, et al. Inflammatory response after laparoscopic versus open resection of colorectal liver metastases: data from the Oslo-CoMet trial. Medicine. 2015;94(42):e1786.
3. Stauffer PR, Goldberg SN. Introduction: thermal ablation therapy. Int J Hyperth. 2004;20:671–7.
4. Vogl TJ, Müller PK, Hammerstingl R, Weinhold N, Mack MG, Philipp C, et al. Malignant liver tumors treated with MR imaging-guided laser-induced thermotherapy: technique and prospective results. Radiology. 1995;196:257–65.
5. Isbert C, Ritz JP, Schilling A, Roggan A, Heiniche A, Wolf KJ, et al. Laser induced thermotherapy (LITT) of experimental liver metastasis-detection of residual tumors using Gd-DTPA enhanced MRI. Lasers Surg Med. 2002;30:280–9.
6. Tranberg KG. Percutaneous ablation of liver tumours. Best Pract Res Clin Gastroenterol. 2004;18:125–45.
7. Steger AC, Lees WR, Shorvon P, Walmsley K, Bown SG. Multiple-fibre low-power interstitial laser hyperthermia: studies in the normal liver. Br J Surg. 1992;79:139–45.
8. Di Costanzo GG, D'Adamo G, Tortora R, Zanfardino F, Mattera S, Francica G, Pacella CM. A novel needle guide system to perform percutaneous laser ablation of liver tumors using the multifiber technique. Acta Radiol. 2013;54:876–81.
9. Pacella CM, Francica G, Di Lascio FM, Arienti V, Antico E, Caspani B, et al. Long-term outcome of cirrhotic patients with early hepatocellular carcinoma treated with ultrasound guided percutaneous laser ablation: a retrospective analysis. J Clin Oncol. 2009;27:2615–21.
10. Heisterkamp J, Van Hillegersberg R, Sinofsky EL, Ijzermans JNM. Interstitial laser photocoagulation with four cylindrical diffusing fibre tips: importance of mutual fibre distance. Lasers Med Sci. 1999;14:216–20.
11. Vogl TJ, Straub R, Eichler K, Woitaschek D, Mack MG. Malignant liver tumors treated with MR imaging guided laser-induced thermotherapy: experience with complications in 899 patients (2,520 lesions). Radiology. 2002;225:367–77.
12. Vogl TJ, Dommermuth A, Heinle B, Nour-Eldin NE, Lehnert T, Eichler K, et al. Colorectal cancer liver metastases: long-term survival and progression-free survival after thermal ablation using magnetic resonance-guided laser-induced interstitial thermotherapy in 594 patients: analysis of prognostic factors. Investig Radiol. 2014;49:48–56.
13. Ahrar K, Gowda A, Javadi S, Borne A, Fox M, McNichols R, et al. Preclinical assessment of a 980-nm diode laser ablation system in a large animal tumor model. J Vasc Interv Radiol. 2010;21:555–61.
14. Pacella CM, Bizzarri G, Francica G, Bianchini A, De Nuntis S, Pacella S, et al. Percutaneous laser ablation in the treatment of hepatocellular carcinoma with small tumors: analysis of factors affecting the achievement of tumor necrosis. J Vasc Interv Radiol. 2005;16:1447–57.
15. Francica G, Petrolati A, Di Stasio E, Pacella S, Stasi R, Pacella CM. Effectiveness, safety and local progression after percutaneous laser ablation foe HCC nodules ≤ 4 cm are not affected by tumor location. Am J Roentgenol. 2012;199:1393–401.
16. Kariyama K, Nouso K, Wakuta A, Kishida M, Nishimura M, Wada N, et al. Percutaneous radiofrequency ablation for treatment of hepatocellular carcinoma in the caudate lobe. Am J Roentgenol. 2011;197:W571–5.
17. Saraireh HA, Bilal M, Singh S. Role of endoscopic ultrasound in liver disease: where do we stand in 2017? World J Hepatol. 2017;9:1013–21.
18. Di Matteo F, Grasso R, Pacella CM, Martino M, Pandolfi M, Rea R, et al. EUS-guided Nd:YAG laser ablation of a hepatocellular carcinoma in the caudate lobe. Gastrointest Endosc. 2011;73:632–6.
19. Jiang T, Tian G, Bao H, Chen F, Deng Z, Li J, Chai W. EUS dating with laser ablation against the caudate lobe or left liver tumors: a win-win proposition? Cancer Biol Ther. 2018;19:145–52.
20. http://globocan.iarc.fr/old/FactSheets/cancers/liver-new.asp.
21. Giorgio A, Tarantino L, de Stefano GN, Catalano O, Cusati B, Del Viscovo LA, Caturelli E. Interstitial laser photocoagulation under ultrasound guidance of liver tumors: results in 104 treated patients. Eur J Ultrasound. 2000;11:181–8.
22. Pacella CM, Bizzarri G, Cecconi P, Caspani B, Magnolfi F, Bianchini A, et al. Hepatocellular carcinoma: long-term results of combined treatment with laser thermal ablation and transcatheter arterial chemoembolization. Radiology. 2001;219:669–78.
23. Francica G, Iodice G, Delle Cave M, Sarrantonio R, Lapiccirella G, Molese V, et al. Factors predicting complete necrosis rate after ultrasound guided percutaneous laser thermoablation of small hepatocellular carcinoma tumors in cirrhotic patients: a multivariate analysis. Acta Radiol. 2007;48:514–9.
24. Pacella CM, Bizzarri G, Francica G, Forlini G, Petrolati A, Valle D, et al. Analysis of factors predicting survival in patients with hepatocellular carcinoma treated with percutaneous laser ablation. J Hepatol. 2006;44:902–9.
25. Di Costanzo GG, Tortora R, D'Adamo G, De Luca M, Lampasi F, Addario L, et al. Radiofrequency ablation versus laser ablation for the treatment of small hepatocellular carcinoma in cirrhosis: a randomized trial. J Gastroenterol Hepatol. 2015;30:559–65.
26. Eichler K, Zangos S, Gruber-Rouh T, Vogl TJ, Mack MG. Magnetic resonance-guided laser-induced thermotherapy in patients with oligonodular hepatocel-

lular carcinoma: long-term results over a 15-year period. J Clin Gastroenterol. 2012;46:796–801.

27. Kei SK, Rhim H, Choi D, Lee WJ, Lim HK, Kim YS. Local tumor progression after radiofrequency ablation of liver tumors: analysis of morphologic pattern and site of recurrence. Am J Roentgenol. 2008;190:1544–51.

28. Liu CH, Arellano RS, Uppot RN, Debra AES, Gervais A, Mueller PR. Radiofrequency ablation of hepatic tumours: effect of post-ablation margin on local tumour progression. Eur Radiol. 2010;20:877–85.

29. Shiina S, Teratani T, Obi S, Sato S, Tateishi R, Fujishima T, et al. A randomized controlled trial of radiofrequency ablation with ethanol injection for small hepatocellular carcinoma. Gastroenterology. 2005;129:122–30.

30. Francica G, Petrolati A, Di Stasio E, Pacella S, Stasi R, Pacella CM. Influence of ablative margin on local tumor progression and survival in patients with HCC < / = 4 cm after laser ablation. Acta Radiol. 2012;53:394–400.

31. Teratani T, Yoshida H, Shiina S, Obi S, Sato S, Tateishi R, et al. Radiofrequency ablation for hepatocellular carcinoma in so-called high-risk locations. Hepatology. 2006;43:1101–8.

32. Morisco F, Camera S, Guarino M, Tortora R, Cossiga V, Vitiello A, et al., Italian Liver Cancer (ITA.LI.CA) Group. Laser ablation is superior to TACE in large sized hepatocellular carcinoma: a pilot case-control study. Oncotarget. 2018;9:17483–90.

33. Zangos S, Eichler K, Balzer JO, Straub R, Hammerstingl R, Herzog C, et al. Large-sized hepatocellular carcinoma (HCC): a neoadjuvant treatment protocol with repetitive transarterial chemoembolization (TACE) before percutaneous MR-guided laser-induced thermotherapy (LITT). Eur Radiol. 2007;17:553–63.

34. Pompili M, Pacella CM, Francica G, Angelico M, Tisone G, Craboledda P, et al. Percutaneous laser ablation of hepatocellular carcinoma in patients with liver cirrhosis awaiting liver transplantation. Eur J Radiol. 2010;74:e6–e11.

35. Arienti V, Pretolani S, Pacella CM, Magnolfi F, Caspani B, Francica G, et al. Complications of laser ablation for hepatocellular carcinoma: a multicentre study. Radiology. 2008;246:947–55.

36. Schlag PM, Benhidjeb T, Stroszczynski C. Resection and local therapy for liver metastases. Best Pract Res Clin Gastroenterol. 2002;16:299–317.

37. Hackl C, Neumann P, Gerken M, Loss M, Klinkhammer-Schalke M, Schlitt HJ. Treatment of colorectal liver metastases in Germany: a ten-year population-based analysis of 5772 cases of primary colorectal adenocarcinoma. BMC Cancer. 2014;14:810.

38. Nikfarjam M, Vijayaragavan M, Malcontenti-Wilson C, Christophi C. Progressive microvascular injury in liver and colorectal liver metastases following laser induced focal hyperthermia therapy. Lasers Surg Med. 2005;37:64–73.

39. Lin WX, Fifis T, Malcontenti-Wilson C, Nikfarjam M, Muralidharan V, Nguyen L, Christophi C. Induction of Th1 Immune responses following laser ablation in a murine model of colorectal liver metastases. J Transl Med. 2011;9:83.

40. Vogl TJ, Wissniowski TT, Naguib NNN, Hammerstingl RM, Mack MG, Münch S, et al. Activation of tumor-specific T lymphocytes after laser-induced thermotherapy in patients with colorectal liver metastases. Cancer Immunol Immunother. 2009;58:1557–63. https://doi.org/10.1007/s00262-009-0663-1.

41. Wong SL, Mangu PB, Choti MA, Crocenzi TS, Dodd GD III, Dorfman GS, et al. American Society of Clinical Oncology 2009 clinical evidence review on radiofrequency ablation of hepatic metastases from colorectal cancer. J Clin Oncol. 2010;28:493–508.

42. Gillams A, Goldberg N, Ahmed M, Bale R, Breen D, Callstrom M, et al. Thermal ablation of colorectal liver metastases: a position paper by an international panel of ablation experts, The Interventional Oncology Sans Frontiers meeting 2013. Eur Radiol. 2015;25:3438–54.

43. Vogl TJ, Straub R, Eichler K, Söllner O, Mack MG. Colorectal carcinoma metastases in liver: laser-induced interstitial thermotherapy—local tumor control rate and survival data. Radiology. 2004;230:450–8.

44. Puls R, Langner S, Rosenberg C, Hegenscheid K, Kuehn JP, Noeckler K, Hosten N. Laser ablation of liver metastases from colorectal cancer with MR thermometry: 5-year survival. J Vasc Int Radiol. 2009;20:225–34.

45. Fiedler VU, Schwarzmaier HJ, Eickmeyer F, Müller FP, Schoepp C, Verreet PR. Laser-induced interstitial thermotherapy of liver metastases in an interventional 0.5 Tesla MRI system: technique and first clinical experiences. J Magn Reson Imaging. 2001;13:729–37.

46. Pacella CM, Valle D, Bizzarri G, Pacella S, Brunetti M, Maritati R, et al. Percutaneous laser ablation in patients with isolated unresectable liver metastases from colorectal cancer: results of a phase II study. Acta Oncol. 2006;45:77–83.

47. Tombesi P, Di Vece F, Sartori S. Laser ablation for hepatic metastases from neuroendocrine tumors. Am J Roentgenol. 2015;204:W732–2.

48. Pacella CM, Nasoni S, Grimaldi F, Di Stasio E, Misischi I, Bianchetti S, Papini E. Laser ablation with or without chemoembolization for unresectable neuroendocrine liver metastases: a pilot study. Int J Endocr Oncol. 2016;3:97–107.

49. Vogl TJ, Naguib NN, Zangos S, Eichler K, Hedayati A, Nour-Eldin NEA. Liver metastases of neuroendocrine carcinomas: interventional treatment via transarterial embolization, chemoembolization and thermal ablation. Eur J Radiol. 2009;72(3):517–28.

50. Frilling A, Sotiropoulos GC, Li J, Kornasiewicz O, Plöckinger U. Multimodal management of neuroendocrine liver metastases. HPB. 2010;12:361–79.

51. Mack MG, Straub R, Eichler K, Söllner O, Lehnert T, Vogl TJ. Breast cancer metastases in liver: laser-

induced interstitial thermotherapy—local tumor control rate and survival data. Radiology. 2004;233:400–9.

52. Vogl TJ, Farshid P, Naguib NN, Zangos S. Thermal ablation therapies in patients with breast cancer liver metastases: a review. Eur Radiol. 2013;23:797–804.

53. Vogl TJ, Jost A, Nour-Eldin NA, Mack MG, Zangos S, Naguib NNN. Repeated transarterial chemoembolisation using different chemotherapeutic drug combinations followed by MR-guided laser-induced thermotherapy in patients with liver metastases of colorectal carcinoma. Br J Cancer. 2012;106:1274–9.

54. Vogl TJ, Naguib NN, Nour-Eldin NEA, Mack MG, Zangos S, Abskharon JE, Jost A. Repeated chemoembolization followed by laser-induced thermotherapy for liver metastasis of breast cancer. Am J Roentgenol. 2011;196:W66–72.

Retroperitoneal and Abdominal Lesions Laser Ablation

Giovanni Mauri, Tian'an Jiang, Qiyu Zhao, and Weilu Chai

5.1 Introduction

The retroperitoneum is the part of the abdomen which is bounded anteriorly by the posterior parietal peritoneum, posteriorly by the transversalis fascia, and laterally by the lateroconal ligaments. The retroperitoneum contains the adrenals, kidneys and ureters, the duodenal loop and the pancreas, the great vessels with their branches and associated lymph node chains, and the ascending and descending portions of the colon, including the caecum. Clinically, retroperitoneal tumors are insidious in onset with few early manifestations, so that they reach a large size by the time of diagnosis: in 80% of cases they are large enough to be palpable. Refractory abdominal pain is the commonest presentation, probably attributable to the invasion to solar plexus. Metastatic retroperitoneal, peritoneal, and nodal disease diffusion are one of the signs of advanced stage or terminal stage of malignancy, which is usually recurrence of a urological, gynaecological, hepatic, pancreatic, or gynaecological tumor. An effective local con-

trol of metastatic disease might represent a way to improve the survival time and the quality of life in patients with advanced stage disease [1].

Surgical resection of retroperitoneal tumors at the time of initial diagnosis offers the most curative potential and largest survival benefit. However, most retroperitoneal tumors are invasive and cannot be resected completely for the constraints of their proximity to vital structures in the abdominal cavity and adjacent compartments. Therefore, in a large majority of cases, it is very difficult to obtain clear microscopic margins, limiting the treatment to an R1 or even R2 resection. Supplemental treatment modalities including radiation therapy, ablation, and chemotherapy have been used in addition to surgical resection to provide more definitive local control of retroperitoneal neoplasms that are not amenable to an R0 resection [2]. Local ablative therapies such as radiofrequency ablation (RFA), microwave ablation (MWA), cryoablation, and irreversible electroporation (IRE) have been reported to be minimally invasive modalities in the palliative treatment of solid tumors in a variety of organs, RFA remaining the most common one [3–10]. More recently, there are interesting data about the use of these thermal and non-thermal techniques in the percutaneous treatment of adenocarcinoma [10]. Also, percutaneous ultrasound-guided LA has been reported to be an efficient and extremely well-tolerated treatment modality in a variety of

G. Mauri (✉)
Division of Interventional Radiology, European Institute of Oncology, IRCCS, Milan, Italy
e-mail: giovanni.mauri@ieo.it

T. Jiang · Q. Zhao · W. Chai
Department of Ultrasound, First Affiliated Hospital, College of Medicine, Zhejiang University, Hangzhou, China

© Springer Nature Switzerland AG 2020
C. M. Pacella et al. (eds.), *Image-guided Laser Ablation*, https://doi.org/10.1007/978-3-030-21748-8_5

different organs and diseases [11–20]. To date, the introduction of curvilinear endoscopic ultrasound (EUS) probes has made possible the booming development of EUS-guided fine-needle aspiration (FNA) [21, 22]. Subsequently, EUS-guided fine-needle injection (FNI), especially the EUS-guided ethanol injection, emerged as a new method for the chemoablation of pancreatic cysts or hepatic tumors [23, 24]. Guided by a needle puncture, laser fiber is inserted at different angles and allows multiple punctures. It has been reported that EUS-guided LA remains a feasible alternative in the situations where the target is hard to reach or where there is a lack of an appropriate puncture route from the percutaneous approach [25–33].

Also, in some cases, small peritoneal implants or nodal metastases can develop after primary surgical resection. These lesions are often detected when still of small dimensions, but can be located in very difficult anatomical locations and/or very close to critical anatomical structures. LA, with the application of very thin devices and very precise energy delivery, might represent the ideal ablation method in this setting.

5.2   Patient Selection

A proper patients' selection is crucial for successful application of laser ablation. Multidisciplinary discussion of each case and deep discussion of the therapeutic proposal with the patient are of paramount importance. As a general rule, LA can be proposed in patients with a limited number of small metastatic lymph nodes in the retroperitoneum or peritoneum or peritoneal localizations, which are not responding to chemotherapy or radiotherapy [2]. LA can be proposed with a curative intent, in order to

eradicate all visible disease locations, or with a palliative intent, in order to reduce the tumor burden or palliate symptoms of the progressing disease [11]. Patients are generally excluded by LA in case of severe comorbidities or coagulation disorders [2].

5.3   LA Procedure

Immediately prior to LA procedure, contrast-enhanced ultrasound (CEUS) imaging or contrast-enhanced CT (CECT) is generally used to thoroughly asses the vascularization of the lesion and its relationship with adjacent structures.

The best approach to the lesion can be established case by case, according to the technical availability and operators' experience. Particularly, the percutaneous approach with US or CT guidance is generally considered the first option when feasible [11], while the EUS approach is reserved to lesions in difficult anatomical locations which can be hardly reached through the percutaneous approach.

General anesthesia is suggested for this kind of procedures, as it allow for a better control of the patients' movement and respiratory excursions, which are considered crucial in this scenario. Furthermore, pain control is extremely better with the patient in general anesthesia, and difficult puncture to deliver local anesthesia is avoided. For US and CT approach, standard techniques can be used. Fusion of preacquired imaging datasets and virtual navigation can be extremely useful in this setting. For EUS-guided procedures, a curvilinear echoendoscope can be used to visualize the lesion through the gastric wall.

LA with a wavelength of 1064 nm with bare fibers (300-μm, quartz-core) with a flat tip is generally used for these treatments. 1.5 m long laser fibers can be used for percutaneous applications, and 3.0 m long fibers for EUS-guided ablations. Fibers are inserted through fine needle (22-gauge), into the end of the sheath, and carefully advanced out of the needle tip for 5 mm. Multiple laser fibers can be inserted simultaneously, and up to four simultaneous laser applications can be performed. The number, length, and arrangement of needles or fibers in the percutaneous approach are determined in accordance with the tumors' size, shape, and location. Real-time ultrasound and subsequent CT acquisitions are used to avoid critical structures such as the pancreas, bowel, vessels, and bile ducts [11].

In transgastric approach, a single-fiber technique with multipuncture LA is generally adopted. The lesion is directly punctured via the adjacent gastrointestinal walls, taking care that the tip of the guiding needle is at least 10 mm away from the distal borderline of the lymph node. Once the fibers are accurately positioned in the desired place, the laser is turned on at a power of 3.0–5.0 W, and a total energy of 1200–1800 J is applied for each single illumination. Procedure is monitored in real time with US when feasible, in order to depict the gas forming during ablation enclosing the whole lesion. CEUS and CECT can be used before patient awakening in order to establish the success of the treatment, to establish if additional ablation is needed, and to depict early signs of complications (Fig. 5.1).

5.4 Results

A recent systematic review of the literature on thermal ablation of retroperitoneal lesions identified 398 patients with 491 retroperitoneal tumors treated with various ablative devices with the percutaneous approach, with good results and few complications. Until now, the evidence is sparse, and several different methods includ-

ing radiofrequency ablation, cryoablation, high-intensity focused ultrasound, and even irreversible electroporation have been applied with good results. In the still limited experiences reported on percutaneous application of laser ablation in the treatment of retroperitoneal lesions, good results and few complications (limited to mild discomfort and fever) were reported. In recent years, EUS-guided laser ablation of pancreatic neuroendocrine and hepatocellular carcinoma has been successfully performed and reported. In the short-term follow-up, contrast-enhanced CT suggested that the ablated zone was uniformly hypoattenuated without any enhancement, leading to the conclusion that EUS-guided LA is an effective and safe method for EUS-accessible solid tumors. Artifon et al. presented their innovative work with EUS-guided alcohol ablation of a left adrenal metastasis in a patient with non-small cell lung cancer, further highlighting the safety of this approach for retroperitoneal ablations [34].

In 2016, Mou et al. evaluated the US-guided LA to unresectable retroperitoneal and hepatic portal lymph nodes from hepatic cancer. The local response rate at 6-month follow-up was 75% and the abdominal pain score decreased significantly in all patients [35]. Percutaneous LA has also been reported to be tolerable for those patients with poor general condition or the one with lesions located at high-risk position, and this is particularly due to the fact that the guiding needle is thinner than in other ablation modalities [2]. The application details of EUS-guided laser ablation to retroperitoneal metastasis, including adrenal metastasis, were also described. Some advantages of this technique appear to be extremely interesting. First, the technique conquered the dilemma of applying percutaneous puncture to a difficult target, which increases the risk of injuring the adjacent tissues. EUS-guided LA switched the puncture orientation to avoid the

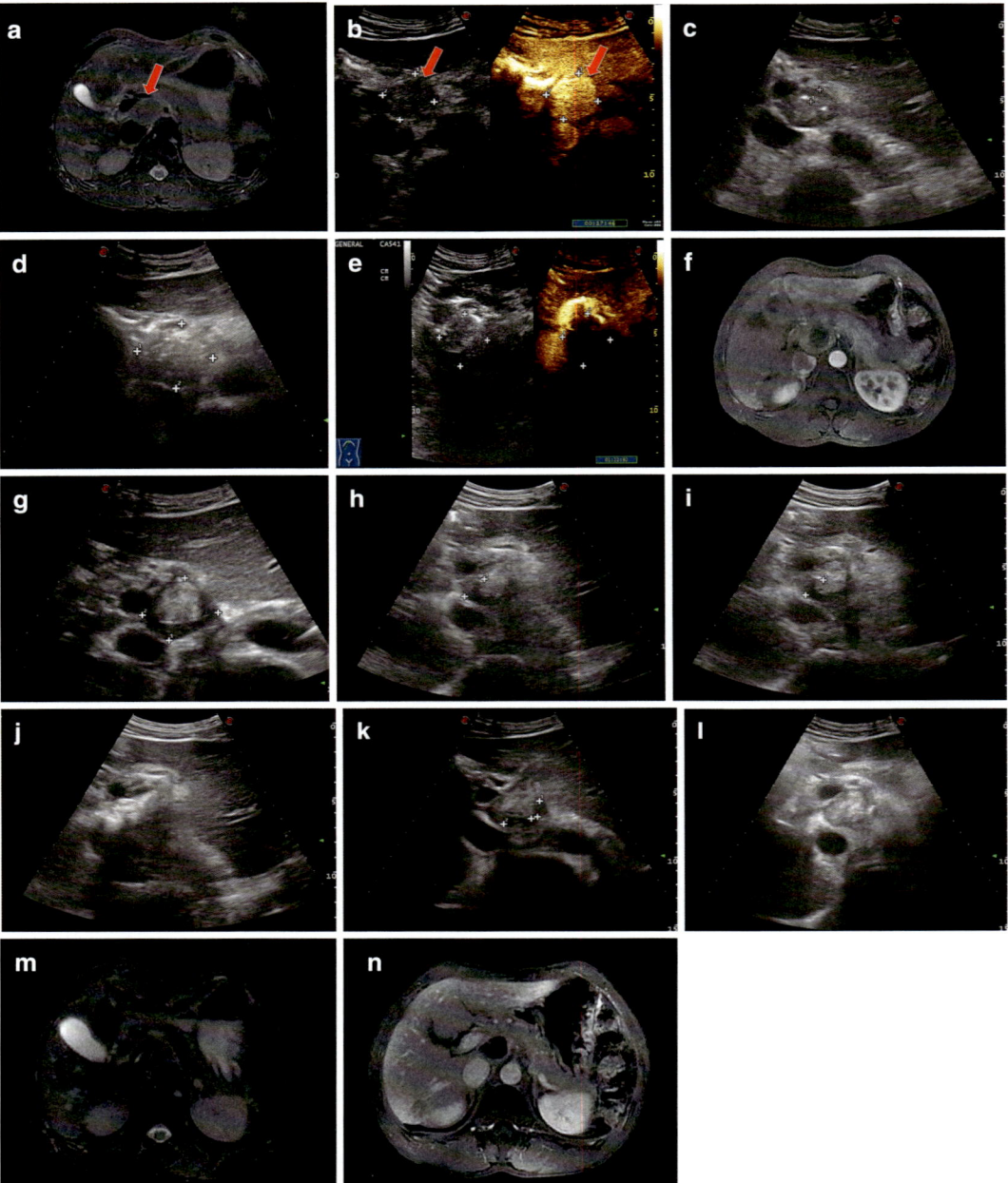

Fig. 5.1 Ultrasound-guided percutaneous laser ablation (LA) of retroperitoneal metastatic tumors from hepatocellular carcinoma (HCC). The AFP was 1389.9 ng/mL. (**a**) T2-weighted magnetic resonance imaging (MRI) showed a hyperintensity lesion (*red arrow*) located at retroperitoneal space. (**b**) Preoperative contrast-enhanced ultrasonography (CEUS) showed that the retroperitoneal lesion (*red arrows*) was hyper-enhanced at arterial phase. (**c**) Two fibers were inserted across the liver into the lesion. A total of 3200 J was transmitted. (**d**) Gas formation during ablation is enclosing the whole lesion. (**e**) In postoperative CEUS, the target was completely non-enhanced. (**f**) Two months after the first period of LA T1-weighted MRI showed that the tumor was recurrent adjacent to the ablation zone. (**g**) In ultrasound image, the recurrent lesion was presented as a hypoechoic zone. AFP was reduced to 446.8 ng/mL. (**h**) The laser fiber was inserted into the right part the recurrent lesion. (**i**) The laser fiber was inserted into the rear part of the recurrent lesion. (**j**) The right and rear parts of the recurrent hypoechoic lesion were totally ablated. (**k**) Two fibers were used to ablate the left and rear parts of recurrent lesion. (**l**) Right after the third ablation, the target hypoechoic lesion was completely ablated. (**m**) Two months after ablation, the AFP was reduced to 109.5 ng/mL. (**n**) MRI revealed that the retroperitoneal lesion was completely ablated

important structures in the puncture route to left adrenal lesions. Second, given its minimal invasiveness, EUS-guided LA was easily performed with short application time, a low risk of collateral damage and good patient tolerance. Finally, the EUS-guided laser fiber could be inserted from multiple angles to ablate the different parts of the tumor. The intraoperative CEUS might help detect residual lesions and direct the fiber placement in the next step [36–38].

5.5   Discussion

Surgical resection, chemotherapy, radiotherapy, and, more recently, thermal ablation have become standard treatments for retroperitoneal and peritoneal lesions. Particularly, R0 dissection is generally recommended whenever feasible, even if the frequency of associated surgical complications still approaches 10% [2, 3]. However, some lesions are not manageable with surgery and in some cases are even not sensitive to radiotherapy or chemotherapy. Some patients whose general condition is poor cannot tolerate chemotherapy, radiotherapy, or surgery, and treatment options are limited for these patients. Image-guided thermal ablation might represent a further therapeutic option for achieving local tumor control in these cases.

The commonly used percutaneous ablation modalities, which include RFA, MWA, cryoablation, and LA, were reported to be applied in retroperitoneal and adrenal metastasis. In a study by Arellano et al., image-guided percutaneous RFA was proposed as a possible alternative to currently available therapies to treat recurrent metastatic disease due to endometrial carcinoma [39]. When the primary foci in liver have been removed, Gao et al. suggested RFA was a supplemental method for the retroperitoneal metastatic lymph nodes from HCC, which was free from the heat-sink effect of adjacent aorta and IVC [40]. In 2014, Wang et al. reported that CT-guided radioactive ^{125}I seed implantation is showing good palliative pain relief with acceptable short-term effects, which has proved to be a relatively uncomplicated

treatment option for symptomatic retroperitoneal metastatic lymph nodes [33]. Other authors reported that CT-guided percutaneous cryoablation was a broadly safe, effective local cancer control option for retroperitoneal metastatic lesions, hepatic non-resectable tumors, or recurrent soft tissue carcinoma [41–43]. Recently, the newly developed non-thermal ablation technique, whose acronym is IRE, was used to supplement primary surgical resection of locally advanced pelvic and retroperitoneal tumors. It helps to provide better local control by margin enhancement where complete macroscopic margins were obtained [44]. Furthermore, it has been reported that RFA might prolong survival in patients with retroperitoneal metastasis, even with controllable hematogenous metastasis [45–50]. The advantages of these minimally invasive therapies are short hospitalization, low morbidity, and acceptable complications. As in adrenal metastasis, image-guided thermal ablation was also effective for local tumor control without major complication and with a low morbidity rate related to the procedure [51–53].

Percutaneous US/CT-guided LA has been reported to be a minimally invasive and extremely well-tolerated procedure without severe complications [54]. We believe that the main advantage of applying laser ablation is the use of very thin needles, which are less traumatic and can be handled more easily by the operator to reach difficult sites. On the other hand, lasers with a wavelength of 1064 nm were used because the penetration of light is optimal in the near infrared spectrum. This type of laser has been commonly used in interstitial ablation because it can target the needle in virtually any plane. The laser destruction of tissue including tissue protein denaturation, coagulative necrosis, tissue liquefaction, vaporization, and carbonization occurs very rapidly. Although part of the heat is removed by blood flow, the size of the affected area is still around 12–15 mm in diameter when 3 W of power were used for 10 min with a single device [2, 36, 37, 55] and around 4 cm using four devices [55–57].

In HCC ablation, the ideal candidates for LA are those with well-differentiated histology, non-

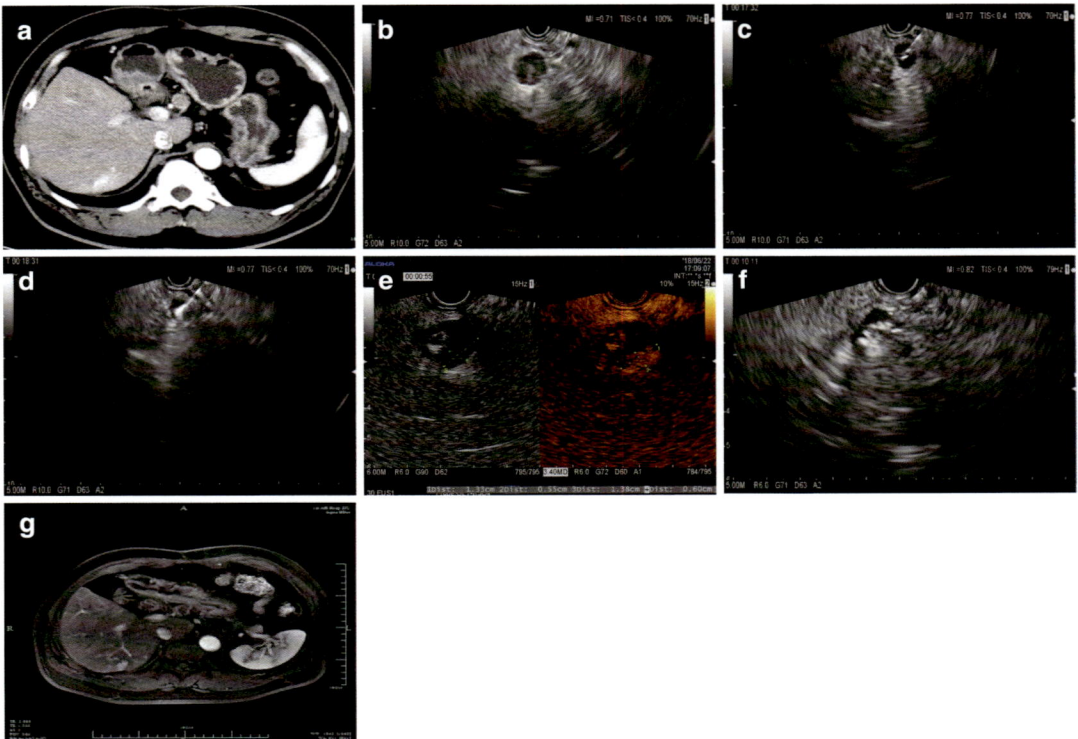

Fig. 5.2 Endoscopic ultrasound (EUS)-guided LA to retroperitoneal metastatic tumor from HCC. The AFP was 124 ng/mL. (**a**) Contrast-enhanced computed tomography (CT) revealed a retroperitoneal lesion adjacent to the posterior wall of the stomach. (**b**) In EUS scanning, a hypoechoic retroperitoneal lesion was revealed. (**c**) EUS-guided LA was performed to ablate the retroperitoneal lesion. (**d**) Gas forming during LA ablation. (**e**) One month after the maneuver, the US examination showed residual tissue of 1.4 × 0.6 cm. The AFP was 101 ng/mL. (**f**) The residual lesion was covered by hyperechoic zone during second ablation. (**g**) In follow-up, the ablation zone was completely ablated

infiltrating growth, naive tumors, a first treatment session, and normal bilirubin levels [13, 58, 59]. Previous studies demonstrated that LA retained an equal ablation efficacy to that of RFA, and the published complete response rate ranged from 82% to 97% [60]. When certain tumors are in close proximity to gastrointestinal structures, the visualization via EUS is more direct and distinct than percutaneous US (Fig. 5.2). With the introduction and development of EUS-guided needle-based interventions, its application to hepatic, pancreatic, and gastrointestinal stromal tumors gained popularity, providing an alternative approach to percutaneous thermal ablation.

5.6   Conclusions

Image-guided laser ablation, applied through the percutaneous or endoscopic route, can represent a safe and effective strategy to manage retroperitoneal and peritoneal lesions, and even to treat metastatic lymph nodes and adrenal metastases (Fig. 5.3), particularly in patients not suitable for surgical resection or not manageable with radiation therapy or chemotherapy. Even if the reported results are promising, they still are limited and have to be considered preliminary, and further studies on larger populations with longer follow-up are necessary.

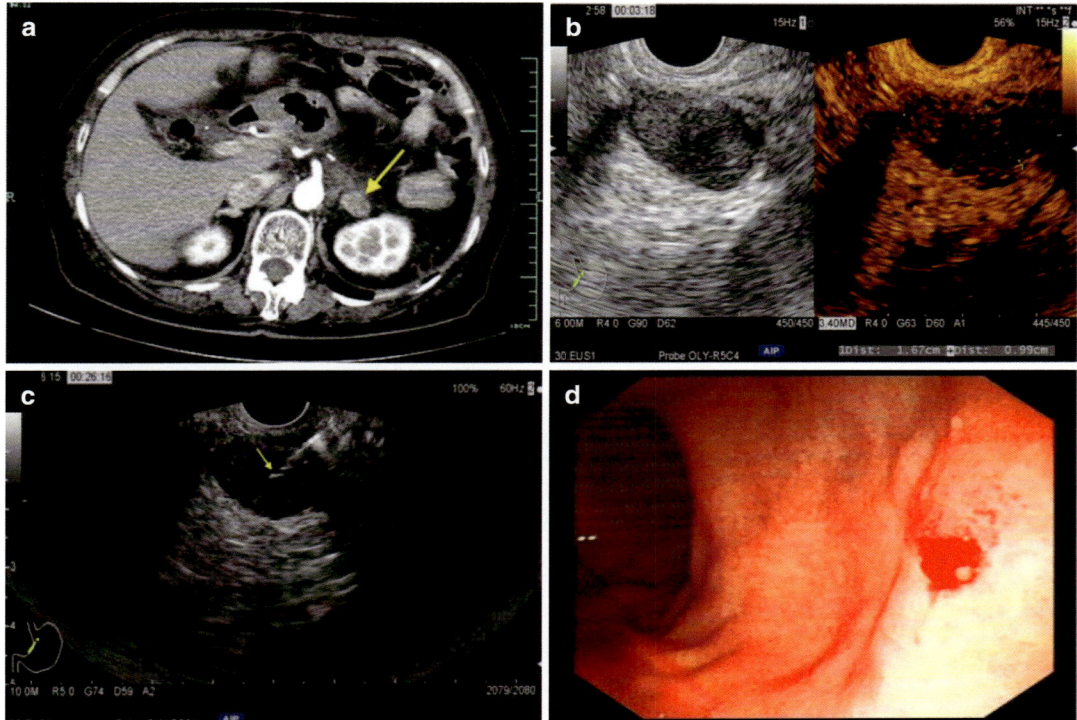

Fig. 5.3 Case of EUS-guided LA in left adrenal metastasis. (**a**) Pre-ablation CT scan discovered a low-density mass in the region of the left adrenal gland, and it was irregularly enhanced during the contrast arterial phase (*yellow arrow*). (**b**) Under the EUS transgastric scanning, a hypoechoic mass with a size of 1.7 × 1.0 cm was seen in the splenonephric space and irregularly hyper-enhanced in the venous phase of CEUS. (**c**) A LA fiber (*yellow arrow*) was inserted through the 22-gauge needle into the mass, and the exposure length of the bare fiber was 1.0 cm. (**d**) The puncture points were checked to rule out bleeding and perforation at the end of LA

References

1. Allan PLP. Clinical ultrasound. Edinburgh: Churchill Livingstone; 2011.

2. Yun M, Zhao Q, Zhong L, Chen F, Jiang T. Preliminary results of ultrasound-guided laser ablation for unresectable metastases to retroperitoneal and hepatic portal lymph nodes. World J Surg Oncol. 2016;14:165.

3. Wong SL, Mangu PB, Choti MA, Crocenzi TS, Dodd GD 3rd, Dorfman GS, et al. American Society of Clinical Oncology 2009 clinical evidence review on radiofrequency ablation of hepatic metastases from colorectal cancer. J Clin Oncol. 2010;28(3):493–508.

4. Shyn PB, Mauri G, Alencar RO, Tatli S, Shah SH, Morrison PR, et al. Percutaneous imaging-guided cryoablation of liver tumors: predicting local progression on 24-hour MRI. AJR Am J Roentgenol. 2014;203(2):W181–91.

5. Zampino MG, Magni E, Ravenda PS, Cella CA, Bonomo G, Della Vigna P, et al. Treatments for colorectal liver metastases: a new focus on a familiar concept. Crit Rev Oncol Hematol. 2016;108:154–63.

6. Monfardini L, Orsi F, Caserta R, Sallemi C, Della Vigna P, Bonomo G, et al. Ultrasound and cone beam CT fusion for liver ablation: technical note. Int J Hyperth. 2018, 35:1–5.

7. Mauri G, Nicosia L, Varano GM, Shyn P, Sartori S, Tombesi P, et al. Unusual tumour ablations: report of difficult and interesting cases. Ecancermedicalscience. 2017;11:733.

8. Mauri G, Cova L, De Beni S, Ierace T, Tondolo T, Cerri A, et al. Real-time US-CT/MRI image fusion for guidance of thermal ablation of liver tumors undetectable with US: results in 295 cases. Cardiovasc Intervent Radiol. 2015;38(1):143–51.

9. Mainini AP, Monaco C, Pescatori LC, De Angelis C, Sardanelli F, Sconfienza LM, et al. Image-guided thermal ablation of benign thyroid nodules. J Ultrasound. 2017;20(1):11–22.

10. D'Onofrio M, Ciaravino V, De Robertis R, Barbi E, Salvia R, Girelli R, et al. Percutaneous ablation of pancreatic cancer. World J Gastroenterol. 2016;22(44):9661–73.

11. Pacella CM, Stasi R, Bizzarri G, Pacella S, Graziano FM, Guglielmi R, et al. Percutaneous laser ablation of unresectable primary and metastatic adrenocortical carcinoma. Eur J Radiol. 2008;66(1):88–94.

12. Pacella CM, Valle D, Bizzarri G, Pacella S, Brunetti M, Maritati R, et al. Percutaneous laser ablation in patients with isolated unresectable liver metastases from colorectal cancer: results of a phase II study. Acta Oncol. 2006;45(1):77–83.

13. Pacella CM, Francica G, Di Lascio FM, Arienti V, Antico E, Caspani B, et al. Long-term outcome of cirrhotic patients with early hepatocellular carcinoma treated with ultrasound-guided percutaneous laser ablation: a retrospective analysis. J Clin Oncol. 2009;27(16):2615–21.

14. Pacella CM, Mauri G, Achille G, Barbaro D, Bizzarri G, De Feo P, et al. Outcomes and risk factors for complications of laser ablation for thyroid nodules: a multicenter study on 1531 patients. J Clin Endocrinol Metab. 2015;100(10):3903–10.

15. Tombesi P, Di Vece F, Sartori S. Laser ablation for hepatic metastases from neuroendocrine tumors. AJR Am J Roentgenol. 2015;204(6):W732.

16. Mauri G, Cova L, Ierace T, Baroli A, Di Mauro E, Pacella CM, et al. Treatment of metastatic lymph nodes in the neck from papillary thyroid carcinoma with percutaneous laser ablation. Cardiovasc Intervent Radiol. 2016;39(7):1023–30.

17. Pacella CM, Mauri G, Cesareo R, Paqualini V, Cianni R, De Feo P, et al. A comparison of laser with radiofrequency ablation for the treatment of benign thyroid nodules: a propensity score matching analysis. Int J Hyperth. 2017;33(8):911–9.

18. Patelli G, Ranieri A, Paganelli A, Mauri G, Pacella CM. Transperineal laser ablation for percutaneous treatment of benign prostatic hyperplasia: a feasibility study. Cardiovasc Intervent Radiol. 2017;40(9):1440–6.

19. Sartori S, Mauri G, Tombesi P, Di Vece F, Bianchi L, Pacella CM. Ultrasound-guided percutaneous laser ablation is safe and effective in the treatment of small renal tumors in patients at increased bleeding risk. Int J Hyperth. 2018;35(1):19–25.

20. Mauri G, Nicosia L, Della Vigna P, Varano GM, Maiettini D, Bonomo G, et al. Percutaneous laser ablation for benign and malignant thyroid diseases. Ultrasonography. 2019;38(1):25–36.

21. Artifon EL, Franzini TA, Kumar A, Matsura PF, Furuya CK Jr, Ishioka S, et al. EUS-guided FNA facilitates the diagnosis of retroperitoneal endometriosis. Gastrointest Endosc. 2007;66(3):620–2.

22. Tian G, Bao H, Li J, Jiang T. Systematic review and meta-analysis of diagnostic accuracy of endoscopic ultrasound (EUS)-guided fine-needle aspiration (FNA) using 22-gauge and 25-gauge needles for pancreatic masses. Med Sci Monit. 2018;24:8333–41.

23. Park JK, Song BJ, Ryu JK, Paik WH, Park JM, Kim J, et al. Clinical outcomes of endoscopic ultrasonography-guided pancreatic cyst ablation. Pancreas. 2016;45(6):889–94.

24. Paik WH, Seo DW, Dhir V, Wang HP. Safety and efficacy of EUS-guided ethanol ablation for treating small solid pancreatic neoplasm. Medicine (Baltimore). 2016;95(4):e2538.

25. Hu YH, Tuo XP, Jin ZD, Liu Y, Guo Y, Luo L. Endoscopic ultrasound (EUS)-guided ethanol injection in hepatic metastatic carcinoma: a case report. Endoscopy. 2010;42(Suppl 2):E256–7.

26. Di Matteo F, Grasso R, Pacella CM, Martino M, Pandolfi M, Rea R, et al. EUS-guided Nd:YAG laser ablation of a hepatocellular carcinoma in the caudate lobe. Gastrointest Endosc. 2011;73(3):632–6.

27. Nakaji S, Hirata N, Iwaki K, Shiratori T, Kobayashi M, Inase M. Endoscopic ultrasound (EUS)-guided ethanol injection for hepatocellular carcinoma dif-

ficult to treat with percutaneous local treatment. Endoscopy. 2012;44(Suppl 2 UCTN):E380.

28. Di Matteo F, Picconi F, Martino M, Pandolfi M, Pacella CM, Schena E, et al. Endoscopic ultrasound-guided Nd:YAG laser ablation of recurrent pancreatic neuroendocrine tumor: a promising revolution? Endoscopy. 2014;46(Suppl 1 UCTN):E380–1.

29. Zhang WY, Li ZS, Jin ZD. Endoscopic ultrasound-guided ethanol ablation therapy for tumors. World J Gastroenterol. 2013;19(22):3397–403.

30. Yoon WJ, Brugge WR. Endoscopic ultrasonography-guided tumor ablation. Gastrointest Endosc Clin N Am. 2012;22(2):359–69, xi.

31. Jiang TA, Deng Z, Tian G, Zhao QY, Wang WL. Efficacy and safety of endoscopic ultrasonography-guided interventional treatment for refractory malignant left-sided liver tumors: a case series of 26 patients. Sci Rep. 2016;6:36098.

32. Ji YB, Varadarajulu S. Endoscopic ultrasound-guided management of pancreatic pseudocysts and walled-off necrosis. Clin Endosc. 2014;47:429–43.

33. Wang Z, Lu J, Gong J, Zhang L, Xu Y, Song S, et al. CT-guided radioactive ^{125}I seed implantation therapy of symptomatic retroperitoneal lymph node metastases. Cardiovasc Intervent Radiol. 2014;37(1):125–31.

34. Artifon EL, Lucon AM, Sakai P, Gerhardt R, Srougi M, Takagaki T, et al. EUS-guided alcohol ablation of left adrenal metastasis from non-small-cell lung carcinoma. Gastrointest Endosc. 2007;66(6):1201–5.

35. Mou Y, Zhao Q, Zhong L, Chen F, Jiang T. Preliminary results of ultrasound-guided laser ablation for unresectable metastases to retroperitoneal and hepatic portal lymph nodes. World J Surg Oncol. 2016;14(1):165.

36. Jiang T, Deng Z, Tian G, Chen F, Bao H, Li J, et al. Percutaneous laser ablation: a new contribution to unresectable high-risk metastatic retroperitoneal lesions? Oncotarget. 2017;8(2):2413–22.

37. Tian G, Jiang T. US-guided percutaneous laser ablation of refractory metastatic retroperitoneal lesions: a care-compliant case report. Medicine (Baltimore). 2017;96(15):e6597.

38. Jiang T, Chai W. Endoscopic ultrasonography (EUS)-guided laser ablation (LA) of adrenal metastasis from pancreatic adenocarcinoma. Lasers Med Sci. 2018;33(7):1613–6.

39. Arellano RS, Flanders VL, Lee SI, Mueller PR, Gervais DA. Imaging-guided percutaneous radiofrequency ablation of retroperitoneal metastatic disease in patients with gynecologic malignancies: clinical experience with eight patients. AJR Am J Roentgenol. 2010;194(6):1635–8.

40. Gao F, Gu Y, Huang J, Zhao M, Wu P. Radiofrequency ablation of retroperitoneal metastatic lymph nodes from hepatocellular carcinoma. Acad Radiol. 2012;19(8):1035–40.

41. Littrup PJ, Bang HJ, Currier BP, Goodrich DJ, Aoun HD, Heilbrun LK, et al. Soft-tissue cryoablation in diffuse locations: feasibility and intermediate term outcomes. J Vasc Interv Radiol. 2013;24(12):1817–25.

42. Mu F, Niu L, Li H, Liao M, Li L, Liu C, et al. Percutaneous comprehensive cryoablation for metastatic hepatocellular cancer. Cryobiology. 2013;66(1):76–80.

43. Li J, Fan W, Niu L, Yang JY. Percutaneous computed tomography-guided cryoablation for recurrent malignant primary retroperitoneal tumors: initial experience of 39 patients. J Vasc Interv Radiol. 2016;27:S81.

44. Underhill CE, Walsh NJ, Bateson BP, Mentzer C, Kruse EJ. Feasibility and safety of irreversible electroporation in locally advanced pelvic and retroperitoneal tumors. Am Surg. 2016;82(9):e263–5.

45. Araujo LH, Gouveia HR, Freitas Ede Q, Pedras FV, Luz JH. Hepatic transarterial chemoembolization and retroperitoneal lymph node radiofrequency ablation in the multidisciplinary approach of an overt metastatic leiomyosarcoma. Cancer Imaging. 2013;13:123–7.

46. Gervais DA, Arellano RS, Mueller PR. Percutaneous radiofrequency ablation of nodal metastases. Cardiovasc Intervent Radiol. 2002;25(6):547–9.

47. Zhao M, Li X, Wang J, Li W, Huang Z. Retroperitoneal schwannoma treated with percutaneous computed tomography-guided radiofrequency ablation. J Neurosurg Spine. 2012;17(2):173–6.

48. Keil S, Bruners P, Brehmer B, Mahnken AH. Percutaneous radiofrequency ablation for treatment of recurrent retroperitoneal liposarcoma. Cardiovasc Intervent Radiol. 2008;31(Suppl 2):S213–6.

49. Monfardini L, Varano GM, Foa R, Della Vigna P, Bonomo G, Orsi F. Local recurrence of renal cancer after surgery: prime time for percutaneous thermal ablation? Cardiovasc Intervent Radiol. 2015;38(6):1542–7.

50. Molina R, Alvarez M, Capilla J, Paez A. Radiofrequency-treated recurrence of urothelial carcinoma of the upper urinary tract after nephroureterectomy. Korean J Urol. 2014;55(12):844–6.

51. Carrafiello G, Lagana D, Recaldini C, Giorgianni A, Ianniello A, Lumia D, et al. Imaging-guided percutaneous radiofrequency ablation of adrenal metastases: preliminary results at a single institution with a single device. Cardiovasc Intervent Radiol. 2008;31(4):762–7.

52. Welch BT, Callstrom MR, Carpenter PC, Wass CT, Welch TL, Boorjian SA, et al. A single-institution experience in image-guided thermal ablation of adrenal gland metastases. J Vasc Interv Radiol. 2014;25(4):593–8.

53. Wood BJ, Abraham J, Hvizda JL, Alexander HR, Fojo T. Radiofrequency ablation of adrenal tumors and adrenocortical carcinoma metastases. Cancer. 2003;97(3):554–60.

54. Arienti V, Pretolani S, Pacella CM, Magnolfi F, Caspani B, Francica G, et al. Complications of laser ablation for hepatocellular carcinoma: a multicenter study. Radiology. 2008;246(3):947–55.

55. Pacella CM, Bizzarri G, Francica G, Bianchini A, De Nuntis S, Pacella S, et al. Percutaneous laser ablation in the treatment of hepatocellular carcinoma

with small tumors: analysis of factors affecting the achievement of tumor necrosis. J Vasc Interv Radiol. 2005;16(11):1447–57.

56. Di Costanzo GG, D'Adamo G, Tortora R, Zanfardino F, Mattera S, Francica G, et al. A novel needle guide system to perform percutaneous laser ablation of liver tumors using the multifiber technique. Acta Radiol. 2013;54(8):876–81.

57. Di Costanzo GG, Francica G, Pacella CM. Laser ablation for small hepatocellular carcinoma: state of the art and future perspectives. World J Hepatol. 2014;6(10):704–15.

58. Caspani B, Ierardi AM, Motta F, Cecconi P, Fesce E, Belli L. Small nodular hepatocellular carcinoma treated by laser thermal ablation in high risk locations: preliminary results. Eur Radiol. 2010;20(9): 2286–92.

59. Francica G, Petrolati A, Di Stasio E, Pacella S, Stasi R, Pacella CM. Effectiveness, safety, and local progression after percutaneous laser ablation for hepatocellular carcinoma nodules up to 4 cm are not affected by tumor location. AJR Am J Roentgenol. 2012;199(6):1393–401.

60. Di Costanzo GG, Tortora R, D'Adamo G, De Luca M, Lampasi F, Addario L, et al. Radiofrequency ablation versus laser ablation for the treatment of small hepatocellular carcinoma in cirrhosis: a randomized trial. J Gastroenterol Hepatol. 2015;30(3):559–65.

Sergio Sartori, Paola Tombesi, Francesca Di Vece,
Claudio Maurizio Pacella, Qiyu Zhao,
and Giovanni Mauri

6.1 Kidney Tumors: Treatment Strategies for T1a Renal Cell Carcinoma

Renal cell carcinoma (RCC) represents 3.8% of all adult cancers in the Western world. RCC can be sporadic or congenital, with congenital cases linked to specific gene mutations. The detection rate of RCC has increased over the last 10 years by approximately 1.7 per year, mainly due to the increased number of incidentally diagnosed cases during diagnostic cross-sectional studies for other diseases [1]. The vast majority of serendipitously diagnosed RCCs are asymptomatic, and of small dimensions, mostly in T1a stage. Conversely, clinical presentation of advanced tumors includes hematuria, pain from local infiltration, or symptoms from metastatic spread. The 5-year survival rate is 91.8% for localized disease and 12.1% for advanced disease. The most important prognostic factors include tumor grade, local extent, and the presence of nodal or distant metastases at presentation [1]. Contrast-enhanced computed tomography (CECT) and magnetic resonance imaging (MRI) play a central role in the detection and characterization of renal lesions, as well as in the staging of the disease.

The treatment options for RCC depend on tumor stage, according to TNM classification and staging. The first therapeutic option for stage T1a and T1b tumors is partial or radical nephrectomy [2]. Partial nephrectomy (open or laparoscopic) is preferred whenever possible, as total nephrectomy may often impact on renal function [3]. As a consequence, radical nephrectomy is usually reserved to centrally located tumors or stage II–III tumors. Focusing on T1a RCC, therapeutic strategies include surgical approach, active surveillance, and ablation therapy [2, 4]. Given that both partial and radical resections offer comparable long-term oncological results for T1a RCC, nephron-sparing surgical technique is largely preferred in order to preserve renal function [5–8]. According to the European Association of Urology's guidelines, partial nephrectomy is strongly recommended for patients affected by T1a RCC [9].

Since the majority of small RCCs grow slowly (mean growth rate is about 3 mm per year) and may be followed up easily with cross-sectional

S. Sartori (✉) · P. Tombesi · F. Di Vece
Section of Interventional Ultrasound, St. Anna
Hospital, Ferrara, Italy
e-mail: srs@unife.it

C. M. Pacella
Department of Diagnostic Imaging and Interventional
Radiology, Regina Apostolorum Hospital,
Albano Laziale, Rome, Italy

Q. Zhao
Department of Ultrasound, The First Affiliated
Hospital, College of Medicine, Zhejiang University,
Hangzhou, China

G. Mauri
Division of Interventional Radiology, European
Institute of Oncology, IRCCS, Milan, Italy

© Springer Nature Switzerland AG 2020
C. M. Pacella et al. (eds.), *Image-guided Laser Ablation*,
https://doi.org/10.1007/978-3-030-21748-8_6

imaging over time, active surveillance has been reported to be a valid alternative to nephrectomy [10, 11]. However, a non-negligible number of small tumors (approximately 20%) cannot present this slow-growing pattern and, on the contrary, can grow aggressively [12, 13]. Moreover, data from the National Swedish Kidney Cancer Register pointed out that 11% of tumors 3–4 cm in diameter had either nodal or distant metastases, and only tumors smaller than 1 cm had neither nodal nor distant spread [14]. Therefore, unanimous consensus on active surveillance has not been reached, because at present there are no diagnostic tools which can suggest proceeding to surveillance or starting a treatment.

Ablation therapies are included among the treatment strategies for T1a stage RCC [4]. All ablation modalities offer a minimally invasive and nephron-sparing treatment option to patients unfit or refusing surgery. The most extensively used and the best established ablation techniques for renal tumors are radiofrequency ablation (RFA) and cryoablation [15–17]. Focusing on the "hot" thermal ablation techniques, RFA is the most experienced modality, and it is widely employed for liver tumors [18]. In the treatment of renal tumors, RFA has been reported to achieve up to 100% complete ablation for nodules smaller than 3 cm and up to over 90% for nodules 3–5 cm in size, whereas results are significantly worse (<25%) for tumors larger than 5 cm [15]. The European Society for Medical Oncology (ESMO) guidelines state that ablation can be considered an effective option in patients with small cortical tumors <3 cm, high surgical risk, solitary kidney, compromised renal function, hereditary, or multiple bilateral RCC [19]. According to the current evidence, the Cardiovascular and Interventional Radiological Society of Europe (CIRSE) guidelines claim that ablation treatments represent a valid option for T1a RCCs, with excellent long-term (>5 years) technical and functional outcomes, and very low complication rates. Moreover, stating the feasibility of such a therapeutic option, the CIRSE guidelines suggest that active surveillance should be reserved to patients not suitable to ablation due to age or comorbidities [4].

Table 6.1 Indications and contraindications for RCC ablation [4]

Indication for treatment with ablation are the following:
– Presence of comorbidities that would increase the risk of surgical intervention (advanced COPD, heart failure)
– Single functioning kidney
– Impaired renal function (GFR < 60 mL/min per 1.73 m^2)
– Presence of more than one small renal tumor
– Patient's choice not to undergo a surgical procedure
Contraindications are the following:
– Uncorrectable coagulopathy
– Extensive spinal deformity that would not permit percutaneous access to the lesion (relative contraindication)

Indications and contraindications for RCC ablation according to CIRSE guidelines are reported in Table 6.1.

The CIRSE guidelines also include a quite interesting section focused on the potential role of ablation in patients who are potentially good surgical candidates. Indeed, several studies report comparable results for percutaneous ablation with respect to partial nephrectomy in patients unsuitable for surgery. A single-center retrospective study by Ma et al. reviewed 52 healthy patients, potentially surgical candidates, with T1a RCC who underwent RFA [20]. The authors reported no recurrence after a follow-up period of 3 years and recurrence-free survival of 94.2% at both 5 and 10 years. Such a durable oncologic (and functional) result suggests that RFA could be considered an alternative to surgery for T1a RCC also in potentially surgical candidates.

In the recent years, last-generation microwave ablation (MWA) has been proved to offer some advantages compared with RFA in the treatment of liver tumors, as it allows obtaining larger ablation volumes with adequate safety margins in a shorter time, and is not limited by the heat sink effect, desiccation, or charring [21–23]. Likewise, MWA may be considered a treatment option for large non-surgical RCC, in association with systemic therapy, or in patients who are poor candidates to or refusing systemic therapy. However, even with the more recent technical improvements, the shape of the ablation zone is ovoid instead of spherical, as it would be required for renal tumors [24]. Moreover, a higher risk of pelvicalyceal injury seems to be associated with the use of MWA than with other modalities [24, 25], and according to the CIRSE guidelines, this technology needs further evaluation and at present it should be limited to the more experienced interventional radiologists.

6.2 Laser Ablation

Laser ablation is currently used in many centers to treat primary and metastatic liver cancers, with very good results that are comparable to those of RFA and MWA for either hepatocellular carcinoma or liver metastases from colorectal cancer [26–28], as confirmed by two randomized trials that compared laser ablation and RFA and found no significant differences between the two techniques [27, 29]. Despite these results, laser ablation is by far the less used ablation modality worldwide, and in a way it is often unjustifiably considered the Cinderella among the ablation techniques [30]. It is not surprising, therefore, that laser ablation had not been used to treat RCC until very recent years. Indeed, the studies reported in the literature were sporadic and involved very small series of patients [31–34]. However, at present there is no ideal ablation technique that outclasses the other ones, and as with RFA, MWA, or cryoablation, laser ablation also has peculiar advantages and limitations that can make it more or less suitable to treat liver and renal cancers according to the characteristics of both patients and tumors [30]. The so-called laser-induced interstitial thermotherapy (LITT) uses quartz fibers with flat or cylindrical diffusing tips and water-cooled laser application sheaths to increase the volume of coagulative necrosis while preventing carbonization at the tip of the laser applicator. LITT has been reported to achieve very large ablation areas of up to 50 mm [35–37], which is particularly useful for the treatment of liver metastases that require large safety margins to take care of microscopic disease around the lesions [37]. However, power applica-

tors are nine French in diameter, that is a too large diameter to be considered best suited to percutaneous ablation of renal tumors, and previous earlier experiences with laser ablation of RCC by using LITT under magnetic resonance guidance did actually not achieve exciting results in terms of both outcome and complications [31–34].

Conversely, the multifiber technique proposed by Pacella et al. [38] and improved by Di Costanzo et al. [39] presents some features that make it potentially interesting in the treatment of small renal tumors. It uses 300-μm bare optical fibers that are introduced into the tumor through 21-gauge needles. The diameter of the needles is considerably thinner than RFA electrodes, MWA antennas, cryoablation probes, and LITT sheaths. Thanks to its lower invasiveness, laser ablation with the multifiber technique has been proposed as the first-choice technique to treat patients at high risk of complications, due to the presence of comorbidities or difficult technical access [30, 40, 41]. Each bare-tip fiber provides an almost spherical thermal lesion of 12–15 mm in diameter, and a beam-splitting device or a multisource device allow for the use of up to four fibers at once, simultaneously delivering the light into each single fiber [42, 43]. Therefore, these devices enable to achieve ablation areas from 1 to 4–5 cm in diameter, and consequently to treat tumors ranging from 5–6 mm to 3 cm in diameter obtaining an acceptable safety margin.

It is known that the kidney is a hypervascular organ and for this reason it is considered more at-risk of bleeding than the liver or other organs when interventional procedures are performed [44, 45]. In particular, renal biopsy and thermal ablation are numbered among the four non-vascular interventional procedures with significant risk of bleeding [44], and needle size has been reported to be a risk factor of hemorrhagic complications [46, 47]. Therefore, the use of thinner needles could have some advantage when thermal ablation is performed to treat RCC, in particular, if the risk of bleeding is increased. Quite recently, a retrospective study on the use of laser ablation with the multifiber technique in patients with small RCC and high risk of bleeding reported very interesting results [48]. The patients were considered at increased risk of bleeding because of impairment of coagulation parameters, concomitant antiplatelet therapy that could not be discontinued, or deep location of the tumor that imposed to cross through a sizeable portion of renal parenchyma to reach the target. The largest diameter of the tumors ranged between 11 and 23 mm. All patients underwent laser ablation under conscious sedation with intravenous midazolam and remifentanil, and the laser fibers were introduced into the tumor under ultrasound guidance through 21-gauge Chiba needles. Two laser fibers spaced 12 mm apart were used for lesions with a diameter up to 14 mm (Fig.6.1), and three fibers spaced from 6 to 12 mm apart were used for those with a diameter exceeding 14 mm; the pull-back technique [39, 40] was used if the anteroposterior diameter of the tumors exceeded 12 mm. 1800 J per fiber were delivered into the tumor in 6 min with the laser machine set at a power of 5 W, and further 1800 J were delivered when the pull-back technique was used. Contrast-enhanced ultrasound (CEUS) by using an 8 μL/mL solution of sulfur hexafluoride microbubbles stabilized by a phospholipid shell (SonoVue®; Bracco, Milan, Italy) as a contrast agent was performed about 10 min after the end of the procedure to assess the completeness of the ablation (Fig. 6.2). If residual enhancing foci of tumoral tissue were identified, another one or two laser fibers were inserted into the viable foci under CEUS guidance, and further 1800 J per fiber were delivered to complete the

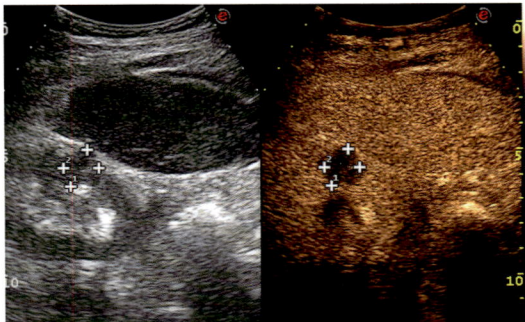

Fig. 6.2 Oblique intercostal CEUS scan performed 10 min after laser ablation showing a 18 × 14 mm non-enhancing zone completely covering the ablated tumor (cross-shaped markers, right side of the split screen)

treatment. Technical success, technical efficacy, primary and secondary efficacy rates, and local tumor progression were defined according to the recommendations of the International Working Group on the Image-guided Tumor Ablation [49]. Complications were classified according to the CIRSE classification system for complications reporting [50]. Technical success was 100%, and just one Grade 1 complication was observed: a small asymptomatic hematoma that spontaneously resolved and did not require any intervention. One-month-technical efficacy was 88.9%; the residual viable tumor foci identified 1 month after laser ablation procedure were successfully treated under CEUS guidance, and secondary efficacy rate was 100%. No local tumor progression was observed during a median follow-up of 26 months (range 11–49 months) [48].

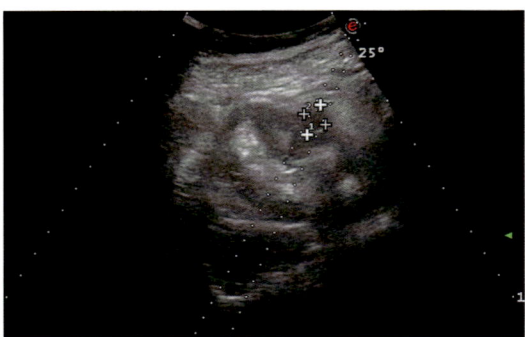

Fig. 6.1 Oblique subcostal ultrasound scan showing a 14 × 9 mm exophytic RCC in the middle third of the right kidney (cross-shaped markers). Two laser fibers spaced 12 mm apart were inserted into the tumor (dotted lines)

6.3   Final Considerations

To date, the experience with laser ablation of renal tumors is quite limited, and cryoablation and RFA (and in the last years MWA in some experienced interventional oncology centers) are currently used worldwide to treat stage T1a RCC. Nevertheless, the above-mentioned and briefly summarized retrospective study suggests that laser ablation is very safe and effective even in at-risk patients [49] and represents a good starting point to investigate its long-term outcomes in prospective studies enrolling larger series of patients with small RCC.

In our opinion, laser ablation can be considered as of now the ablation technique of first choice to treat at-risk patients with small RCC and could represent in the future a valid alternative to cryoablation, RFA, and MWA also in patients with normal coagulation parameters and no increased risk of bleeding.

References

1. http://seer.cancer.gov/statfacts/html/kidrp.html. Accessed Nov 2015.
2. Capitanio U, Montorsi F. Renal cancer. Lancet. 2015;387(10021):894–906.
3. McKiernan J, Simmons R, Kats J, Russo P. Natural history of chronic renal insufficiency after partial and radical nephrectomy. Urology. 2002;59:816–20.
4. Krokidis ME, Orsi F, Katsanos K, Helmberger T, Adam A. CIRSE guidelines on percutaneous ablation of small renal cell carcinoma. Cardiovasc Intervent Radiol. 2017;40:177–91.
5. Huang WC, Elkin EB, Levey AS, Jang TL, Russo P. Partial nephrectomy vs. radical nephrectomy in patients with small renal tumors—is there a difference in mortality and cardiovascular outcomes? J Urol. 2009;181(1):55–61.
6. Zini L, Perrotte P, Capitanio U, Jeldres C, Shariat SF, Antebi E, et al. Radical versus partial nephrectomy: effect on overall and noncancer mortality. Cancer. 2009;115(7):1465–71.
7. Thompson RH, Boorjian SA, Lohse CM, Leibovich BC, Kwon ED, Cheville JC, et al. Radical nephrectomy for T1a renal masses may be associated with decreased overall survival compared with partial nephrectomy. J Urol. 2008;179(2):468–71.
8. Patard JJ, Bensalah KC, Pantuck AJ, Klatte T, Crepel M, Verhoest G, et al. Radical nephrectomy is not superior to nephron sparing surgery in PT1B-PT2N0M0 renal tumors: a matched comparison analysis in 546 cases. Eur Urol Suppl. 2008;7(3):194.
9. Ljungberg B, Bensalah K, Canfield S, Dabestani S, Hofmann F, Hora M, et al. EAU guidelines on renal cell carcinoma: 2014 update. Eur Urol. 2015;67(5):913–24.
10. Chawla SN, Crispen PL, Hanlon AL, Greenberg RE, Chen DY, Uzzo RG. The natural history of observed enhancing renal masses: meta-analysis and review of the world literature. J Urol. 2006;175(2):425–31.
11. Rais-Bahrami S, Guzzo TJ, Jarrett TW, Kavoussi LR, Allf ME. Incidentally discovered renal masses: oncological and perioperative outcomes in patients with delayed surgical intervention. BJU Int. 2009;103:1355–8.
12. Bosniak MA, Birnbaum BA, Krinsky GA, Waisman J. Small renal parenchymal neoplasms: further observations on growth. Radiology. 1995;197:589–97.
13. Oda T, Miyao N, Takahashi A, Yanase M, Masumori N, Itoh N, et al. Growth raters of primary and metastatic lesions of renal cell carcinoma. Int J Urol. 2001;8:473–7.
14. Gudmundsson E, Hellborg H, Lundstam S, Erikson S, Ljungberg B, Swedish Kidney Cancer Quality Register Group. Metastastic potential in renal cell carcinomas ≤7 cm: Swedish Kidney Cancer Quality Register data. Eur Urol. 2011;60(5):975–82.
15. Gervais DA, McGovern FJ, Arellano RS, McDougal WS, Mueller PR. Radiofrequency ablation of renal cell carcinoma. Part 1. Indications, results, and role in patient management over a 6-year period and ablation of 100 tumors. AJR. 2005;185:64–71.
16. Georgiades CS, Rodriguez R. Efficacy and safety of percutaneous cryoablation for stage 1A/B renal cell carcinoma: results of a prospective, single-arm, 5-year study. Cardiovasc Intervent Radiol. 2014;37(6):1494–9.
17. Breen D, Bryant TJ, Abbas A, Shepherd B, McGill N, Andreson JA, et al. Percutaneous cryoablation of renal tumors: outcomes from 171 tumors in 147 patients. BJU Int. 2013;112(6):758–65.
18. McDermott S, Gervais DA. Radiofrequency ablation of liver tumors. Semin InterventRadiol. 2013;30(1):49–55.
19. Escudier B, Porta C, Schmidinger M, Algaba F, PAtard JJ, Khoo V, et al. Renal cell carcinoma: ESMO Clinical Practice Guidelines for diagnosis, treatment and follow-up. Ann Oncol. 2014;25(3):49–56.
20. Ma Y, Bedir S, Cadeddu JA, Gahan JC. Long-term outcomes in healthy adults after radiofrequency ablation of T1a renal tumors. BJU Int. 2014;113:51–5.
21. Boutros C, Somasundar P, Garrean S, Saied A, Espat NJ. Microwave coagulation therapy for hepatic tumors: review of the literature and critical analysis. Surg Oncol. 2010;19:e22–32.
22. Lubner MG, Brace CL, Ziemlewicz TJ, Hinshaw JL, Lee FT Jr. Microwave ablation of hepatic malignancy. Semin Intervent Radiol. 2013;30:56–66.
23. Di Vece F, Tombesi P, Ermili F, Maraldi C, Sartori S. Coagulation areas produced by cool-tip radiofrequency ablation and microwave ablation using a device to decrease back-heating effects: a prospective pilot study. Cardiovasc InterventRadiol. 2014;37:723–9.
24. Knavel EM, Hinshaw JL, Lubner MG, Andreano A, Thomas FW, Lee FT Jr, et al. High-powered gas-cooled microwave ablation: shaft cooling creates an effective stick function without altering the ablation zone. AJR Am J Roentgenol. 2012;198:W260–5.
25. Horn JC, Patel RS, Kim E, Nowakowski FS, Lookstein RA, Fischman AM. Percutaneous microwave ablation of renal tumors using a gas-cooled 2.4-Gh probe: technique and initial results. J Vasc Intervent Radiol. 2014;25:448–53.

26. Pacella CM, Francica G, Di Lascio FM, Arienti V, Antico E, Caspani B, et al. Long-term outcome of cirrhotic patients with early hepatocellular carcinoma treated with ultrasound-guided percutaneous laser ablation: a retrospective analysis. J Clin Oncol. 2009;27:2615–21.

27. Ferrari FS, Megliola A, Scorzelli A, Stella A, Vigni F, Drudi FM, et al. Treatment of small HCC through radiofrequency ablation and laser ablation. Comparison of techniques and long-term results. Radiol Med. 2007;112:377–93.

28. Puls R, Langner S, Rosenberg C, Hegenscheid K, Kuehn JP, Noeckler K, et al. Laser ablation of liver metastases from colorectal cancer with MR thermometry: 5-year survival. J Vasc Radiol. 2009;20:225–34.

29. Di Costanzo GG, Tortora R, D'Adamo G, De Luca M, Lampasi F, Addario L, et al. Radiofrequency ablation versus laser ablation for the treatment of small hepatocellular carcinoma in cirrhosis: a randomized trial. J Gastroenterol Hepatol. 2015;30:559–65.

30. Sartori S, Di Vece F, Ermili F, Tombesi P. Laser ablation of liver tumors: an ancillary technique, or an alternative to radiofrequency and microwave? World J Radiol. 2017;9(3):91–6.

31. Karinimi J, Ojala R, Hellstrom P, Sequeros RB. MRI-guided percutaneous laser ablation of small renal cell carcinoma: Initial clinical experience. Acta Radiol. 2010;51:467–72.

32. De Jode MG, Vale JA, Gedroyc WM. MR-guided laser thermoablation of inoperable renal tumors in an open-configuration interventional MR scanner: preliminary clinical experience in three cases. J Magn Reson Imaging. 1999;10:545–9.

33. Dick EA, Joarder R, De Jode MG, Wragg P, Vale JA, Gedroyc WM. Magnetic resonance imaging-guided laser thermal ablation of renal tumors. BJU Int. 2002;90:814–22.

34. Giesbrandt K, Walser E. MR imaging-guided laser ablation of hepatic and renal tumors. AJR Am J Roentgenol. 2012;198:E642.

35. Huang GT, Wang TH, Sheu JC, Daikuzono N, Sung JL, Wu MZ, et al. Low-power laserthermia for the treatment of small hepatocellular carcinoma. Eur J Cancer. 1991;27:1622–7.

36. Muralidharan V, Malcontenti-Wilson C, Christophi C. Interstitial laser hyperthermia for colorectal liver metastases: the effect of thermal sensitization and the use of a cylindrical diffuser tip on tumor necrosis. J Clin Laser Med Surg. 2002;20:189–96.

37. Vogl TJ, Straub R, Zangos S, Mack MG, Eichler K. MR-guided laser induced thermotherapy (LITT) of liver tumours: experimental and clinical data. Int J Hyperth. 2004;20:713–24.

38. Pacella CM, Bizzarri G, Magnolfi F, Cecconi P, Caspani B, Anelli V, et al. Laser thermal ablation in the treatment of small hepatocellular carcinoma: results in 74 patients. Radiology. 2001;221:712–20.

39. Di Costanzo GG, D'Adamo G, Tortora R, Zanfardino F, Mattera S, Francica G, et al. A novel needle guide system to perform percutaneous laser ablation of liver tumors using the multifiber technique. Acta Radiol. 2013;54:876–81.

40. Pacella CM, Bizzarri G, Francica G, Bianchini A, De Nuntis S, Pacella S, et al. Percutaneous laser ablation in the treatment of hepatocellular carcinoma with small tumors: analysis of factors affecting the achievement of tumor necrosis. J Vasc Interv Radiol. 2005;16:1447–57.

41. Francica G, Petrolati A, Di Stasio E, Pacella S, Stasi R, Pacella CM. Effectiveness, safety, and local progression are not affected by tumor location. AJR Am J Roentgenol. 2012;199:1393–401.

42. Francica G, Petrolati A, Di Stasio E, Pacella S, Stasi R, Pacella CM. Effectiveness, safety, and local progression after percutaneous laser ablation for hepatocellular carcinoma nodules up to 4 cm are not affected by tumor location. AJR Am J Roentgenol. 2012;199:1393–401.

43. Di Costanzo GG, Francica G, Pacella CM. Laser ablation for small hepatocellular carcinoma: State of the art and future perspectives. World J Hepatol. 2014;6:704–15.

44. Taslakian B, Georges Sabaaly M, Al-Kutoubi A. Patient evaluation and preparation in vascular and interventional radiology: what every interventional radiologist should know (part 1: patient assessment and laboratory tests). Cardiovasc Intervent Radiol. 2016;39:325–33.

45. Babaei Jandaghi A, Lebady M, Zamani AA. A randomized clinical trial to compare coaxial and noncoaxial techniques in percutaneous core needle biopsy of renal parenchyma. Cardiovasc Intervent Radiol. 2017;40:106–11.

46. Chunduri S, Whittier WL, Korbert SM. Adequacy and complication rates with 14- vs. 16-gaude automated needles in percutaneous renal biopsy of native kidneys. Semin Dial. 2015;28:E11–!4.

47. Corapi KM, Chen JL, Balk EM, Gordon CE. Bleeding complications of native kidney biopsy: a systematic review and meta-analysis. Am J Kidney Dis. 2012;60:62–73.

48. Sartori S, Mauri G, Tombesi P, Di Vece F, Bianchi L, Pacella CM. Ultrasound-guided laser ablation is safe and effective in the treatment of small renal tumors in patients at increased bleeding risk. Int J Hyperth. 2018;11:1–7. https://doi.org/10.1080/02656736.2018.1468038.

49. Ahmed M, Solbiati L, Brace CL, Breen DJ, Callstrom MR, Charboneau JW, et al. Image-guided tumor ablation: standardization of terminology and reporting criteria—a 10-year update. J Vasc Interv Radiol. 2014;25:1691–705, e4.

50. Filippiadis DK, Binkert C, Pellerin O, Hoffmann RT, Krajina A, Pereira PL. CIRSE quality assurance document and standards for classification of complications: the CIRSE classification system. Cardiovasc Intervent Radiol. 2017;40:1141–6.

Benign Thyroid Nodule Laser Ablation

Enrico Papini, Rinaldo Guglielmi,
Agnese Persichetti, and Claudio Maurizio Pacella

7.1 Introduction

The clinical management of thyroid lesions has been performed for many years by means of physical examination, thyroid radioisotope scan, and surgery. During the last decades, however, the advent of thyroid ultrasonography (US) and fine-needle aspiration biopsy (FNAB) has radically changed the diagnostic approach to thyroid nodular disease. The widespread application of US is now resulting in the detection of solid and cystic thyroid nodules in a large part of the adult population, with a frequency that rises with adult and old age and with female sex and that, in several series, approximate 50% [1–8]. The cytological assessment with US-guided fine-needle aspiration biopsy (US-FNAB) has sharply reduced the need for diagnostic surgery and only a minority of the recently diagnosed lesions undergo thyroidectomy. Most cytologically benign thyroid nodules are asymptomatic, their volume remain nearly unchanging over the years, and go to long-term follow-up without any intervention [9]. Even if the majority of thyroid lesions do not need therapy, a few of them (about 10%) progressively

increase in size and cause local signs or pressure symptoms. Due to the discomfort or the anxiety, a large part of these last lesions are finally dealt with thyroidectomy [10, 11]. Surgery is a well-established treatment and is currently at low risk of major complications. However, the costs of thyroid surgery, the esthetic damage due to the cervical scar (that may be prevented only by rather complicated and expensive trans-axillary or trans-oral surgical approaches [12–15]), the risk of major or minor complications, and the frequent need of life-long substitution therapy should be evaluated when this clinical problem is approached [16, 17]. On the basis of these considerations, various image-guided office-based, minimally invasive procedures have been proposed with the aim of producing a clinically significant debulking of thyroid lesions and a nonsurgical management of benign symptomatic nodules [18].

In 1990, US-guided percutaneous ethanol injection was the first proposed technique for the shrinkage of autonomously functioning thyroid nodules [19]. Due to the side effects of the treatment and its technical limits, percutaneous ethanol injection is presently used only for the treatment of cystic or predominantly fluid lesions that relapse after a prior aspiration [20]. So, since 2000, US-guided minimally invasive techniques based on thermal ablation by means of energy sources (such as laser, radiofrequency, microwave, and high-intensity focused ultrasound) were investigated and are now increasingly

E. Papini (✉) · R. Guglielmi · A. Persichetti
Department of Endocrinology and Metabolism,
Regina Apostolorum Hospital,
Albano Laziale, Rome, Italy

C. M. Pacella
Department of Diagnostic Imaging and Interventional
Radiology, Regina Apostolorum Hospital,
Albano Laziale, Rome, Italy

© Springer Nature Switzerland AG 2020
C. M. Pacella et al. (eds.), *Image-guided Laser Ablation*,
https://doi.org/10.1007/978-3-030-21748-8_7

employed in clinical practice. Among these thermal procedures, laser ablation is the most thoroughly assessed and less invasive technique and currently represents a safe and effective tool for the management of benign and selected malignant thyroid lesions.

7.2 Basic Principles of Laser Treatment

The model for the interstitial laser coagulation of body tissues was first proposed by Bown in 1983 and was subsequently validated in several experimental models [21–24]. Laser light is coherent and monochromatic, is precisely focused on the selected target, and permits the delivery of a considerable amount of energy at a distance through an optical fiber with a silica-based core. The optical fibers are flexible, with a diameter ranging from 300 to 600 μm, and transmit laser light to the tip of the fiber optic [25–27]. When laser light interacts with biological tissues, scattering and absorption occur, and the delivered photons induce rapid heating and thermal injury [23, 25, 28, 29].

Different laser sources and wavelengths are available and various types of fibers, tips, and applicators may be employed. Nd:YAG lasers, operating at 1064 nm, seem most suited for procedures in deep-seated organs because of their superior penetration and absorption properties in perfused soft tissues. Currently, the majority of laser procedures use either Nd:YAG or diode lasers ($\lambda = 800$–980 nm) operating in the range of 2–40 W [25].

Thermal ablation destroys the tissues by increasing their temperature so as to induce irreversible cellular damage. A temperature set at about 40 °C generally does not adversely influence cellular homeostasis while a temperature level of 45 °C results in a greater susceptibility of the cells to the injury induced by physical and chemical agents [24, 30]. An irreversible cellular damage occurs only when cells are maintained at a temperature value of 46 °C for 1 h, and the damage appears with ever-increasing quickness as the temperature level further rises [31, 32]. At

a temperature level between 60 and 100 °C, a rapid coagulation of the proteins takes place with irreversible injury of enzymes, nucleic acids, and proteins, followed by cellular death over the course of a few days [22–24, 30, 33–36]. Critical temperature at the margin of the coagulative zone has been shown to range from 30 to 77 °C for normal tissue and from 41 to 64 °C for neoplastic tissues [37–39], with relevant variation of the thermal dose required to induce cell death different tissues [37]. On the other hand, a temperature value greater than 105 °C is followed by tissue carbonization and vaporization, changes that obstacle a total ablation due to the insulating effect on energy diffusion of thermal energy [32, 40–43]. On the basis of these effects, laser treatment results in a zone of coagulative necrosis with well-defined margins, a well-predictable size, and the destruction of all the cells in the ablated area.

7.3 Technique and Devices

Laser sources are variable but the most used is a 820 nm diode or a 1064 nm neodymium-yttrium-aluminium garnet (Nd:YAG) laser [25, 44–46]. Applicators of different gauge [44–48] may be used for the insertion in the target lesion and are preferentially represented by flexible 21G (<1 mm in diameter) spinal needles [47]. The commonly employed laser equipment is a 1064 nm continuous wave Nd:YAG source, operated with an output power that ranges from 3 to 5 W, and a flat-tipped quartz optical fiber with a 300-μm diameter. Laser ablation may be performed either under US guidance (with the use of a dedicated device) or assistance (with a freehand technique) by means of a last-generation US system equipped with a high-frequency linear transducer (7.5–15 MHz).

The treatment is usually performed on the patient in supine position with hyperextended neck. An accurate local anesthesia with xylocaine is performed on the skin entry site, along the planned needle tract, and on the thyroid capsule. In the case of anxiety, a mild sedation may be given with diazepam intramuscularly or by mouth. Under US monitoring, the spinal needle is inserted into the target thyroid lesion, in most cases along its longest axis. Treatments are generally performed with a fixed-power protocol (usually with a 3 W output) while the illumination time changes according to the planned ablation volume. Usually, the illumination time ranges from a minimum of 400 s to a maximum of 600 s with a total energy delivery of 1200–1800 J per optical fiber. The use as applicators of thin and minimally traumatic spinal needles allows a precise and safe positioning of one or more needles depending on the volume, shape, and location of the nodule. When multiple applicators are employed, they should be separated by a space of at least 0.8 cm and placed next to each other on the same plane to better allow the simultaneous real time control of two optical fibers. The fiber tip should be positioned at a minimum safety distance of 5–10 mm from the critical structures of the neck. In case of lesions close to the carotid vessels or the trachea wall, as for cancer recurrences in the thyroid bed, a preliminary hydro-dissection with saline solution may be performed to separate the target from the vital structure. From one to three illuminations may be performed during the same session retracting the needle with a "pullback" technique [47]. At US monitoring, the area under ablation is visualized as an echogenic zone that gradually enlarges during the illumination, and the treatment is concluded when the area of hyper-echogenicity due to tissue evaporation is stationary in size [44, 45, 49–53]. A reliable evaluation of the real size of the ablated area is achieved a few hours after treatment with the intravenous injection of a second-generation ultrasound contrast medium or, less precisely, with the use of color- or power-doppler. Notably, the zone of coagulative necrosis attains its maximum size about 72 h after the ablation [54], because the cellular injury and the occlusion of the vessels that supply the tissue fully develop during the days following the treatment. Figure 7.1a–f shows a representative case of a predominantly solid cold nodule before treatment (a, b), during the ablation maneuver (c, d), and 12 months after treatment (e, f).

7.4 Thyroid Lesions Suitable for Laser Ablation

Thyroid nodules are suitable for laser ablation in the presence of the following criteria: (a) single thyroid nodule or multinodular goiter with an evidently dominant lesion; (b) hypo- or isofunctioning appearance at radioisotope thyroid scan; (c) progressive growth associated with either local compression symptoms or esthetic concern; and (d) consistently benign cytological reports at two FNAs. As the risk of overlooking a thyroid malignancy should be carefully prevented, the presence of suspicious US findings is a partial contraindication to laser ablation even in the case of benign cytological findings.

Thyroid nodules with solid, spongiform, or nearly completely solid structure are successfully ablated while pseudocystic lesions should be drained of the fluid component immediately before laser illumination [53]. Notably, laser ablation is an effective treatment also for pseudocystic nodules that repeatedly relapse after percutaneous ethanol injection.

Before treatment, withdrawal of antiplatelet therapy for at least 72 h is suggested, unless the patient is at high risk of cardiovascular events, while the anticoagulant treatment with NAO drugs may be stopped 24 h before laser ablation. Prothrombin time, partial thromboplastin time, and complete blood cell count should be assessed before the procedure. A preliminary direct laryngoscopy should be routinely performed [47]. Finally, the patient should be informed that a regular US follow-up is appropriate even after a successful minimally invasive treatment and the disappearance of local symptoms.

7.5 Clinical Results in Hypofunctioning Thyroid Nodules

Several preliminary experimental tests were performed in the 1990s, first in laboratory on liver tissue and thereafter in vivo on animal models [55–57] and ex vivo on freshly resected thyroid glands [58]. The initial feasibility study in humans

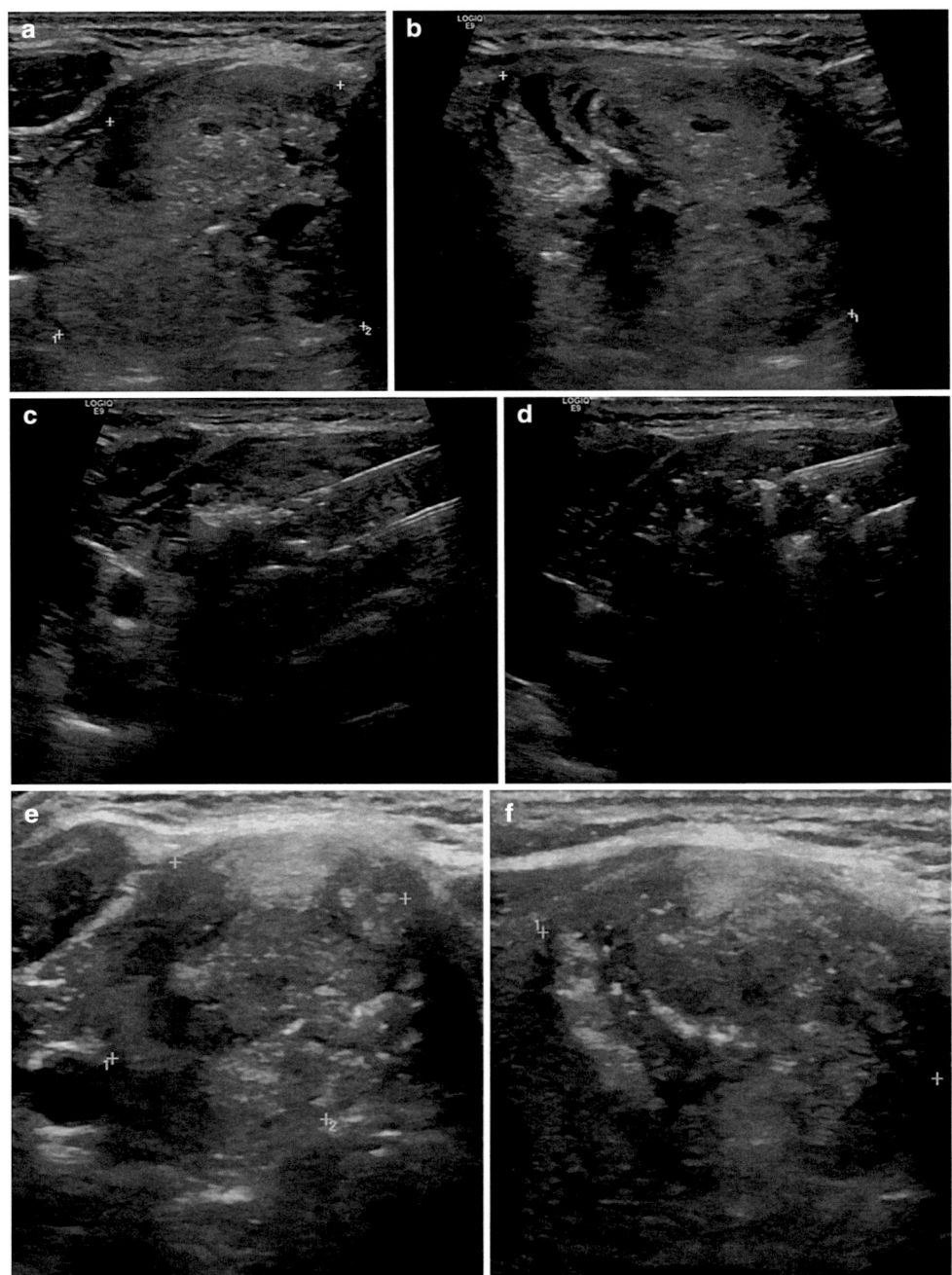

Fig. 7.1 (**a**, **b**) Representative case of solid nodule treated with laser ablation (LA). (**a**) US axial scan and (**b**) longitudinal scan—showing the nodule with a fluid component ≥20% of the volume at baseline before the treatment. (**c**, **d**) LA performed with two fibers and only one pull-back. The US longitudinal scan (**c**) shows two thin 21G introducers spaced 1 cm apart from each other in the deepest part of the target nodule during the first illumination. In (**d**) US imaging shows the second illumination of the nodule. The laser fibers positioned along the long axis of the nodule are retracted about

1 cm for a second illumination to cover the entire volume of the nodule. This technique is also known as "pull-back technique," which has the advantage of reducing the number of direct nodule punctures, the invasiveness of the procedure, and the discomfort for the patients. During the procedure, it develops gas (*visible both in c and d*) for temperatures above 100 °C with consequent boiling of the aqueous component of the nodule. (**e**, **f**) The two US scans in **e** (*axial*) and in **f** (*longitudinal*) show the volumetric reduction 12 months after treatment equal to 68% compared to the volume at baseline

on the use of image-guided percutaneous thermal ablation for the treatment of thyroid nodules was published in 2000 [58]. The histological examination confirmed the geometrical shape of tissue damage and its relationship with the delivered energy that was previously observed in experimental models [58]. Subsequent cytological and histological studies on 15 cold thyroid nodules that were sampled or resected 12 months after ablation treatment consistently demonstrated a well-defined area of coagulative necrosis with signs of inflammatory reaction in the ablated areas [59]. No evidence of malignant change was observed in thyroid lesions resected 24 months after laser treatment [60].

During the last years, several case reports [49, 61] and non-randomized [44–47, 62–64] and randomized studies [48, 50, 65, 66] have been performed on the treatment of thyroid lesions with US-guided laser ablation. All these data consistently confirmed the clinical value, good tolerability, and substantial safety of laser thermal ablation for thyroid nodular disease. The reported volume decrease at 12 months ranged from 43% to 84% [65, 67] (Table 7.1). Volume reduction was persistent, as follow-up studies demonstrated that the mean nodule volume decrease remained at 48% and 51% versus baseline size at the 3-[64] and 5-year [52] controls. In 2014, an Italian multicenter prospective randomized trial, performed with a single ablation session and fixed treatment parameters, showed a nodule volume decrease between 49% and 60% 3 years after laser treatment [66]. Accordingly, only a minority (9%) of the treated nodules demonstrated a partial regrowth at 3 years after treatment [64]. These findings were further confirmed by an externally monitored multicenter retrospective study on a series of 1531 patients [70] that demonstrated an up to nearly 80% decrease of thyroid nodules volume after one or more treatments in large size lesions. Notably, in these controlled studies, the vast majority of patients treated with laser ablation reported in a visual-analogue questionnaire the disappearance or the relevant amelioration of their local compression symptoms or esthetic damage and defined the procedure as fairly well tolerated [50, 52, 65, 66].

7.6 Clinical Results in Hyperfunctioning Thyroid Nodules

Several studies on laser treatment of small series of hyperfunctioning thyroid nodules reported the control of thyroid hyperfunction and the disappearance of the previously hyperfunctioning area at post-ablation thyroid scintigraphy [49, 62, 75]. However, at least two other trials showed that laser ablation did not constantly result in normalization of serum TSH levels and that repeated laser treatments were required to achieve satisfactory results [47, 61, 76]. These findings were confirmed by a prospective randomized study on 30 hyperfunctioning nodules associated with hyperthyroidism and suppression of normal thyroid tissue. Treatments were performed either with a single thermal ablation session or with a therapeutic radioiodine dose. Follow-up demonstrated that laser treatment and ^{131}I therapy resulted in a similar nodule size decrease but also that thermal ablation was less effective in the control of hyperthyroidism because induced serum TSH normalization in only about 50% of patients [77]. As a whole, the available evidence demonstrates the clinical efficacy of thermal ablation for the treatment of small size, solitary, and mildly hyperfunctioning nodules [63, 76, 78]. Since functionally satisfactory results are attained only when about 80% of the volume of the hyperfunctioning nodule is ablated [79], clinical results are unsatisfactory in toxic nodular goiter or large size toxic nodules, and in these cases the normalization of thyroid function usually necessitates repeated treatment sessions the favorable results are [61] (Table 7.2). Laser ablation, however, may be of use in selected cases of

Table 7.1 Clinical outcomes of patients with symptomatic benign cold thyroid nodules treated with laser ablation (major series)

Author	Pts/nodules no.	RCT	US pattern[a] solidity	Baseline vol (mL (mean))	Laser source	Major complication no. (%)	Minor complication no. (%)	FU	Volume reduction (% (mean))
Dossing et al. [44]	16		≥80	10.0	820 diode	0	0	6	46
Spiezia et al. [62]	5/5		>80	11.1	Nd:YAG	1 (8.3)[b]	0	12	61
Pacella et al. [47]	8/8		≥80	22.7	Nd:YAG	2 (8.3)[c]	0	6	63
Papini et al. [68]	20 vs. 20[d]		≥80	24.1	Nd:YAG	0	0	6	64
Dossing et al. [50]	15 vs. 15[d]	Yes	≥80	8.2	820 diode	0	0	6	44med
Dossing et al. [51]	10/10		≥70	9.6	820 diode	0	0	12	57 med
Dossing et al. [51]	15 vs. 15[e]	Yes	≥80	10.1/10.7	820 diode	0	0	6	45 vs. 58med
Gambelunghe et al. [48]	5 vs. 5[d]	Yes	≥80	8.2	Nd:YAG	0	0	30 weeks	44
Cakir et al. [45][f]	15/12[f]		≥80	11.9	810 diode	0	1(7.6)	12	82
Papini et al. [65]	21 vs. 21 vs. 20[g]	Yes	≥80	11.7/13.6/12.1	Nd:YAG	0	0	12	>40
Valcavi et al. [64]	122/122[h]		≥80	23.1	Nd:YAG	3 (2.5)	20(16.3)	36	48
Dossing et al. [52]	78/78	Yes	≥80	8.2	820 diode	0	0	67	51med
Amabile et al. [46]	51/51[i]		≥80	53.5	980 diode	0	0	12	82
Gambelunghe et al. [69]	20 vs. 20[j]		≥80	15/14	Nd:YAG	0	2 (5)	36	+11/57
Gambelunghe et al. [69]	50 vs. 50[k] [100]	Yes	≥80	21/21	Nd:YAG	0–1(0.02)[b]	0	6	55/56 med
Papini et al. [66]	101 vs. 99[l]	Yes	≥80	12	Nd:YAG	1 (1)[b]	0	36	57
Achille et al. [67]	45/45		≥80	24	Nd:YAG	1(2.5)[b]	0	12	84
Pacella et al. [70]	1531/1534		≥80	27	Nd:YAG	8 (0.5)	9 (0.6)	12	73
Negro et al. [71]	64/64		≥80	15.7	Nd:YAG	4/56 (7.1)[b]	0	48	56

Mauri et al. [72]	31/315[m]	–	20.3	Nd.YAG	1 (0.02)[b]	0	12	70
Pacella et al. [73]	449/449[132][n]	≥80	21.5	Nd:YAG	–	–	12	63
Oddo et al. [74]	14/14	≥80	19	Nd:YAG	0	1 (7.1)	12	58

Pts patients

[a]Uniformly solid or predominantly solid with not more than 20% fluid component

[b]Transient dysphonia

[c]Transient dysphonia lasting 24 and 48 h, respectively

[d]Pts treated with single LA session vs. pts under observation

[e]15 pts with cold nodules treated with one laser session vs. 15 pts treated with radioiodine therapy

[f]One patient had taken 300 mg acetyl salicylic acid daily for 1 year

[g]Pts treated with laser energy vs. patients treated with L–T4 or no treated

[h]The energy was delivered continuously while retracting the applicators in a single session

[i]The energy was delivered continuously while extracting the needle in multiple sessions

[j]Retrospective comparison between a group treated with low amount of energy and one treated with a high amount of energy

[k]Retrospective comparison between patients treated with local anesthetic and patients treated without local anesthetic

[l]101 pts treated with LA vs. 99 under observation

[m]Retrospective comparison study

[n]Retrospective study of comparison using propensity score system

Table 7.2 Clinical outcomes of patients with symptomatic benign hot thyroid nodules treated with laser ablation (major series)

Author	Nodules no.	RCT	US pattern solidity ≥ 80	Baseline vol (mL (mean))	Lasers source	Total energy load or J/mL (mean)	Number of session (mean)	FU months	Volume reduction % (mean)	TSH changes (%)[a]	Hormones changes (%)[a]
Dossing et al. [49]	1		Solid	8.2	820 diode	1950	1	9	40	N[b]	N[b]
Spiezia et al. [62]	7		Solid	3.2	Nd:YAG		1	12	74	N[c]	7/7 (100)
Pacella et al. [47]	16		Solid	7.9	Nd:YAG	816 (J/mL)	2.7	6	62	5/16(31)	5/16 (31)
Gambelunghe et al. [48]	8		Solid	8.2	Nd:YAG	1900 (J/mL)	1	30 weeks	44	8/8(100)	8/8 (100)
Barbaro et al. [76]	18		Solid	21.1	Nd:YAG		3	12	59	N[d]	
Dossing et al. [77]	14 vs. 15	Yes[e]	Solid	10.6/11.2	820 diode	217 (J/mL)	1	6	44/47	7/14–15/15 (50–100)	N[f]
Valcavi et al. [63]	1		Solid	2.5	Nd:YAG		1	–	95	N[f]	N[f]
Rotondi et al. [61]	1		Solid	55.0	980 diode		4	10	91	N[g]	N[g]
Amabile et al. [46]	26		Solid	55.3	980 diode	379 (J/mL)	3.2 cycle	12	82	23/26 (88)	–
Gambelunghe et al. [78]	82		Solid	12 (5–118)	Nd:YAG	7200 J (median)	1	12	42	N[h] (53)	N[h]

no. stands for number of nodules

[a]Improvement rate (%)

[b]N = Normalization of serum TSH and peripheral hormones within 2 months who remained normal during additional 9 months

[c]N = Normalization: no recurrence of hyperthyroidism up to 12 months

[d]N = Normalization: after a time ranging from 3–6 weeks to 2–3 months, all patients with single AFTN (*n* = 8) and 5 pts (50%) of 10 with multinodular goiter had improvement of serum levels of FT3 and FT4 and a complete normalization of TSH that remained unaltered during follow-up

[e]RCT comparing a single radioiodine dose and a single laser therapy

[f]N = Complete normalization of TSH and peripheral hormones

[g]N = Six months after LA, normalization of TSH and thyroid hormones that remained so throughout a 30-month follow-up

[h]The percentage of patients who discontinued metimazole therapy was reduced by increasing the initial volume of the toxic nodule. In nodules with a volume less than 5 mL, all patients were able to suspend methimazole; this percentage was reduced to 90.2% in nodules with a volume between 5 and 15 mL, 61.1% in those with volume 15–25 mL, and only 28.5% in nodules larger than 25 mL

large toxic nodules for a combined treatment with radioiodine. A prospective trial [80] randomized 15 cases of large hyperfunctioning nodules treated with laser ablation followed by ^{131}I with a similar number of matched patients treated with radioiodine only. The combined treatment resulted in a faster decrease of nodule volume and in a more rapid control of hyperthyroidism and pressure symptoms than the therapy with radioiodine only.

7.7 Clinical Results in Cystic Thyroid Lesions

Few data are available on the use of thermal ablation for cystic thyroid lesions. A prospective study randomly assigned 44 prevalently cystic thyroid nodules to simple drainage or to fluid aspiration without delay followed by laser treatment [53]. A greater than 50% volume decrease and the improvement of pressure symptoms was demonstrated in 15 of 22 (68%) of patients in the thermal ablation group and only in 4 of 22 (18%) cases in the aspiration alone group at the 6-month control. Moreover, thermal ablation induced a relevant shrinkage of the solid part of the predominantly cystic lesion (from 1.8 to 1.0 mL), while in the aspiration only group, the solid part was substantially unchanged (Table 7.3). The procedure was well tolerated, no complications were observed and thyroid function was unchanged.

Percutaneous ethanol injection is the first-line nonsurgical treatment for thyroid cysts and predominantly cystic nodules because of its low expense, safety, and rapidity [81]. So, thermal ablation is selectively appropriate for the treatment of cystic lesions (mostly due to persistent bleeding) that relapse after percutaneous ethanol injection and for mixed nodules with a relevant fluid component both to prevent fluid refilling and to achieve a satisfactory shrinkage of the solid portion of the nodule.

7.8 Complications and Side Effects of Laser Treatment

The technique of image-guided laser treatment is rather simple and is usually well tolerated. A modest cervical pain, some neck swelling, and, rarely, a low fever are described by the patients after the ablation, may persist 24–48 h, and are effectively controlled by the administration of analgesics by mouth.

Minor complications are uncommon and include a more protracted neck and local inflammation pain that persist more than 48 h [47, 68]. Cervical bleeding and skin burn are definitely uncommon events [70, 82]. Relevant neck oedema sometimes associated with cystic change and rupture of the treated lesion have been occasionally reported [64]. Transitory hyperthyroidism or late hypothyroidism is unusual [64].

Major complications are rare and are due to an incorrect or overzealous technique of treatment. No relevant changes besides a modest fibrosis were reported in the cervical tissues surrounding the treated nodule in patients who eventually underwent surgery because of the coexistence of cytologically suspicious areas [59, 60].

An adequate training is anyway necessary before starting the laser procedure. Up to now, the single most relevant complication was a case of injury of the trachea that necessitated surgical repair, induced by the incorrect insertion of the laser fiber by an untrained operator

Table 7.3 Clinical outcomes of patients with symptomatic benign cystic thyroid nodules treated with laser ablation

Author	Pts nodules no.	RCT	US pattern	Baseline volume	Laser source	Major complication no. (%)	Minor complication no. (%)	FU	Volume reduction % (mean)
Dossing et al. [53]	22 vs. 22[a]	Yes	Cystic	11.8	820 diode	0	0	36	57

[a]22 pts treated with aspiration followed by LA session vs. 22 pts aspiration without LA session

[83]. Indeed, in a series of 122 procedures performed by physicians in the initial part of their learning curve, laryngeal nerve injury was observed in 1.6% of patients [64]. Conversely, a trial performed in four centers with specific expertise in minimally invasive procedures showed a definitely low risk of complications [66]. A spontaneously resolving case of vocal cord paresis was observed (<1%) and the use of analgesics for more than 24 h was required in a minority (5%) of patients [66].

A very low incidence (0.5%) of side effects and complications was confirmed in the large multicenter retrospective Italian study that collected over 1500 thyroid lesions treated by operators with specific expertise in the field [70]. More generally, a recent analysis in order to evaluate the incidence of complications of the entire population treated with LA in the various centers has documented an incidence of major complications of 0.7% and 1.4% of the minor complications [84] (Table 7.1).

As a general rule, the presence of severe pain during the laser procedure is a useful warning symptom that may prevent the risk of periprocedural complications. So, if the patient complains of an increasing pain, laser firing should be discontinued, the position of the fibers should be controlled, and the procedure should be performed after a careful repositioning of the fiber tip within the target nodule [47, 67, 69, 70, 76].

7.9 Conclusions for Clinical Practice

The occurrence of thyroid nodular disease in the general population is definitely high and the number of benign lesions that are growing or become symptomatic is accordingly increasing. In these cases, a timely and appropriate use of thermal ablation is followed by the modification of the natural history of growing benign nodules. So, the nonsurgical treatment of nodules that are cause of concern avoids the unfavorable influence of thyroidectomy on the quality of life (due to the esthetic damage and the long-term substitution therapy), decreases the direct and indirect costs of treatment, and allows a more appropriate use of surgical facilities.

Various image-guided thermal techniques, with different modalities of action, are now accessible. US-guided laser ablation is the most thoroughly assessed and less invasive of these techniques and may be safely used by operators with expertise in the field of thyroid US and US-guided FNA. However, a specific training and an initial tutorship are appropriate for decreasing the potential risk of complications. A second cytologic assessment of the benign nature of the lesion that is increasing in size is recommended before the ablation treatment to further decrease the risk of overlooking a well-differentiated thyroid cancer.

US-guided laser ablation is recommended for the treatment of solid, or predominantly solid, nonfunctioning thyroid nodules that with time keep growing and become symptomatic or cause cosmetic concern. Laser ablation results in a clinically significant volume decrease and the recovery from pressure symptoms in the vast majority of cases. Volume reduction, as a rule, persists over many years and the procedure can be safely repeated in case of a late, and usually partial, regrowth. Notably, the risk of esthetic cervical injury or thyroid function changes is nearly absent and the risk of periprocedural complications is very low.

Laser ablation may be used for the treatment of small-size hyperfunctioning thyroid nodules that are associated with subclinical hyperthyroidism and do not induce a complete suppression of the surrounding thyroid tissue. In these autonomously functioning nodules, especially in young patients, normalization of serum TSH is achieved without irradiation and no risk of late hypothyroidism.

On the other hand, in large-size hyperfunctioning nodules, laser ablation is generally not cost-effective, due to the need of repeated treatments, in comparison with ^{131}I treatment. So, it should be reserved to patients who cannot access surgical or radioiodine treatments or may be used for a preliminary debulking of huge toxic lesions before ^{131}I therapy.

Finally, laser ablation may be of use for the conclusive treatment of mostly cystic thyroid lesions that repeatedly relapse after percutaneous drainage and ethanol injection. Before thermal ablation, efficacy, complications, and tolerability of laser treatment should be fully explained, discussed with the patient, and weighted against the results and side-effects of traditional management options.

References

1. Mortensen JD, Woolner LB, Bennett WA. Gross and microscopic findings in clinically normal thyroid glands. J Clin Endocrinol Metab. 1955;15(10):1270–80.
2. Carroll BA. Asymptomatic thyroid nodules: incidental sonographic detection. AJR Am J Roentgenol. 1982;138(3):499–501.
3. Harach HR, Franssila KO, Wasenius VM. Occult papillary carcinoma of the thyroid. A "normal" finding in Finland. A systematic autopsy study. Cancer. 1985;56(3):531–8.
4. Tan GH, Gharib H. Thyroid incidentalomas: management approaches to nonpalpable nodules discovered incidentally on thyroid imaging. Ann Intern Med. 1997;126(3):226–31.
5. Wiest PW, Hartshorne MF, Inskip PD, Crooks LA, Vela BS, Telepak RJ, et al. Thyroid palpation versus high-resolution thyroid ultrasonography in the detection of nodules. J Ultrasound Med. 1998;17(8):487–96.
6. Brander AE, Viikinkoski VP, Nickels JI, Kivisaari LM. Importance of thyroid abnormalities detected at US screening: a 5-year follow-up. Radiology. 2000;215(3):801–6.
7. Frates MC, Benson CB, Charboneau JW, Cibas ES, Clark OH, Coleman BG, et al. Management of thyroid nodules detected at US: Society of Radiologists in Ultrasound consensus conference statement. Radiology. 2005;237(3):794–800.
8. Gharib H, Papini E. Thyroid nodules: clinical importance, assessment, and treatment. Endocrinol Metab Clin N Am. 2007;36(3):707–35, vi.
9. Durante C, Costante G, Lucisano G, Bruno R, Meringolo D, Paciaroni A, et al. The natural history of benign thyroid nodules. JAMA. 2015;313(9):926–35.
10. Cooper DS, Doherty GM, Haugen BR, Kloos RT, Lee SL, Mandel SJ, et al. Revised American Thyroid Association management guidelines for patients with thyroid nodules and differentiated thyroid cancer. Thyroid. 2009;19(11):1167–214.
11. Gharib H, Papini E, Paschke R, Duick DS, Valcavi R, Hegedus L, et al. American Association of Clinical Endocrinologists, Associazione Medici Endocrinologi, and European Thyroid Association medical guidelines for clinical practice for the diagnosis and management of thyroid nodules: executive summary of recommendations. J Endocrinol Invest. 2010;33(5 Suppl):51–6.
12. Piccoli M, Mullineris B, Santi D, Gozzo D. Advances in robotic transaxillary thyroidectomy in Europe. Curr Surg Rep. 2017;5(8):17.
13. Aidan P, Arora A, Lorincz B, Tolley N, Garas G. Robotic thyroid surgery: current perspectives and future considerations. ORL J Otorhinolaryngol Relat Spec. 2018;80(3–4):186–94.
14. Shan L, Liu J. A systemic review of transoral thyroidectomy. Surg Laparosc Endosc Percutan Tech. 2018;28(3):135–8.
15. Materazzi G, Fregoli L, Papini P, Bakkar S, Vasquez MC, Miccoli P. Robot-assisted transaxillary thyroidectomy (RATT): a series appraisal of more than 250 cases from Europe. World J Surg. 2018;42(4):1018–23.
16. Bergenfelz A, Jansson S, Kristoffersson A, Martensson H, Reihner E, Wallin G, et al. Complications to thyroid surgery: results as reported in a database from a multicenter audit comprising 3,660 patients. Langenbeck's Arch Surg. 2008;393(5):667–73.
17. Watt T, Hegedus L, Groenvold M, Bjorner JB, Rasmussen AK, Bonnema SJ, et al. Validity and reliability of the novel thyroid-specific quality of life questionnaire, ThyPRO. Eur J Endocrinol. 2010;162(1):161–7.
18. Gharib H, Hegedus L, Pacella CM, Baek JH, Papini E. Clinical review:nonsurgical, image-guided, minimally invasive therapy for thyroid nodules. J Clin Endocrinol Metab. 2013;98(10):3949–57.
19. Bennedbaek FN, Karstrup S, Hegedus L. Percutaneous ethanol injection therapy in the treatment of thyroid and parathyroid diseases. Eur J Endocrinol. 1997;136(3):240–50.
20. Paschke R, Hegedus L, Alexander E, Valcavi R, Papini E, Gharib H. Thyroid nodule guidelines: agreement, disagreement and need for future research. Nat Rev Endocrinol. 2011;7(6):354–61.
21. Bown SG. Phototherapy in tumors. World J Surg. 1983;7(6):700–9.
22. Matthewson K, Coleridge-Smith P, O'Sullivan JP, Northfield TC, Bown SG. Biological effects of intrahepatic neodymium:yttrium-aluminum-garnet laser photocoagulation in rats. Gastroenterology. 1987;93(3):550–7.
23. Thomsen S. Pathologic analysis of photothermal and photomechanical effects of laser-tissue interactions. Photochem Photobiol. 1991;53(6):825–35.
24. Muller G, Roggan A. Laser-induced interstitial thermotherapy. Bellingham, WA: SPIE-The International Society for Optical Engineering; 1995.
25. Stafford RJ, Fuentes D, Elliott AA, Weinberg JS, Ahrar K. Laser-induced thermal therapy for tumor ablation. Crit Rev Biomed Eng. 2010;38(1):79–100.
26. Ahrar K, Gowda A, Javadi S, Borne A, Fox M, McNichols R, et al. Preclinical assessment of a 980-nm diode laser ablation system in a large animal tumor model. J Vasc Interv Radiol. 2010;21(4):555–61.
27. Ahmed M, Brace CL, Lee FT Jr, Goldberg SN. Principles of and advances in percutaneous ablation. Radiology. 2011;258(2):351–69.
28. Trembley H, Ryan T, Strohbehn J. Interstitial hyperthermia: physics, biology, and clinical aspects. Hyperthermia and oncology. Utrecht: VSP; 1992. p. 11–98.
29. Jacques SL. Laser-tissue interactions. Photochemical, photothermal, and photomechanical. Surg Clin North Am. 1992;72(3):531–58.
30. Heisterkamp J, van Hillegersberg R, Ijzermans JN. Critical temperature and heating time for coagulation damage: implications for interstitial laser coagulation (ILC) of tumors. Lasers Surg Med. 1999;25(3):257–62.
31. Larson TR, Bostwick DG, Corica A. Temperature-correlated histopathologic changes following microwave thermoablation of obstructive tissue in

patients with benign prostatic hyperplasia. Urology. 1996;47(4):463–9.

32. Goldberg SN, Gazelle GS, Halpern EF, Rittman WJ, Mueller PR, Rosenthal DI. Radiofrequency tissue ablation: importance of local temperature along the electrode tip exposure in determining lesion shape and size. Acad Radiol. 1996;3(3):212–8.

33. Zervas NT, Kuwayama A. Pathological characteristics of experimental thermal lesions. Comparison of induction heating and radiofrequency electrocoagulation. J Neurosurg. 1972;37(4):418–22.

34. Goldberg SN, Gazelle GS, Compton CC, Mueller PR, Tanabe KK. Treatment of intrahepatic malignancy with radiofrequency ablation: radiologic-pathologic correlation. Cancer. 2000;88(11):2452–63.

35. Nikfarjam M, Muralidharan V, Christophi C. Mechanisms of focal heat destruction of liver tumors. J Surg Res. 2005;127(2):208–23.

36. Nikfarjam M, Malcontenti-Wilson C, Christophi C. Focal hyperthermia produces progressive tumor necrosis independent of the initial thermal effects. J Gastrointest Surg. 2005;9(3):410–7.

37. Mertyna P, Hines-Peralta A, Liu ZJ, Halpern E, Goldberg W, Goldberg SN. Radiofrequency ablation: variability in heat sensitivity in tumors and tissues. J Vasc Interv Radiol. 2007;18(5):647–54.

38. Mertyna P, Dewhirst MW, Halpern E, Goldberg W, Goldberg SN. Radiofrequency ablation: the effect of distance and baseline temperature on thermal dose required for coagulation. Int J Hyperthermia. 2008;24(7):550–9.

39. Mertyna P, Goldberg W, Yang W, Goldberg SN. Thermal ablation a comparison of thermal dose required for radiofrequency-, microwave-, and laser-induced coagulation in an ex vivo bovine liver model. Acad Radiol. 2009;16(12):1539–48.

40. Dachman A, Smith M, Burris J, VanDeMerwe W. Interstitial laser ablation in experimental models and in clinical use. Semin Interv Radiol. 1993;10:101–12.

41. McGahan JP, Browning PD, Brock JM, Tesluk H. Hepatic ablation using radiofrequency electrocautery. Investig Radiol. 1990;25(3):267–70.

42. Nolsoe CP, Torp-Pedersen S, Burcharth F, Horn T, Pedersen S, Christensen NE, et al. Interstitial hyperthermia of colorectal liver metastases with a US-guided Nd-YAG laser with a diffuser tip: a pilot clinical study. Radiology. 1993;187(2):333–7.

43. McGahan JP, Dodd GDI. Radiofrequency ablation of the liver: current status. AJR Am J Roentgenol. 2001;176:3–16.

44. Dossing H, Bennedbaek FN, Karstrup S, Hegedus L. Benign solitary solid cold thyroid nodules: US-guided interstitial laser photocoagulation—initial experience. Radiology. 2002;225(1):53–7.

45. Cakir B, Topaloglu O, Gul K, Agac T, Aydin C, Dirikoc A, et al. Effects of percutaneous laser ablation treatment in benign solitary thyroid nodules on nodule volume, thyroglobulin and anti-thyroglobulin levels, and cytopathology of nodule in 1 yr follow-up. J Endocrinol Investig. 2006;29(10):876–84.

46. Amabile G, Rotondi M, Pirali B, Dionisio R, Agozzino L, Lanza M, et al. Interstitial laser photo-coagulation for benign thyroid nodules: time to treat large nodules. Lasers Surg Med. 2011;43(8):797–803.

47. Pacella CM, Bizzarri G, Spiezia S, Bianchini A, Guglielmi R, Crescenzi A, et al. Thyroid tissue: US-guided percutaneous laser thermal ablation. Radiology. 2004;232(1):272–80.

48. Gambelunghe G, Fatone C, Ranchelli A, Fanelli C, Lucidi P, Cavaliere A, et al. A randomized controlled trial to evaluate the efficacy of ultrasound-guided laser photocoagulation for treatment of benign thyroid nodules. J Endocrinol Investig. 2006;29(9):RC23–6.

49. Dossing H, Bennedbaek FN, Hegedus L. Ultrasound-guided interstitial laser photocoagulation of an autonomous thyroid nodule: the introduction of a novel alternative. Thyroid. 2003;13(9):885–8.

50. Dossing H, Bennedbaek FN, Hegedus L. Effect of ultrasound-guided interstitial laser photocoagulation on benign solitary solid cold thyroid nodules—a randomised study. Eur J Endocrinol. 2005;152(3):341–5.

51. Dossing H, Bennedbaek FN, Hegedus L. Effect of ultrasound-guided interstitial laser photocoagulation on benign solitary solid cold thyroid nodules: one versus three treatments. Thyroid. 2006;16(8):763–8.

52. Dossing H, Bennedbaek FN, Hegedus L. Long-term outcome following interstitial laser photocoagulation of benign cold thyroid nodules. Eur J Endocrinol. 2011;165(1):123–8.

53. Dossing H, Bennedbaek FN, Hegedus L. Interstitial laser photocoagulation (ILP) of benign cystic thyroid nodules—a prospective randomized trial. J Clin Endocrinol Metab. 2013;98(7):E1213–7.

54. Nikfarjam M, Muralidharan V, Malcontenti-Wilson C, Christophi C. Progressive microvascular injury in liver and colorectal liver metastases following laser induced focal hyperthermia therapy. Lasers Surg Med. 2005;37(1):64–73.

55. Pacella CM, Rossi Z, Bizzarri G, Papini E, Marinozzi V, Paliotta D, et al. Ultrasound-guided percutaneous laser ablation of liver tissue in a rabbit model. Eur Radiol. 1993;3:26–32.

56. Pacella CM, Papini E, Fabbrini R, Bizzarri G, Anelli V, Rinaldi G, et al. Ultrasound-guided percutaneous interstitial laser ablation of thyroid nodules. In: Feasibility study: E.C.R.'95—European Congress Radiology, Vienna, 5–10 Mar 1995.

57. Pacella CM, Papini E, Bizzarri G, Anelli V, Crescenzi A, Pacella S. Ultrasound-guided (US) percutaneous interstitial laser photo-coagulation of thyroid tissue. Feasibility study (abstract). In: RSNA, editor. 84th Scientific assembly and annual meeting, Chicago, IL, 29 Nov–4 Dec 1998.

58. Pacella CM, Bizzarri G, Guglielmi R, Anelli V, Bianchini A, Crescenzi A, et al. Thyroid tissue: US-guided percutaneous interstitial laser ablation—a feasibility study. Radiology. 2000;217(3):673–7.

59. Piana S, Riganti F, Froio E, Andrioli M, Pacella CM, Valcavi R. Pathological findings of thyroid nodules after percutaneous laser ablation: a series of 22 cases with cyto-histological correlation. Endocr Pathol. 2012;23(2):94–100.

60. Cakir B, Ugras NS, Gul K, Ersoy R, Korukluoglu B. Initial report of the results of percutaneous laser

ablation of benign cold thyroid nodules: evaluation of histopathological changes after 2 years. Endocr Pathol. 2009;20(3):170–6.

61. Rotondi M, Amabile G, Leporati P, Di Filippo B, Chiovato L. Repeated laser thermal ablation of a large functioning thyroid nodule restores euthyroidism and ameliorates constrictive symptoms. J Clin Endocrinol Metab. 2009;94(2):382–3.

62. Spiezia S, Vitale G, Di Somma C, Pio Assanti A, Ciccarelli A, Lombardi G, et al. Ultrasound-guided laser thermal ablation in the treatment of autonomous hyperfunctioning thyroid nodules and compressive nontoxic nodular goiter. Thyroid. 2003;13(10): 941–7.

63. Valcavi R, Bertani A, Pesenti M, Al Jandali Rifa'Y LR, Frasoldati A, Formisano D, et al. Laser and radiofrequency ablation procedures. In: Baskin HJ, Duick DS, Levine RA, editors. Thyroid ultrasound and ultrasound guided FNA biopsy. 2nd ed. New York: Springer; 2008. p. 191–218.

64. Valcavi R, Riganti F, Bertani A, Formisano D, Pacella CM. Percutaneous laser ablation of cold benign thyroid nodules: a 3-year follow-up study in 122 patients. Thyroid. 2010;20(11):1253–61.

65. Papini E, Guglielmi R, Bizzarri G, Graziano F, Bianchini A, Brufani C, et al. Treatment of benign cold thyroid nodules: a randomized clinical trial of percutaneous laser ablation versus levothyroxine therapy or follow-up. Thyroid. 2007;17(3):229–35.

66. Papini E, Rago T, Gambelunghe G, Valcavi R, Bizzarri G, Vitti P, et al. Long-term efficacy of ultrasound-guided laser ablation for benign solid thyroid nodules. Results of a three-year multicenter prospective randomized trial. J Clin Endocrinol Metab. 2014;99(10):3653–9.

67. Achille G, Zizzi S, Di Stasio E, Grammatica A, Grammatica L. Ultrasound-guided percutaneous laser ablation in treating symptomatic solid benign thyroid nodules: our experience in 45 patients. Head Neck. 2016;38:677–82.

68. Papini E, Guglielmi R, Bizzarri G, Pacella CM. Ultrasound-guided laser thermal ablation for treatment of benign thyroid nodules. Endocr Pract. 2004;10(3):276–83.

69. Gambelunghe G, Bini V, Monacelli M, Avenia N, D'Ajello M, Colella R, et al. The administration of anesthetic in the thyroid pericapsular region increases the possibility of side effects during percutaneous laser photocoagulation of thyroid nodules. Lasers Surg Med. 2013;45(1):34–7.

70. Pacella CM, Mauri G, Achille G, Barbaro D, Bizzarri G, De Feo P, et al. Outcomes and risk factors for complications of laser ablation for thyroid nodules. A multicenter study on 1531 patients. J Clin Endocrinol Metab. 2015;100(10):3903–10.

71. Negro R, Salem TM, Greco G. Laser ablation is more effective for spongiform than solid thyroid nodules. A 4-year retrospective follow-up study. Int J Hyperthrmia. 2016;32:822–8. https://doi.org/10.1080/02656736.2016.1212279.

72. Mauri G, Cova L, Monaco CG, Sconfienza LM, Benedini S, Ambrogi F, Milani V, Baroli A, Ierace T, Corbetta S, Solbiati L. Benign thyroid nodules treatment using percutaneous laser ablation (PLA) and radiofrequency ablation (RFA). Int J Hyperthermia. 2017;33:295–9. https://doi.org/10.1080/02656736.2016.1244707.

73. Pacella CM, Mauri G, Cesareo R, Paqualini V, De Feo P, Gambelunghe G, Raggiunti B, Tina D, Cianni R, Deandrea M, Limone P, Misischi I, Mormile A, Giusti M, Oddo S, Achille G, Di Stasio E, Papini E. A comparison of laser with radiofrequency ablation for the treatment of benign thyroid nodules: a propensity score matching analysis. Int J Hyperthermia. 2017;33:911–9. https://doi.org/10.1080/02656736.2017.1332395.

74. Oddo S, Felix E, Mussap M, Giusti M. Quality of life in patients treated with percutaneous laser ablation for non-functioning benign thyroid nodules: a prospective single-center study. Korean J Radiol. 2018;19(1):175–84.

75. Cakir B, Gul K, Ugras S, Ersoy R, Topaloglu O, Agac T, et al. Percutaneous laser ablation of an autonomous thyroid nodule: effects on nodule size and histopathology of the nodule 2 years after the procedure. Thyroid. 2008;18(7):803–5.

76. Barbaro D, Orsini P, Lapi P, Pasquini C, Tuco A, Righini A, et al. Percutaneous laser ablation in the treatment of toxic and pretoxic nodular goiter. Endocr Pract. 2007;13(1):30–6.

77. Dossing H, Bennedbaek FN, Bonnema SJ, Grupe P, Hegedus L. Randomized prospective study comparing a single radioiodine dose and a single laser therapy session in autonomously functioning thyroid nodules. Eur J Endocrinol. 2007;157(1):95–100.

78. Gambelunghe G, Stefanetti E, Colella R, Monacelli M, Avenia N, De Feo P. A single session of laser ablation for toxic thyroid nodules: three-year follow-up results. Int J Hyperthermia. 2018;34:1–5.

79. Pacella CM, Mauri G. Is there a role for minimally invasive thermal ablations in the treatment of autonomously functioning thyroid nodules? Int J Hyperthermia. 2018;34:1–3.

80. Chianelli M, Bizzarri G, Todino V, Misischi I, Bianchini A, Graziano F, et al. Laser ablation and 131-Iodine: a 24-month pilot study of combined treatment for large toxic nodular goitre. J Clin Endocrinol Metab. 2014;99:E1283–6.

81. Guglielmi R, Pacella CM, Bianchini A, Bizzarri G, Rinaldi R, Graziano FM, et al. Percutaneous ethanol injection treatment in benign thyroid lesions: role and efficacy. Thyroid. 2004;14(2):125–31.

82. Cakir B, Gul K, Ersoy R, Topaloglu O, Korukluoglu B. Subcapsular hematoma complication during percutaneous laser ablation to a hypoactive benign solitary thyroid nodule. Thyroid. 2008;18(8):917–8.

83. Di Rienzo G, Surrente C, Lopez C, Quercia R. Tracheal laceration after laser ablation of nodular goitre. Interact Cardiovasc Thorac Surg. 2010;14(1):115–6.

84. Pacella CM. Image-guided thermal ablation of benign thyroid nodules. J Ultrasound. 2017;20(4):347–9.

Laser Ablation of Thyroid Cancer and Metastatic Lymph Nodes

8

Tian'an Jiang, Luigi Solbiati, Weiwei Zhan,
and Giovanni Mauri

8.1   Introduction

Increasing incidence of malignant tumors in the neck, thyroid cancer in particular, has been reported worldwide while the mortality has remained stable [1–3]. The rise in thyroid cancer incidence (over 10/100,000 women in high incidence areas), along with an increase in the incidence of papillary thyroid microcarcinomas (PTMCs), has been commonly attributed to increased detection of the disease whereas the decline in mortality is likely due to changes in risk factor exposure, diagnosis, and treatment of the disease. Neck metastases do not exclusively derive from head and neck tumors. According to the literature, the incidence of cervical metastasieis from esophageal and breast cancer is estimated to be 14.5% and 4%, respectively [4, 5].

T. Jiang (✉)
Department of Ultrasound, First Affiliated Hospital,
College of Medicine, Zhejiang University,
Hangzhou, China
e-mail: tiananjiang@zju.edu.cn

L. Solbiati
Department of Biomedical Sciences, Humanitas
University, Milan, Italy

W. Zhan
Department of Ultrasound, Rui Jin Hospital, School
of Medicine, Shanghai Jiao Tong University,
Ruijin, China

G. Mauri
Division of Interventional Radiology, European
Institute of Oncology, IRCCS, Milan, Italy

Willner et al. [6] reported that the 2 and 5 years of survival rate in supraclavicular lymph nodes metastasis patients was 56% and 28%, respectively.

The increased detection rate has then brought about the increased need for proper treatment. Surgical resection has long been considered the first-line treatment for malignant tumors in the neck. However, the invasiveness of surgery increases incidence of complications due to proximity of the tumor to various critical structures in the neck. Incidence of recurrent laryngeal nerve injury, for example, reached up to 25% after prophylactic radical neck dissection in the United States [7]. Post-surgery hypothyroidism in treating thyroid lesions requires life-long use of substitute medications. Scar of the incision also fails to meet the need for beauty. It became evident that ^{131}I therapy also results in shrinkage of the thyroid gland, even if hyperthyroidism persists. Percutaneous ethanol injection is cheap, and it may reduce the volume of benign thyroid nodules [8]; however, possible limitations are the difficulty of inducing a well-defined area of necrosis and the need of multiple sessions for complete ablation that is unsuitable for the treatment of neoplastic lesions. Minimally invasive ablation therapies have therefore replaced surgery as optimal treatments for tumors in the neck under many circumstances. With fewer complications, less recovery time, and better repeatability, thermal ablation has been recommended to treat benign

© Springer Nature Switzerland AG 2020
C. M. Pacella et al. (eds.), *Image-guided Laser Ablation*,
https://doi.org/10.1007/978-3-030-21748-8_8

thyroid nodules and recurrent thyroid cancers since 2012 [9]. Among these methods, laser thermal ablation was confirmed as a nonsurgical procedure that induced better-shaped ablation lesions for small tumors in the neck and lowered the risk of major complications than that reported with other thermal treatments due to the use of fine needles and less energy for the treatment of solid or complex thyroid lesions [10–13]. Studies further clarified the possibility and benefits of applying laser ablation for treating primary malignant tumors in the neck. The 2015 ATA guidelines no longer acknowledged the benefits of prophylactic central compartment lymph node dissection but recommended active surveillance for low-risk papillary thyroid microcarcinoma management based on the results of previous trials and reflections on overtreatment [7, 14–18]. Among patients under surveillance, however, disease progression such as size enlargement of the tumor and novel appearance of lymph-node metastasis still occurred in a small proportion of cases [16, 17]. The presence of supraclavicular metastases is associated with an unfavorable prognosis and the development of distant metastases [18, 19]. Laser ablation provides us with an alternative method to achieve tumor-free status while reducing the risk of potential harm caused by overtreatment. The aim of this chapter is therefore to describe the technique and the results of LA in the treatment of thyroid carcinoma and other malignant tumors in the neck.

8.2   Technique and Devices

Because of minimal invasive access and low complications rate, laser thermal ablation has been studied and applied in treatment of benign lesions [20–25] and also in a variety of primary and secondary malignant thyroid tumors for combination therapy [22–25]. Before thermal ablation, malignancies in all patients were ruled out by means of US evaluation. After being carefully sterilized, 1.0–1.5 mL of 2% lidocaine hydrochloride was injected step by step into superficial tissue [26]. A 21-gauge spinal needle was inserted into the center of thyroid lesions with US guidance, and

Nd:YAG laser operating at 1.064 µm is used [27]. The size, shape, and location of the nodules played the key role in determining the number of needles and their arrangement. The optical fiber was inserted through the sheath of the needle, and about 5-mm-long fiber was in direct contact with the tissue [26]. At US monitoring, the needle and fiber tips were always clearly visualized as hyperechoic spots. A single bare fiber releases 1800 J output power of 3–5 W to the tissue, producing an almost spherical lesion with a maximum diameter of 12–16 mm when illuminated for 4–6 min [28]. The area targeted is small so multiple ablations are required to cover the tumor volume and as many as four fibers may be activated simultaneously to ablate larger tumors with a distance between tips of 15 mm [29]. At the end of the treatment, the treated area appeared as an irregular and ill-defined hyperechoic zone that progressively decreased over time. Because the proximity of the surrounding vital structures made it dangerous to attempt complete necrosis of lesions in the neck, the volume of ablated tissue was limited Thus, talking with the patient during surgery could whether there was injury or not.

8.3   Results

8.3.1   Primary Thyroid Cancers

The overwhelming majority of patients with thyroid cancer will be recommended surgical excision, no matter that the primary disease or recurrence in the thyroid after initial treatment. RFA and MWA had significant clinical application in treating solitary papillary thyroid microcarcinoma and locally metastatic well-differentiated thyroid carcinomas [30, 31]. Compared to other thermal ablation techniques, LA appears to have some advantages due to a very small needle (21 gauge) used in a complex region (Fig. 8.1). Moreover, the thermal energy deployed in LA is precise to obtain a small ablation volume. Thus it could theoretically minimize the risk of injuring structures in the neck. Pacella et al. [19] firstly reported a case of a 75-year-old woman with a rapidly progressive anaplastic thyroid carcinoma.

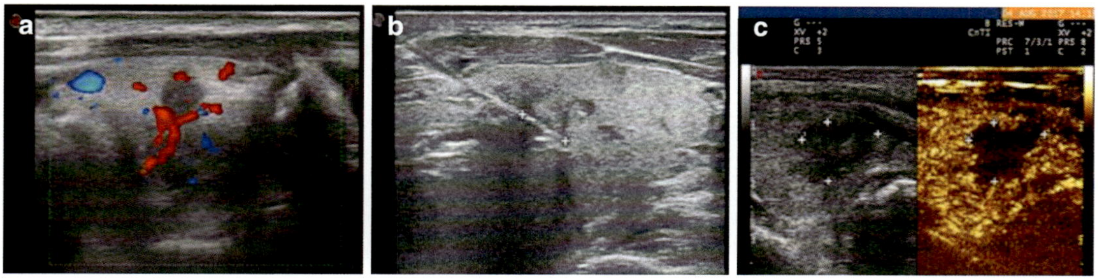

Fig. 8.1 Laser ablation of right thyroid papillary carcinoma treated with a power of 5.0 W. (**a**) An 5 × 5 mm hypoechoic nodule on the right lobe of thyroid proven to be papillary carcinoma. (**b**) A 21-gauge laser fiber was inserted through the nodule. (**c**) One day after LA treatment, CEUS confirmed that the nodule was completely ablated without any contrast enhancement

The volume of the tumor and local symptoms reduced significantly and kept stability during the following 4 months, after performed a large area of ablation along with a subsequent external beam radiation therapy associated with chemotherapy. Papini et al. [32] reported the use of laser ablation for an 81-year-old woman with a papillary microcarcinoma (<1 cm papillary thyroid carcinoma). The patient had decompensated liver cirrhosis and renal failure and had undergone recent surgery followed by external beam radiotherapy for breast cancer. A solitary 8 × 7 × 7 mm^3 hypoechoic nodule with microcalcifications was found in the right thyroid lobe at neck US examination. Two 21-gauge spinal needles were inserted and 3600 J of energy with an output power of 3 W was delivered for 10 min, and the lesion became smaller in size than on initial presentation at 24 months US follow-up examination. Valcavi et al. [33] also used percutaneous LA to treat three microcarcinomas in the operating room under general anesthesia immediately before surgical removal. This study demonstrates that conventional histology showed destructured and carbonized tissue as well as a complete lack of viability on immunohistochemical analysis of the surgical specimens, meaning LA is a technically feasible option for the complete destruction of cytology-proven PTMC. In 2017, a retrospective study [34] was conducted in 30 patients with single PTMC. At the 12-month follow-up, the mean values of maximum diameter and volume (2.6 mm and 9.1 mm^3, respectively) were significantly smaller than that at pre-ablation (4.8 mm

and 43.7 mm^3, respectively); 10 (33.3%) ablation zones had disappeared, and 20 (66.67%) ablation zones remained scar-like lesions. Most of the cases (29/30) were completely ablated with a single LA, which was for no more than 350 s. FNAB of the ablated zones at 1, 6, and 12 months demonstrated necrotic material and inflammatory cells without viable neoplastic cells. The results of the studies showed that LA for complete destruction of a small-sized PTMC was technically feasible without extra-glandular spread or nodal metastases.

8.3.2 Recurrent Thyroid Cancers

Recurrent thyroid cancer occurs in up to 20% and 59% of patients with papillary thyroid cancer after operation, radioactive iodine therapy, or thyroid hormone therapy [35]. Reoperation is difficult due to scar tissue formation which leads to a high risk of complications. Both percutaneous ethanol and thermal ablation techniques have been reported in the setting of palliation of recurrent thyroid cancer. A recent meta-analysis compared RFA and percutaneous ethanol in 270 patients and 415 thyroid nodules, concluding that both approaches were acceptable with between 53% and 69% of lesions disappearing completely [36]. Dupuy et al. [37] reported 8 patients with recurrent thyroid cancer were treated by RFA as outpatients and no recurrent disease at the treatment site was detected, with a mean follow-up of 10.3 months, but a minor skin burn and 1 vocal cord paralysis occurred while the hoarseness did not completely resolve after 2 months. Zhou et al. [38] reported a retrospective study of 21 patients with 27 recurrent PTC lesions who underwent LA. The volume reduction and complete disappearance rate of the treated tumors were 98.9% and 85.2%, respectively, at final follow-up visit. The mean largest diameter and the average baseline volume were reduced from 7.5 ± 2.8 mm and 105.4 ± 114 mm^3 to 0.4 ± 1 mm and 0.8 ± 2.4 mm^3 at the final follow-up, concluding that LA is effective for the treatment of recurrent PTCs with a beneficial success rate. Although LA is unlikely to alter the clinical course, particularly for those patients with recurrent nodal disease in the neck, it may become a primary choice of treatment for recurrent thyroid cancers in selected patients who are ineligible for surgery and/or prefer not to have further surgery.

8.3.3 Nodal Metastases

Treatment is based on repeated surgery and/or repeated radioiodine ablation to metastatic lymph node. However, most metastatic lymph nodes may have lost their ability to uptake radioiodine. Furthermore, cervical nodal recurrence may occur in up to 30% of patients after initial treatment. Thus, finding less-invasive alternatives may be more meaningful. Percutaneous minimally invasive treatments have a good advantage which can be performed several times without increased technical difficulties due to the previous treatments. PEI and RFA have been introduced to obtain good local control of treated lymph nodes. However, this is off-set by an often higher complication rate [30, 37, 39, 40]. The efficacy of LA was similar to that of radioiodine treatment for patients with metastatic lymph node [41]. LA was performed in a prospective and observational study of 21 metastatic lymph nodes in 17 patients who underwent radical thyroid resection; the largest diameters and volumes post-LA significantly decreased compared to pre-LA [42]. Mauri et al. [43] reported there were 24 patients previously treated with thyroidectomy, neck dissection, and radioiodine therapy. All 46

lymph nodes showed positive in FDG-PET/CT before LA. 86.9% of lymph nodes demonstrated complete ablation at 30 ± 11 months, and five patients underwent successfully a second ablation session. LA likely represents a new effective therapy for the treatment of cervical lymph node metastases in the neck and for reducing the morbidity of a second surgical operation. Figure 8.2 shows images of a 79-year-old patient with left metastatic cervical lymph node from papillary carcinoma successfully treated with thin-needle laser technique.

8.3.4 Safety and Complications

Complications and side effects are minimal in LA. The treatment was well tolerated at the present study [23]. Ninety eight (80.3%) out of one hundred and twelve patients reported a mild sensation of pain and regional discomfort. In patients with intense intraoperative local pain, radiating to the jaw, teeth, chest, or back, the laser was turned off which could be explained by thyroid capsule thermal damage, and regional discomfort, and self-limited neck swelling that were resolved without treatment within 2 weeks after LA. Prednisone administration was prolonged to reduce persisting pain. When a few of the patients complained of voice changes caused by recurrent laryngeal nerve injury, the "hydrodissection technique" may play an important role between the mass and the expected location of the recurrent laryngeal nerve. Some researchers reported a decreased serum thyroid-stimulating hormone level and increased free thyroxin possibly because of transient thyroid tissue damage by LA [40, 44]. In the two patients who experienced post-operative laryngeal dysfunction, reduction in vocal cord motility occurred 12–24 h after LA; direct laryngoscopy demonstrated vocal cord palsy. An additional course of corticosteroids (oral prednisone 25 mg for 2 weeks, 12.5 mg for 2 weeks, and 5 mg for 2 weeks) was administered, and vocal cord motility recovered after 6–10 weeks [23]. In the event of vagal symptoms with bradycardia occurred when the patient has no history of cardiovascular disease, the bed was tilted in

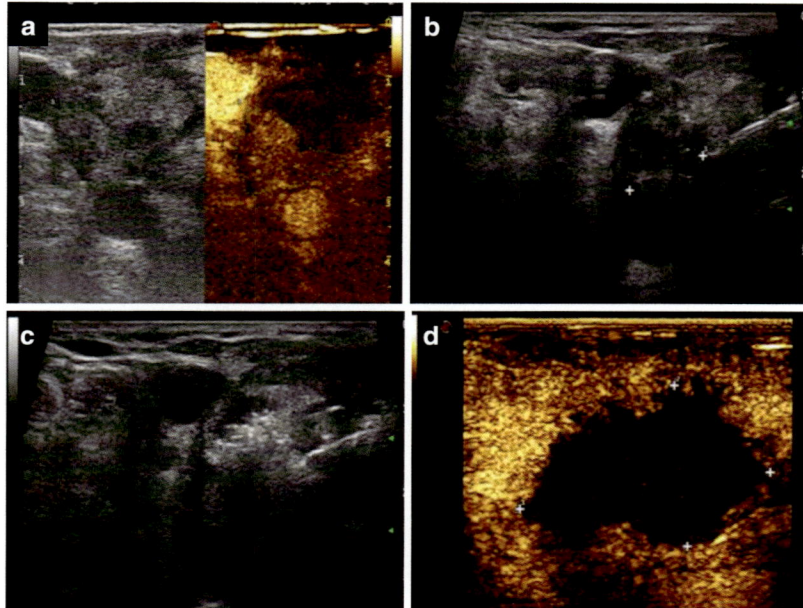

Fig. 8.2 Laser treatment for left cervical metastasis of thyroid papillary carcinomas. A 79-year-old woman underwent total thyroidectomy due to proven thyroid papillary carcinoma in 2009. An enlarged lymph node in the left cervical was confirmed to be metastasis by FNA in 2015 and treated with RFA. (**a**) In 2016, local recurrence (delineated in green circle) was appeared as hyperechoic area in CEUS and confirmed by pathology. (**b**) A 21-gauge laser fiber was inserted into the lesion with a 5 mm distance between margin and tip of the needle. (**c**) Target area was gradually covered by bubbles of gas expanding during the treatment. (**d**) One day after the treatment, CEUS confirmed that the nodule was completely ablated

Trendelenburg position and LA was temporarily interrupted until spontaneous recovery; otherwise further treatment must be taken immediately.

References

1. Lim H, Devesa SS, Sosa JA, et al. Trends in thyroid cancer incidence and mortality in the United States, 1974–2013. JAMA. 2017;317:1338–48.
2. Davies L, Welch HG. Current thyroid cancer trends in the United States. JAMA Otolaryngol Head Neck Surg. 2014;140:317–22.
3. La Vecchia C, Malvezzi M, Bosetti C, et al. Thyroid cancer mortality and incidence: a global overview. Int J Cancer. 2015;136:2187–95.
4. Tachimori Y, Ozawa S, Numasaki H, et al. Supraclavicular node metastasis from thoracic esophageal carcinoma: a surgical series from a Japanese multi-institutional nationwide registry of esophageal cancer. J Thorac Cardiovasc Surg. 2014;148:1224–9.
5. Sproson EL, Herd MK, Spedding AV, Brennan PA, Puxeddu R. Treatment of breast adenocarcinoma metastasis to the neck: dedifferentiation of the tumor as suggested by hormone markers. Head Neck. 2012;34:1095–9.
6. Willner J, Kiricuta IC, Kölbl O. Locoregional recurrence of breast cancer following mastectomy: always a fatal event? Results of univariate and multivariate analysis. Int J Radiat Oncol Biol Phys. 1997;37:853–63.
7. Haugen BR. 2015 American Thyroid Association Management guidelines for adult patients with thyroid nodules and differentiated thyroid cancer: what is new and what has changed? Cancer-Am Cancer Soc. 2017;123:372–81.
8. Na DG, Lee JH, Jung SL, et al. Radiofrequency ablation of benign thyroid nodules and recurrent thyroid cancers: consensus statement and recommendations. Korean J Radiol. 2012;13:117–25.
9. Pacella CM, Mauri G, Achille G, Barbaro D, et al. Outcomes and risk factors for complications of laser ablation for thyroid nodules: a multicenter study on 1531 patients. J Clin Endocr Metab. 2015;100:3903–10.
10. Gharib H, Hegedüs L, Pacella CM, et al. Clinical review:nonsurgical, image-guided, minimally invasive therapy for thyroid nodules. J Clin Endocrinol Metab. 2013;98:3949–57.

11. Yang YL, Chen CZ, Zhang XH. Microwave ablation of benign thyroid nodules. Future Oncol. 2014;10:1007–14.

12. Baek JH, Lee JH, Sung JY, et al. Complications encountered in the treatment of benign thyroid nodules with US-guided radiofrequency ablation: a multicenter study. Radiology. 2012;262:335–42.

13. Gharib H, Papini E, Garber JR, et al. American Association of Clinical Endocrinologists, American College of Endocrinology, and Associazione Medici Endocrinologi Medical guidelines for clinical practice for the diagnosis and management of thyroid nodules—2016 update. Endocr Pract. 2016;22:1–60.

14. Sugitani I, Toda K, Yamada K, et al. Three distinctly different kinds of papillary thyroid microcarcinoma should be recognized: our treatment strategies and outcomes. World J Surg. 2010;34:1222–31.

15. Ito Y, Miyauchi A, Kihara M, et al. Patient age is significantly related to the progression of papillary microcarcinoma of the thyroid under observation. Thyroid. 2014;24:27–34.

16. Tuttle RM, Fagin JA, Minkowitz G, et al. Natural history and tumor volume kinetics of papillary thyroid cancers during active surveillance. JAMA Otolaryngol. 2017;143:1015–20.

17. Viola D, Materazzi G, Valerio L, et al. Prophylactic central compartment lymph node dissection in papillary thyroid carcinoma: clinical implications derived from the first prospective randomized controlled single institution study. J Clin Endocr Metab. 2015;100:1316–24.

18. Pergolizzi S, Settineri N, Santacaterina A, et al. Ipsilateral supraclavicular lymph node metastases from breast cancer as only site of disseminated disease. Chemotherapy alone vs. induction chemotherapy to radical radiation therapy. Ann Oncol. 2001;12:1091–5.

19. Van den Sangen MJC, Coebergh JW, et al. Detection, treatment, and outcome of isolated supraclavicular recurrence in 42 patients with invasive breast carcinoma. Cancer. 2003;98:11–7.

20. Higuchi N, Bleier AR, Jolesz FA, et al. Magnetic resonance imaging of the acute effects of interstitial neodymium:YAG laser irradiation on tissues. Investig Radiol. 1992;27:814–21.

21. Pacella CM, Rossi Z, Bizzarri G, et al. Ultrasound-guided percutaneous laser ablation of liver tissue in a rabbit model. Eur Radiol. 1993;3:26–32.

22. Pacella CM, Bizzarri G, Spiezia S, et al. Thyroid tissue: US-guided percutaneous laser thermal ablation. Radiology. 2004;232:272–80.

23. Valcavi R, Riganti F, Bertani A, et al. Percutaneous laser ablation of cold benign thyroid nodules: a 3-year follow-up study in 122 patients. Thyroid. 2010;20:1253–61.

24. Papini E, Bizzarri G, Pacella CM. Percutaneous laser ablation of benign and malignant thyroid nodules. Curr Opin Endocrinol Diabetes Obes. 2008;15:434–9.

25. Nixon IJ, Angelos P, Shaha AR, et al. Image-guided chemical and thermal ablations for thyroid disease: review of efficacy and complications. Head Neck. 2018;40:2103–15.

26. Pacella CM, Bizzarri G, Guglielmi R, et al. Thyroid tissue: US-guided percutaneous interstitial laser ablation—a feasibility study. Radiology. 2000;217:673–7.

27. Wyman A, Duffy S, Sweetland HM, et al. Preliminary evaluation of a new high-power diode laser. Lasers Surg Med. 1992;12:506–9.

28. Tranberg KG. Percutaneous ablation of liver tumours. Best Pract Res Clin Gastroenterol. 2004;18:125–45.

29. Pacella CM, Bizzarri G, Cecconi P, et al. Hepatocellular carcinoma: long-term results of combined treatment with laser thermal ablation and transcatheter arterial chemoembolization. Radiology. 2001;219:669–78.

30. Kim JH, Yoo WS, Park YJ, et al. Efficacy and safety of radiofrequency ablation for treatment of locally recurrent thyroid cancers smaller than 2 cm. Radiology. 2015;276:909–18.

31. Yue W, Wang S, Yu S, et al. Ultrasound-guided percutaneous microwave ablation of solitary T1N0M0 papillary thyroid micro-carcinoma: initial experience. Int J Hyperth. 2014;30:150–7.

32. Papini E, Guglielmi R, Gharib H, et al. Ultrasound-guided laser ablation of incidental papillary thyroid microcarcinoma: a potential therapeutic approach in patients at surgical risk. Thyroid. 2011;21(8):917–20.

33. Valcavi R, Piana S, Bortolan GS, et al. Ultrasound-guided percutaneous laser ablation of papillary thyroid microcarcinoma: a feasibility study on three cases with pathological and immunohistochemical evaluation. Thyroid. 2013;23(12):1578–82.

34. Zhou W, Jiang S, Zhan W, et al. Ultrasound-guided percutaneous laser ablation of unifocal T1N0M0 papillary thyroid microcarcinoma: preliminary results. Eur Radiol. 2017;27:2934–40.

35. Kim BM, Kim MJ, Kim EK, et al. Controlling recurrent papillary thyroid carcinoma in the neck by ultrasonography-guided percutaneous ethanol injection. Eur Radiol. 2008;18:835–42.

36. Suh CH, Baek JH, Choi YJ, et al. Efficacy and safety of radiofrequency and ethanol ablation for treating locally recurrent thyroid cancer: a systematic review and meta-analysis. Thyroid. 2016;26:420–8.

37. Dupuy DE, Monchik JM, Decrea C, et al. Radiofrequency ablation of regional recurrence from well-differentiated thyroid malignancy. Surgery. 2001;130:971–7.

38. Zhou W, Zhang L, Zhan W, et al. Percutaneous laser ablation for treatment of locally recurrent papillary thyroid carcinoma <15 mm. Clin Radiol. 2016;71:1233–9.

39. Maxon HR 3rd, Englaro EE, Thomas SR, et al. Radioiodine-131 therapy for well-differentiated thyroid cancerda quantitative radiation dosimetric approach: outcome and validation in 85 patients. J Nucl Med. 1992;33:1132e6.

40. Monchik JM, Donatini G, Iannuccilli J, Dupuy DE. Radiofrequency ablation and percutaneous etha-

nol injection treatment for recurrent local and distant well-differentiated thyroid carcinoma. Ann Surg. 2006;244:296–304.

41. Vannucchi G, Covelli D, Perrino M, et al. Ultrasoundguided percutaneous ethanol injection in papillary thyroid cancer metastatic lymph-nodes. Endocrine. 2014;47:648–51.

42. Zhang L, Zhou W, Zhan W. Role of ultrasound in the assessment of percutaneous laser ablation of cervical metastatic lymph nodes from thyroid carcinoma. Acta Radiol. 2018;59:434–40.

43. Mauri G, Cova L, Ierace T, et al. Treatment of metastatic lymph nodes in the neck from papillary thyroid carcinoma with percutaneous laser ablation. Cardiovasc Intervent Radiol. 2016;39:1023–30.

44. Gambelunghe G, Fede R, Bini V, et al. Ultrasound-guided interstitial laser ablation for thyroid nodules is effective only at high total amounts of energy: results from a three-year pilot study. Surgery. 2013;20:345–50.

Parathyroid Diseases Laser Ablation

9

Tian'an Jiang, Luigi Solbiati, Weiwei Zhan, and Giovanni Mauri

9.1 Introduction

Parathyroid diseases can be divided into illnesses that cause hyperparathyroidism (HPT) and hypoparathyroidism, and the major disease of parathyroid glands is the overactivity of one or more of the parathyroid lobes, which make too much parathyroid hormone (PTH). This is called hyperparathyroidism. Long-term HPT is associated with complications such as hypercalcemia, osteoporosis, kidney stones, and various other symptoms. Hyperparathyroidism can be classified into primary hyperparathyroidism (PHPT) and secondary hyperparathyroidism (SHPT).

PHPT is the third most common endocrine disorder, with an incidence of 0.03% in the general population; furthermore, its incidence increases with age [1–3]. In PHPT, there is a lack of a known or recognized stimulus, and one or more parathyroid glands secrete excess parathyroid hormone. Single gland adenoma is the most common cause (75–85%); multi-gland adenoma arises in a substantial proportion (two glands in 2–12% of cases, three glands in 1–2%, and four or more in 1–15%); and parathyroid carcinoma is rare (1%) [2]. SHPT is a frequently encountered problem in the treatment of patients with the end-stage chronic renal disease, affecting approximately one in three patients undergoing long-term dialysis [4–7].

Although disease progression can be managed by using medical therapy, such as orally active vitamin D sterols, intravenous vitamin D analogs, and cinacalcet, surgical treatment may still be the standard therapy in patients with severe HPT [8, 9]. Nevertheless, surgical parathyroidectomy has risks such as permanent hypoparathyroidism and those caused by anesthesia, especially in older patients [10]. As a result, some patients of advanced age may reject the surgical approach due to the perceived higher surgical risks. Some younger patients are also unwilling to undergo resection for cosmetic reason since this would leave a surgical scar on the neck [3]. Minimally invasive alternative is desirable compared with traditional surgical treatment and would have potential advantages such as reduced risks, faster recovery, less side effects, and, ideally, lower cost, which could

T. Jiang (✉)
Department of Ultrasound, First Affiliated Hospital, College of Medicine, Zhejiang University, Hangzhou, China
e-mail: tiananjiang@zju.edu.cn

L. Solbiati
Department of Biomedical Sciences, Humanitas University, Milan, Italy

W. Zhan
Department of Ultrasound, Rui Jin Hospital, School of Medicine, Shanghai Jiao Tong University, Ruijin, China

G. Mauri
Division of Interventional Radiology, European Institute of Oncology, IRCCS, Milan, Italy

© Springer Nature Switzerland AG 2020
C. M. Pacella et al. (eds.), *Image-guided Laser Ablation*, https://doi.org/10.1007/978-3-030-21748-8_9

benefit the patients who decline surgery or for whom surgery is considered inappropriate.

In recent years, various percutaneous ablation modalities have been developed for use in patients with locally treatable causes of HPT, such as percutaneous ethanol injection (PEI), high-intensity focused ultrasound treatment (HIFU) [11], microwave ablation (MWA) [12], radiofrequency ablation (RFA) [13–15] and laser ablation (LA) [1, 3, 15, 16].

Ultrasound-guided PEI has proved to be useful in treating HPT in highly selected patients. Nevertheless, because of the need for repeated treatments, the incidence of relapse, and side effects, PEI is not considered a first-line therapy for HPT [1]. Other nonsurgical therapies, such as HIFU and RFA, have been more recently proposed. However, clinical experience with these techniques is still too limited [1]. LA is a minimally invasive technique that has been proposed over a decade ago as a possible therapy for patients with HPT [1, 3, 16]. Laser ablation provides a photothermal tumor destruction technique that can destroy solid tumor in parenchymal organs. Laser energy is transmitted through the thin optic fibers and causes a well-defined area of coagulative necrosis, which results in the destruction of tumor tissue by direct heating while limiting damage to surrounding structures. The aim of this chapter is to describe the technique and the results of LA in the treatment of HPT.

9.2　Technique and Devices

9.2.1　Patient Selection and Indications for Treatment

Inclusion criteria:

(a) Age $\geq$ 18 years.
(b) Uncontrolled HPT with adequate medical therapy.
(c) Intact PTH level greater than or equal to 400 pg/mL (400 ng/L).
(d) Persistent elevation of total serum calcium values.

(e) At least one enlarged parathyroid gland visualized on sonography and accessible for LA treatment (i.e., no important structures such as a large blood vessel and nerve in the puncture path).
(f) No intractable complication such as cardiac insufficiency or hypertension that could not be controlled with drugs.
(g) US-guided fine-needle aspiration provided pathological confirmation that the lesion was of parathyroid origin.
(h) Surgical treatment that was contraindicated (because of a high risk of general anesthesia or symptoms of acute severe hypercalcemia) or refused (to avoid a postoperative scar on the neck).

Exclusion criteria:

(a) Intact PTH level less than 400 pg/mL (400 ng/L).
(b) Medication effectiveness (controlled HPT with adequate medical therapy).
(c) US examination showing no hyperplastic parathyroid glands.
(d) Abnormal coagulation function tests.
(e) Intractable complications such as cardiac insufficiency or hypertension that could not be controlled with drugs.

9.2.2　Laser Ablation Procedures

The patients are in the supine position with the neck extended. Routine disinfection and draping of the neck are performed. In order to maximize the possibility of complete necrosis and reduce the incidence of complications, ultrasonography and CEUS should be performed before LA to determine the size and blood supply of the parathyroid gland and evaluate the surrounding tissues.

Before LA is performed, intravenous access should be obtained by means of an antecubital vein. Patients are given minimal to moderate sedation with midazolam and fentanyl before LA. The patient is conscious throughout the procedure to allow the assessment of vocal cord function. If the patient experiences hoarseness of voice during the procedure, LA should be stopped immediately and laryngoscopy performed to assess vocal cord mobility.

Local anesthesia is carried out with 2% lidocaine under US guidance to the skin, subcutaneous tissues, muscles, and tissues adjacent to the parathyroid gland, particularly those situated posteriorly. Then, a 21-gauge Chiba needle is placed carefully into the target parathyroid lesion using a freehand-guided technique. The needle core is removed, and a plane-cut quartz optical fiber (diameter: 300-µm) is advanced through the needle sheath and positioned in the parathyroid nodule. The sheath is withdrawn to leave the bare optic fiber tip in direct contact with the parathyroid tissue. The LA procedure is performed with an output power of 3.0 W delivered for 3–10 min depending on lesion

volume (3 min for lesions <1 mL in volume, and increasing progressively with lesion volume up to a maximum of 10 min). The central portion of the nodular area is monitored continuously with ultrasonography to prevent overablation. The LA session must end when the entire parathyroid gland becomes hyperechogenic. After ablation, CEUS is performed 10 min after LA to assess the vascularity of the nodule. If the nonenhanced zone at CEUS covers the ablated gland, the ablation is considered complete. If there is nodular enhancement inside a gland, an additional LA session is conducted immediately with the aim of obtaining a lack of enhancement throughout the entire nodule. Figure 9.1 shows all the phases of a percutaneous treatment of an increased volume parathyroid successfully treated with laser technique.

Fig. 9.1 (**a**) Axial US image shows an enlarged parathyroid gland behind the inferior portion of the right lobe of the thyroid gland. (**b**) CEUS demonstrated hyperenhancement of the parathyroid nodule before LA. (**c**) Ultrasonography image showing a 21-gauge needle inserted into the parathyroid (**d**) Axial US image shows hyperechoic area emerging inside nodule during the LA procedure. (**e**) The color Doppler image obtained 1 h after ablation showed no flow signalin the ablated area. (**f**) CEUS image obtained 1 h after ablation shows nonenhancing area covering nodule, which suggests that complete ablation was achieved with LA

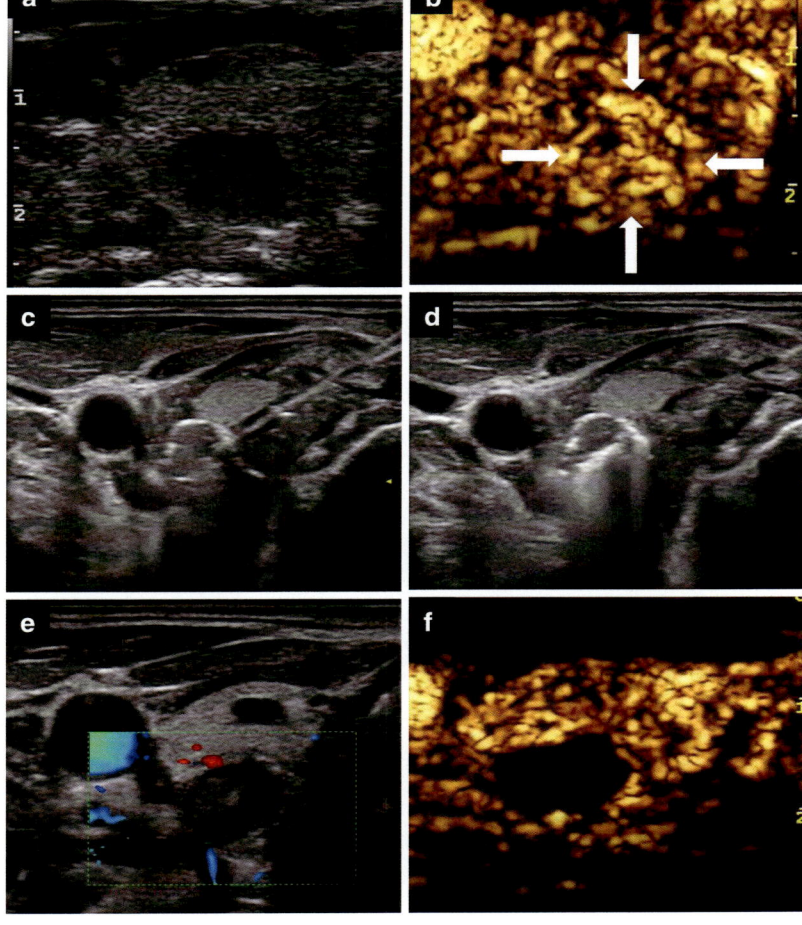

9.2.3 Follow-Up and Outcome Measures

Patients should be closely monitored for possible complications such as fever, skin burns, and pain within 24 h after percutaneous LA treatment. Serum biochemical profiles, including parathyroid hormone, calcium, phosphate, and alkaline phosphatase (ALP) levels, should be studied before LA and 1 day, 6 months, and 12 months after LA. Follow-up US is performed 1, 6, and 12 months after LA therapy to evaluate changes in parathyroid gland size.

9.3 Results

We conducted a study to evaluate the safety and efficacy of LA as a nonsurgical treatment for primary parathyroid adenoma [3]. Surgery was contraindicated in, or refused by, the included patients. No immediate enhancement of the lesion on CEUS after LA was considered "complete ablation." Nodule size, serum calcium, and parathyroid hormone level were compared before and after LA. Complete ablation was achieved in all patients treated ($n = 21$) with 1 ($n = 20$) or 2 ($n = 1$) sessions. Our study demonstrated that nodule volume decreased from 0.93 ± 0.58 mL at baseline to 0.53 ± 0.38 and 0.48 ± 0.34 mL at 6 and 12 months after LA ($P<0.05$). At 1 day, 6 months, and 12 months after LA, serum PTH decreased from 15.23 ± 3.00 pmol/L at baseline to 7.41 ± 2.79, 6.95 ± 1.78, and 6.90 ± 1.46 pmol/L. Serum calcium decreased from 3.77 ± 0.77 mmol/L at baseline to 2.50 ± 0.72, 2.41 ± 0.37, and 2.28 ± 0.26 mmol/L, respectively ($P<0.05$). At 12 months, the success rate of treatment (normalization of PTH and serum calcium) reached 81%. No serious complications were observed.

9.4 Final Considerations

Surgical treatment remains the current standard therapy in symptomatic primary and secondary hyperparathyroidism. However, its drawbacks include the risks associated with the use of general anesthesia, the need for a long incision, and possible recurrent laryngeal nerve injury and scar formation. As a result, it is difficult for doctors to advise individual patients on the trade-off between the advantages and disadvantages of surgery. For these reasons, a nonsurgical option would be preferable for treating HPT.

In recent years, various percutaneous ablation modalities have been developed; important advantages of LA over other techniques are precise control of the ablation parameters and the ability to achieve a small and precise ablative area using small needles, thereby minimizing damage to surrounding tissues. Several retrospective studies have shown that LA is a safe and effective treatment of PTH.

In 2001, Bennedbaek et al. [16] first described the successful use of LA in a single PHPT patient with severe hypercalcaemia. Normal serum calcium level was achieved after the second treatment and the PTH level became normal two months after the third treatment. No side effects were encountered. These preliminary results suggested that US-guided LA is a feasible, minimally invasive technique for focal parathyroid tumor ablation and could be a useful nonsurgical alternative for selected patients with PHP. These results were later partially confirmed by a second study conducted on three patients, in which only one in three patients showed long-term remission of HPT after LA [17].

In our opinion, it is crucial to carefully evaluate the extent of ablation that can tell us that the whole gland has been truly and completely ablated. This data has not always been carefully evaluated by other authors [1]. The site and the size of the lesion are such that it is not always possible to have this information. Probably the use of CEUS could be of considerable help to evaluate the completeness of the ablation maneuver (absence of enhancement) [3]. However, it must be emphasized that only a careful and long follow-up of at least 3 years and perhaps even more can give us real guarantees that the maneuver has indeed been successful. In fact, the absence of enhancement does not mean a vitality of all adenomatous cells.

In light of the data available in the literature, the limits of the other techniques experimented in this field, such as HIFU [18] and radiofrequency [19], appear evident to us. This is not the place for an open and in-depth discussion on this comparison, which would have the limits of a comparison between different populations and only with literature data. In other words, it is not possible at the present state of research to plan direct and controlled comparisons. However, we can say, as already highlighted earlier in this chapter, that the laser technique has all the characteristics to be effectively used in this particular field of research.

In conclusion, LA is safe and effective for managing HPT. It may represent a nonsurgical alternative for patients with refractory drug-resistant HPT or HPT patients who refuse or cannot undergo parathyroidectomy.

References

1. Andrioli M, Riganti F, Pacella CM, Valcavi R. Long-term effectiveness of ultrasound-guided laser ablation of hyperfunctioning parathyroid adenomas: present and future perspectives. AJR Am J Roentgenol. 2012;199(5):1164–8.
2. Fraser WD. Hyperparathyroidism. Lancet. 2009; 374(9684):145–58.
3. Jiang T, Chen F, Zhou X, Hu Y, Zhao Q. Percutaneous Ultrasound-Guided Laser Ablation with Contrast-Enhanced Ultrasonography for Hyperfunctioning Parathyroid Adenoma: A Preliminary Case Series. Int J Endocrinol. 2015;2015:673604.
4. Tentori F, Wang M, Bieber BA, Karaboyas A, Li Y, Jacobson SH, et al. Recent changes in therapeutic approaches and association with outcomes among patients with secondary hyperparathyroidism on chronic hemodialysis: the DOPPS study. CJASN. 2015;10(1):98–109.
5. Saunders RN, Karoo R, Metcalfe MS, Nicholson ML. Four gland parathyroidectomy without reimplantation in patients with chronic renal failure. Postgrad Med J. 2005;81(954):255–8.
6. Drueke TB. Cell biology of parathyroid gland hyperplasia in chronic renal failure. JASN. 2000;11(6): 1141–52.
7. Hargrove GM, Pasieka JL, Hanley DA, Murphy MB. Short- and long-term outcome of total parathyroidectomy with immediate autografting versus subtotal parathyroidectomy in patients with end-stage renal disease. Am J Nephrol. 1999;19(5): 559–64.
8. Younes M, Belghali S, Zrour-Hassen S, Bejia I, Touzi M, Bergaoui N. Complete reversal of tumoral calcinosis after subtotal parathyroidectomy in a hemodialysis patient. Joint BoneSpine. 2008;75(5): 606–9.
9. Raggi P, Chertow GM, Torres PU, Csiky B, Naso A, Nossuli K, et al. The ADVANCE study: a randomized study to evaluate the effects of cinacalcet plus low-dose vitamin D on vascular calcification in patients on hemodialysis. Nephrol Dial Transplant. 2011;26(4):1327–39.
10. Torres PU, Prie D, Beck L, Friedlander G. New therapies for uremic secondary hyperparathyroidism. J Ren Nutr. 2006;16(2):87–99.
11. Kovatcheva RD, Vlahov JD, Stoinov JI, Kirilov GG, Krivoshiev SG, Arnaud F, et al. High-intensity focussed ultrasound (HIFU) treatment in uraemic secondary hyperparathyroidism. Nephrol Dial Transplant. 2012;27(1):76–80.
12. Cao XL, Cheng ZG, Yu XL, Han ZY, Liang P. Ultrasound-guided percutaneous microwave ablation of parathyroid adenoma. JVIR. 2016;27(12):1929–31.
13. Xu SY, Wang Y, Xie Q, Wu HY. Percutaneous sonography-guided radiofrequency ablation in the management of parathyroid adenoma. Singap Med J. 2013;54(7):e137–40.
14. Kim BS, Eom TI, Kang KH, Park SJ. Radiofrequency ablation of parathyroid adenoma in primary hyperparathyroidism. J Med Ultrason. 2014;41(2): 239–43.
15. Peng C, Zhang Z, Liu J, Chen H, Tu X, Hu R, et al. Efficacy and safety of ultrasound-guided radiofrequency ablation of hyperplastic parathyroid gland for secondary hyperparathyroidism associated with chronic kidney disease. Head Neck. 2017;39(3):564–71.
16. Bennedbaek FN, Karstrup S, Hegedus L. Ultrasound guided laser ablation of a parathyroid adenoma. Br J Radiol. 2001;74(886):905–7.
17. Adda G, Scillitani A, Epaminonda P, Di Lembo S, Motta F, Cecconi P, et al. Ultrasound-guided laser thermal ablation for parathyroid adenomas: analysis of three cases with a three-year follow-up. Horm Res. 2006;65(5):231–4.
18. Kovatcheva R, Vlahov J, Stoinov J, Lacoste F, Ortuno C, Zaletel K. US-guided high-intensity focused ultrasound as a promising non-invasive method for treatment of primary hyperparathyroidism. Eur Radiol. 2014;24(9):2052–8.
19. Carrafiello G, Lagana D, Mangini M, Dionigi G, Rovera F, Carcano G, et al. Treatment of secondary hyperparathyroidism with ultrasonographically guided percutaneous radiofrequency thermoablation. Surg Laparosc Endosc Percutan Tech. 2006;16(2):112–6.

Guglielmo Manenti, Giovanni Mauri,
Tommaso Perretta, and Rosaria Meucci

10.1 Introduction

Breast cancer (BC) is the most frequent cancer in women, representing 28.8% of all cancer diagnosis. It is the second most common form of cancer in the world, with an estimated lifetime risk of 1:10 women [1]. Despite the steadily increasing number of newly diagnosed BCs worldwide, breast cancer mortality has decreased in most Western countries in recent years. This could be attributable to the combined effect of early detection of small tumors—due to the introduction of screening programs—and the application in current clinical practice of more effective drug treatments resulting in a significant increase in the survival rate of these patients.

While mastectomy is still performed in some patients (multicentric cancers, unfavorable ratio between tumor size and breast size, nonresponsiveness to neoadjuvant chemotherapy), breast-conserving surgery is nowadays the standard approach for early-stage breast cancers in several countries [2]. Over the past 26 years, six randomized trials have shown that early-stage breast cancer treatment with conservative surgery

and breast radiotherapy in women leads to an overall survival equivalent to mastectomy. More recently, the quadrantectomy with complete axillary dissection followed by whole-breast irradiation has become the cornerstone of breast-conservative surgery [1].

The results of many studies have shown that the outcome of conservative treatment is comparable to mastectomy's, with a reduction in functional and cosmetic limits [3]. Currently, 60–80% of newly diagnosed breast cancer patients receive breast-conservative surgery. If the recommendation of the World Health Organization were adopted and all developed countries planned extensively for mammography screening programs for women aged 50–69, breast cancer would be diagnosed at a very early stage and there would be an increase in breast-conservative treatment. The standard-of-care surgical technique for small, nonpalpable, screening-detected cancers is lumpectomy after mammographically or sonographically guided localization. Sentinel lymph node biopsy (SLNB) is a standard axillary surgery in early-stage breast cancer, if the SLNB result is positive, subsequent axillary lymph node dissection is a routine procedure. Other forms of treatment such as intraoperative radiation therapy as opposed to whole-breast radiation also emerge [4].

The next step in breast-conserving surgery could be local ablation of small breast carcinomas, provided that it is equally effective as lumpectomy, but with fewer complications and a better cosmetic outcome than a lumpectomy.

G. Manenti (✉) · T. Perretta · R. Meucci
Department of Diagnostic Imaging and Interventional Radiology, Tor Vergata University, Rome, Italy

G. Mauri
Division of Interventional Radiology, European Institute of Oncology, IRCCS, Milan, Italy

© Springer Nature Switzerland AG 2020
C. M. Pacella et al. (eds.), *Image-guided Laser Ablation*,
https://doi.org/10.1007/978-3-030-21748-8_10

10.2 Overview of Breast Percutaneous Ablation

A number of efforts in clinical cancer research are currently made to identify effective instrumental approaches, such as minimally invasive surgery, that are cosmetically more acceptable to patients. The breast is a suitable organ for percutaneous treatment, as it is superficially localized in the chest and covered only by skin. Numerous new treatments have been tested in recent years, guided by minimally invasive breast cancer imaging to further reduce invasiveness. These treatments can achieve local tumor ablation through various types of energy [5], which is transmitted to the tumor through a percutaneous approach. The treatment may increase or decrease the temperature in the target tissue area, thus destroying breast cancer cells. Techniques presently used include cryotherapy microwave energy, radiofrequency and laser light (all generated by electromagnetic waves), high-intensity focused ultrasound (through mechanical waves), and irreversible electroporation [6–9]. Within this context, minimally invasive ablation techniques have also progressed, with the goal of achieving outcomes similar to those of breast conservation therapy, but with decreased morbidity, shorter hospitalization stay, and improved cosmetic results (Fig. 10.1).

Minimally invasive methods have also been used for the treatment of breast cancer in inoperable patients and in patients with comorbidities. For patients who are not surgical candidates or who refuse surgery, percutaneous ablation may be an option for palliative or curative settings [10].

10.3 Breast Laser Ablation (LA) Technique

10.3.1 Feasibility and Efficacy

To achieve laser ablation [11] of breast lesions, laser fibers are inserted into the lesion through a needle, and the light energy guided by the fiber is absorbed into the tissue, causing cell death [12] (Figs. 10.2, 10.3, and 10.4). Initial studies aimed at treating breast tumors with laser therapy followed by surgical excision were limited because they typically did not quantify the extent of ablation, but rather reported the absence or presence of ablative changes intended as histological alteration of the tumor and the glandular tissue. Overall, such changes were reported in 90–100% of tumors [13–15]. Hence, only a few studies have properly evaluated the quality of laser therapy ablation followed by excision [16, 17]. These studies show complete ablation rates of 70–100%, improving with experience. In the largest series published [16], 54 patients with tumor size between 5 and 23 mm and various tumor anatomopathological features were enrolled. A continuous-wave 805 nm diode laser was used during the procedure under mammography guidance. A systematic surgery was performed after the procedure revealed complete tumor destruc-

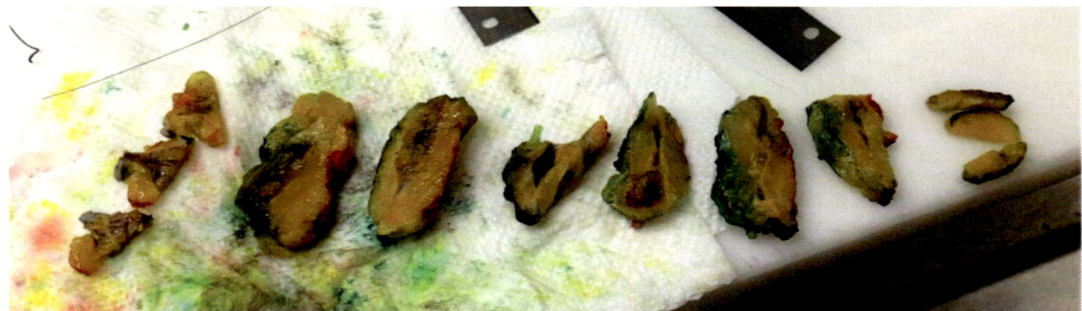

Fig.10.1 Macroscopic 5 mm section of breast tissue after lumpectomy. In the central area, the coagulative necrosis induced by the previous laser ablation is visible

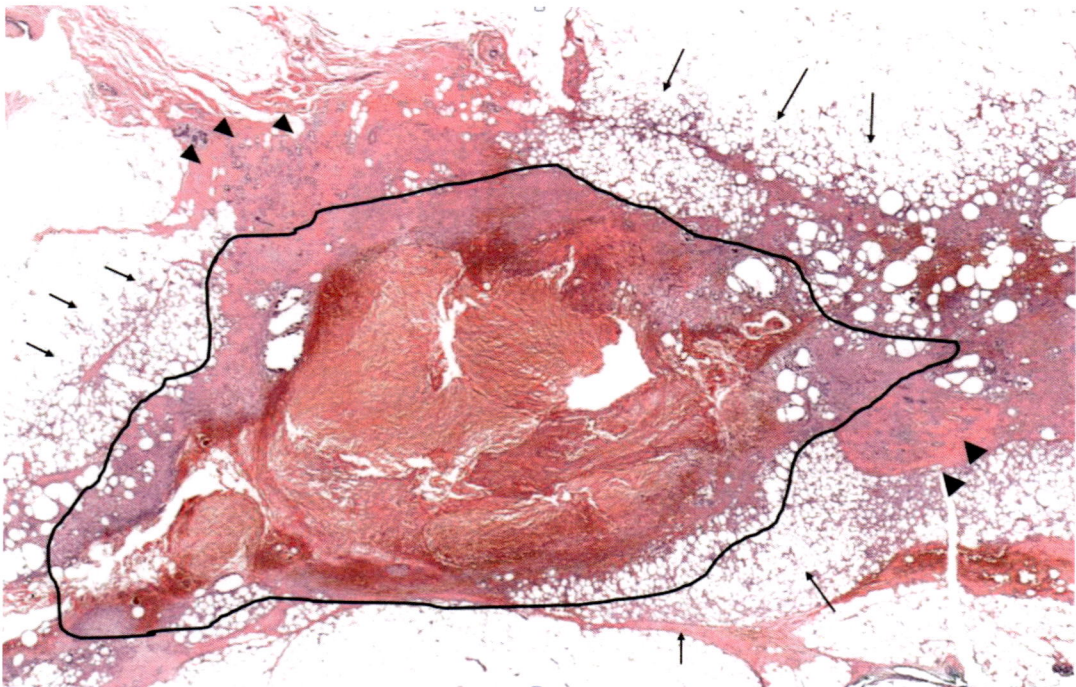

Fig.10.2 Effect of laser ablation procedure. The central area represents the effect of the laser procedure, filled by necrotic debris, erythrocytes, and inflammatory cells, surrounded by lymphocytes and hystiocytes as a reaction to the procedure (surrounded area). Liponecrosis is observed in the surrounding adipose tissue (arrows). Arrowheads show the atypical epithelial ducts on the edges of the area, representing the residual neoplasia

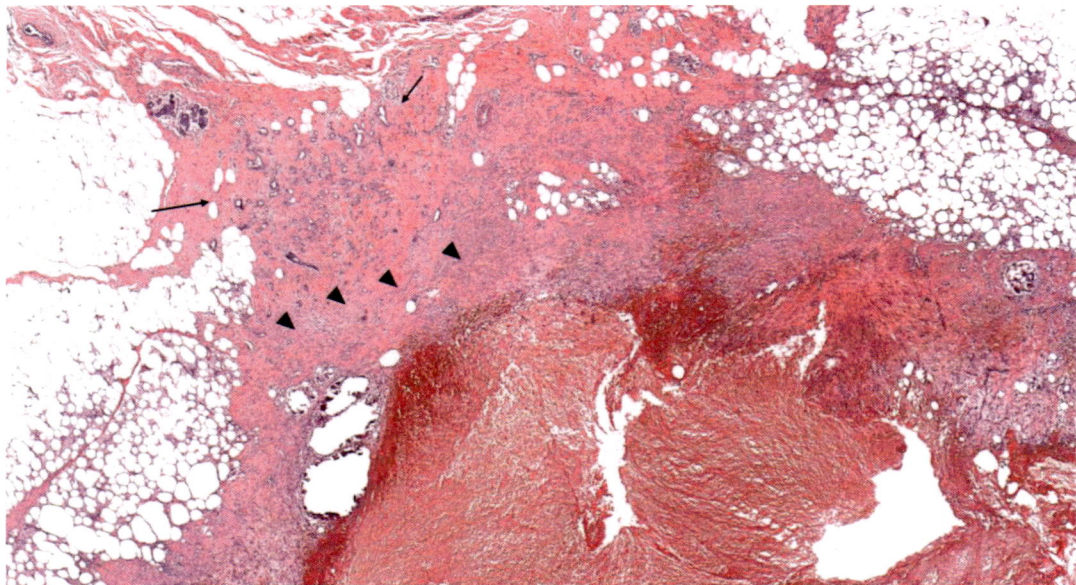

Fig.10.3 At higher magnification (2×), the residual neoplasia (arrows) is better observed compared to flogistic tissue (arrowheads) surrounding the area of the laser ablation

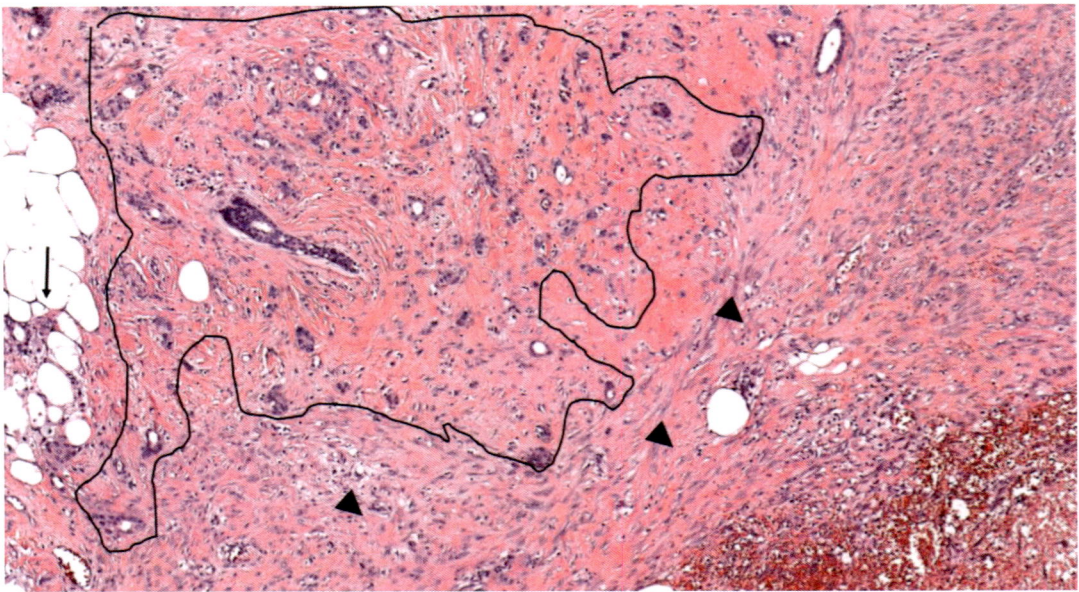

Fig.10.4 At higher magnification (10×), the atypical ducts of the neoplasia (surrounded area) are observed close to reactive stroma and flogistic tissue (arrowheads). On the left, liponecrosis is observed as procedure effect (arrow)

tion in 38 patients (70%) on histopathological examination. Haraldsdottir et al. [18] used also an 805 nm diode laser. This study included tumors measuring less than 30 mm. The procedure was ultrasound-guided. Complete removal was obtained in 3 patients out of 24 patients treated. Van Esser et al. [12] used another laser, the Nd:YAG 1064 nm. Fourteen patients with tumors measuring less than 20 mm were treated under ultrasound guidance. Complete removal was obtained in half of the patients. However, in most of the studies performed on LA of breast carcinomas, the treatment parameters were predetermined. When treatment parameters are predetermined, possible cooling effects of blood flow (heat-sink effect or siphon effect) and differences in density of breast and tumor tissue cannot be taken into account, possibly leading to undertreatment of the tumor tissue. Real-time monitoring and adjusting of the treatment parameters would be ideal for transmitting the amount of energy needed to successfully ablate the target lesion completely. The type of tissue, its density, and its vascularization play a decisive role in obtaining the complete ablation of the tumor tissue, and only a real-time monitoring of ablation

procedure could help to obtain the complete ablation of the tumor mass.

In most studies, the progress of ablation was monitored by ultrasound [12, 15, 19]. The temperature near the tip of the fiber reaches 100 °C, causing the vaporization of the liquid component of the tumor tissue [13, 15] with the consequent production of hyperechogenic gas bubbles, which make monitoring with ultrasound difficult [20]. Similarly, the stereotaxic guide does not allow a good visualization of the treatment area [13, 16].

Although lasers can be placed under ultrasound or stereotactic guidance, Korourian et al. [21] demonstrated that MRI may be more useful. Korourian and colleagues used laser therapy to treat 29 patients under MRI guidance. They found complete ablation in 76% of tumors. They also analyzed the proliferative capability of the excised specimen as a function of distance from the center of the laser and concluded that laser therapy can be effective in tumors 1 cm or smaller [15].

Adverse effects include pain, which can be managed with local anesthesia. Other common complications described in literature are hyperemia and skin burns gaseous rupture of tumor tissue [15, 16, 22]. Moreover, Van Esser et al. have described a pneumothorax in one patient [12]. To avoid complications, many studies suggest to treat "target" lesions localized at least 1 cm from the skin surface and pectoralis muscle [23, 24]. All studies in the literature agree that the size of the "target" lesion is a key factor to obtain a complete ablation [25, 26]. Van Esser et al. [12] investigated the feasibility of ultrasound-guided LA in invasive breast cancers up to 2 cm in size. Overall, the invasive breast cancer was completely ablated in 50% of patients (total $n = 14$). There was a clear association between the success rate of LA and tumor size: cancers were completely ablated in seven (88%) of eight and one (17%) of six patients with a carcinoma <2 cm and ≥2 cm, respectively. These results show that LA can completely ablate small invasive breast carcinomas. Nori et al. [10] assessed the feasibility of ultrasound-guided percutaneous laser ablation as the treatment of small unifocal breast cancer in inoperable elderly patients and in patients who refuse surgery. This study showed that percutaneous laser ablation is a feasible and effective option for selected unresectable breast cancer patients. They obtained complete ablation in patients with small lesions (T1 lesions ≤2 cm).

Previous studies have shown the importance of tumor size to completely ablate breast carcinomas [25, 26]. Notably, the number of fibers used in clinical trials also depends on the size of the lesion. For example, Haraldsdottir et al. [18] used one laser fiber, placed at the center of the tumor, for small tumors (<15 mm; $n = 1/410$) and four laser fibers, positioned a few millimeters from the edge of the tumor, for large tumors. In this study, the dimensions of the lesions ranged from 7 to 55 mm (average 23 mm). So, the rate of necrosis was higher in the small tumor. In order to avoid incomplete treatment, several studies have suggested the use of local ablative methods on well-localized tumors, smaller than 15–20 mm, containing less than 25% of ductal carcinoma in situ (DCIS) cancer in the core biopsy and only minimal calcifications at mammography (higher risk of DCIS). On the other hand, tumors that show lobular differentiation should be excluded from local ablation even in a curative setting [10, 12, 18, 23, 27].

10.3.2 Advantages

There seems to be little difference in local efficacy between percutaneous ablation techniques and laser-heating methods. One advantage of using LA is that the tissue destruction is precise and reproducible and gives a well-controlled lesion with minimal trauma. Furthermore, some studies show that LA can elicit a strong immunologic response against the treated tumor, even if not radically treated [28] (Fig. 10.3). Additionally, the photocoagulation effect of this technique reduces bleeding during the procedure.

To implement percutaneous ablation as the breast-conserving treatment for small carcinomas of the breast, reliable intraoperative imaging is essential to monitor placement of the laser fiber and the effect of treatment. In recent years, a real-time magnetic resonance–guided thermal mapping has become available in the clinic. Laser technology is MR-compatible. A considerable advantage of this technology when used under MR guidance is the possibility of obtaining an accurate temperature map during the procedure that is useful to optimize the treatment and avoid the onset of complications. MR guidance is destined to replace ultrasound and stereotactic guidance as it allows for a real-time monitoring of the procedure, which is challenging with other guidance systems (Figs. 10.5 and 10.6).

Long-term cosmetic results are intuitively expected to be better with percutaneous ablation than breast-conserving surgery, especially with laser technique thanks to the use of thin devices (<1 mm).

10.3.3 Disadvantages

The first issue that limits the clinical use of LA procedures is the need of greater manual skills in free-hand real-time ultrasound guidance compared to ultrasound-guided needle biopsies. With percutaneous ablation, the operator must place the probe in the geometric center of the target lesion, and this may become a technical challenge in the case of subcentimeter lesions, that is, those that are best treated with the technique.

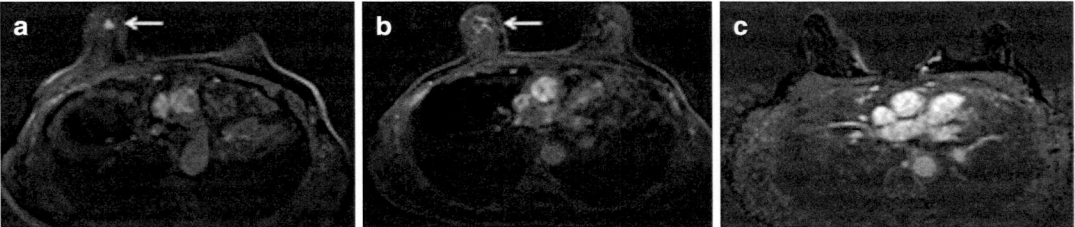

Fig.10.5 A 43-year-old woman who undergoes laser ablation of a right breast lesion. Dynamic Contrast-Enhanced MR 3D T1W axial sequence. Post-processing subtraction of unenhanced images was performed on dynamic contrast-enhanced acquisitions. (**a**) MR exam before laser therapy shows a mass enhancement of the right breast. (**b**) MR exam after 2-week post-procedure shows the effect of laser ablation: a heterogeneous *mass* enhancement with a central necrosis surrounded by a rim enhancement due to flogosis. (**c**) In MR exam after 6 months, no more pathological enhancement was found

Fig. 10.6 A 76-year-old woman who undergoes laser ablation of a right breast lesion (Dmax 21 mm with skin and nipple retraction). Dynamic Contrast-Enhanced MR 3D T1W axial sequence. Post-processing subtraction of unenhanced images was performed on dynamic contrast-enhanced acquisitions. MR exam after 2-week post-procedure shows the effect of laser ablation: a heterogeneous *mass* enhancement with a central necrosis surrounded by a rim enhancement due to flogosis. Still evident are the skin and nipple retraction

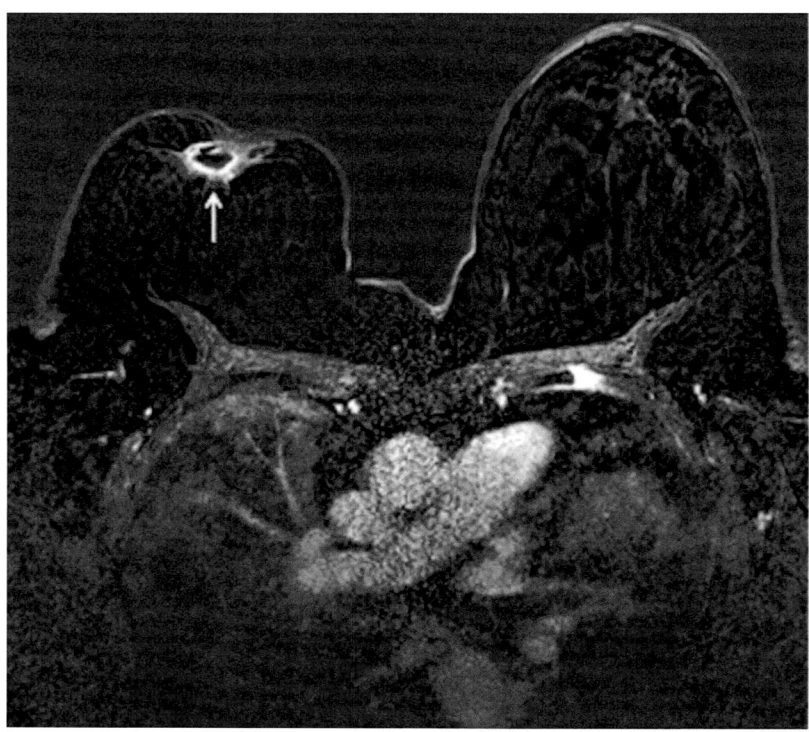

There is no room for error in the placement of an ablative device in the treatment of breast cancer. Imaging-guided percutaneous ablation procedures cannot be performed without the participation of a breast imaging radiologist skilled in percutaneous breast intervention.

Although these techniques are minimally invasive, the disease status in the axilla must be verified by sentinel node mapping and biopsy. Determination of the sentinel node via sentinel lymph node biopsy (SLNB) is important for adequate staging and further treatment. The possibility that local ablation of the tumor tissue disturbs the lymph drainage pattern also exists. In available studies on LA to date, no clear data have been provided on the timing of the SLNB. In the report by Van Esser et al. [12], the SLNB was performed directly before the LA procedure. Another obstacle to the adoption of percutaneous ablation techniques is the ability to show tumor response. Some studies have used MRI or repeated biopsy to assess treatment response [19, 29], whereas others studies have used as the reference standard the subsequent surgical excision [18].

10.4   Follow-Up After LA in Patients That Did Not Undergo Surgery

Another issue not often addressed is the need for stringent follow-up after percutaneous ablation of breast cancer. Nori et al. [10] began clinical follow-up at 1 week, then at 3 months, and every 6 months until the fifth year. Clinical examination assessed the skin and nipple conditions and the clinical size of the treated lesion, if palpable. Radiological follow-up included a weekly US examination from the first and fourth week after the ablation procedure. Follow-up also included bilateral mammography and ultrasound after 6 months from the laser procedure and every 12 months thereafter up to 5 years. Several studies assessed that MRI beyond that is helpful in preoperative tumor size assessment, and patient selection has been relatively successful in showing the presence of residual tumor after laser therapy [29, 30]. Manenti et al. [31] in their feasibility study supported that the validation tests with MRI study aimed to quantifying the results after minimally invasive imaging-guided treatments for breast lesions.

10.5   LA Application in Benign Lesions

One of the first applications of LA in breast lesions was performed in 1999 when Sompracas et al. [32] proposed the use of interstitial laser hyperthermia in breast fibroadenomas as an outpatient procedure. They treated 27 fibroadenomas less than 20 mm with a procedure that was ultrasound-guided. A 1064 nm ND:YAG laser was used. Clinical (40–100%) and ultrasound (20–90%) size reduction of fibroadenomas was obtained. Several years later, another group [33]

described two cases of in situ laser ablation of fibroadenoma and the outcome after 6–8 years of follow-up. They reported a minimally invasive imaging-guided laser treatment of two breast fibroadenoma and long term follow-up in two patients; one with single and the other with multiple bilateral tumors. The treatment is an office-based procedure given under local anesthesia with minimal pain and discomfort. It is esthetically superior to lumpectomy, and follow-up at 3 years shows a significant volume reduction of the fibroadenomas (40–50%).

10.6   Conclusions

To implement this minimally invasive approach, several steps need to be taken. First, the exact tumor size should be reliably assessed. Second, the treatment should be safe and able to completely destroy all tumor tissue (including in situ cancer) locally. Finally, a reliable real-time way to monitor the treatment results should be available. The authors consider that tumors should be carefully selected for treatment by percutaneous ablation. Successful LA of invasive breast cancer seems to be feasible when confined to small (≤2 cm) nonlobular carcinomas without a surrounding extensive in situ component. Importantly, a good visibility with the imaging modality used to guide the procedure is needed. The prospect of performing imaging-guided percutaneous treatment under local anesthesia in an outpatient treatment room is attractive for both patients and treating physicians and has the potential for substantial cost savings.

It is important to bear in mind that experimentation with percutaneous ablation of breast cancer as a replacement for lumpectomy is associated with ethical concerns. Most applications of percutaneous ablation of malignant disease (e.g., prostate cancer, liver and bone metastases) have focused on palliation, not cure, in patients with an otherwise poor prognosis and for whom the therapeutic alternatives cause more risk or are simply not available. In contrast, patients who have participated in testing of percutaneous ablation of small breast cancers already have an excellent prognosis with the current standard treatment of breast conservation, that is, lumpectomy and radiation therapy. Therefore, any percutaneous ablation technique with curative intent must be proved to be at least as effective as the standard treatment, because if the percutaneous ablation procedure fails, the patient's best chance for cure may have been compromised. After percutaneous ablation, the mass is not physically removed so the lesions' margins cannot be assessed pathologically, and complete treatment of the tumor cannot be validated.

Most of the published studies enrolled small groups of patients, so the evidence regarding the value of laser ablation techniques is quite sparse. This limitation is particularly noteworthy when considering not only the technical success but also the efficacy and rate of complications. Hence it is hard to draw reliable conclusions [34].

The authors assume that treatment of early-stage breast cancer (TNM T1a and T1b) with the features described above is the most relevant application of LA. A new interesting field of investigation could be the treatment of small (≤2 cm) breast lesions classified as lesions of uncertain malignant potential (B3) that are a heterogeneous group of abnormalities with a borderline histological spectrum and a variable but low risk of associated malignancy [35].

References

1. American Cancer Society, editor Cancer Facts & Figures; 2016.
2. van Dam PA, Tomatis M, Marotti L, Heil J, Mansel RE, Rosselli Del Turco M, et al. Time trends (2006-2015) of quality indicators in EUSOMA-certified breast centres. Eur J Cancer. 2017;85:15–22.
3. Moran MS, Schnitt SJ, Giuliano AE, Harris JR, Khan SA, Horton J, et al. Society of Surgical Oncology-American Society for Radiation Oncology consensus guideline on margins for breast-conserving surgery with whole-breast irradiation in stages I and II invasive breast cancer. Ann Surg Oncol. 2014;21(3):704–16.
4. Schnitt SJ, Moran MS, Houssami N, Morrow M. The Society of Surgical Oncology-American Society for Radiation Oncology Consensus Guideline on Margins for Breast-Conserving Surgery With Whole-Breast Irradiation in Stages I and II Invasive Breast Cancer: Perspectives for Pathologists. Arch Pathol Lab Med. 2015;139(5):575–7.
5. Zhao Z, Wu F. Minimally-invasive thermal ablation of early-stage breast cancer: a systemic review. Eur J Surg Oncol. 2010;36(12):1149–55.
6. Gardner RA, Vargas HI, Block JB, Vogel CL, Fenn AJ, Kuehl GV, et al. Focused microwave phased array thermotherapy for primary breast cancer. Ann Surg Oncol. 2002;9(4):326–32.
7. Burak WE Jr, Agnese DM, Povoski SP, Yanssens TL, Bloom KJ, Wakely PE, et al. Radiofrequency ablation of invasive breast carcinoma followed by delayed surgical excision. Cancer. 2003;98(7):1369–76.
8. Furusawa H, Namba K, Thomsen S, Akiyama F, Bendet A, Tanaka C, et al. Magnetic resonance-guided focused ultrasound surgery of breast cancer: reliability and effectiveness. J Am Coll Surg. 2006;203(1):54–63.
9. Manenti G, Bolacchi F, Perretta T, Cossu E, Pistolese CA, Buonomo OC, et al. Small breast cancers: in vivo percutaneous US-guided radiofrequency ablation with dedicated cool-tip radiofrequency system. Radiology. 2009;251(2):339–46.
10. Nori J, Gill MK, Meattini I, Delli Paoli C, Abdulcadir D, Vanzi E, et al. The evolving role of ultrasound guided percutaneous laser ablation in elderly unresectable breast cancer patients: a feasibility pilot study. Biomed Res Int. 2018;2018:9141746.
11. Ahmed M, Brace CL, Lee FT Jr, Goldberg SN. Principles of and advances in percutaneous ablation. Radiology. 2011;258(2):351–69.
12. van Esser S, Stapper G, van Diest PJ, van den Bosch MA, Klaessens JH, Mali WP, et al. Ultrasound-guided laser-induced thermal therapy for small palpable invasive breast carcinomas: a feasibility study. Ann Surg Oncol. 2009;16(8):2259–63.
13. Bloom KJ, Dowlat K, Assad L. Pathologic changes after interstitial laser therapy of infiltrating breast carcinoma. Am J Surg. 2001;182(4):384–8.
14. Harries SA, Amin Z, Smith ME, Lees WR, Cooke J, Cook MG, et al. Interstitial laser photocoagulation as a treatment for breast cancer. Br J Surg. 1994;81(11):1617–9.
15. Akimov AB, Seregin VE, Rusanov KV, Tyurina EG, Glushko TA, Nevzorov VP, et al. Nd: YAG interstitial laser thermotherapy in the treatment of breast cancer. Lasers Surg Med. 1998;22(5):257–67.
16. Dowlatshahi K, Francescatti DS, Bloom KJ. Laser therapy for small breast cancers. Am J Surg. 2002;184(4):359–63.
17. Schwartzberg LS, Blair SL. Strategies for the Management of Early-Stage Breast Cancer in Older Women. J Natl Compr Cancer Netw. 2016;14(5 Suppl):647–50.
18. Haraldsdottir KH, Ivarsson K, Gotberg S, Ingvar C, Stenram U, Tranberg KG. Interstitial laser thermotherapy (ILT) of breast cancer. Eur J Surg Oncol. 2008;34(7):739–45.
19. Mumtaz H, Hall-Craggs MA, Wotherspoon A, Paley M, Buonaccorsi G, Amin Z, et al. Laser therapy for

breast cancer: MR imaging and histopathologic correlation. Radiology. 1996;200(3):651–8.

20. Varghese T, Techavipoo U, Zagzebski JA, Lee FT Jr. Impact of gas bubbles generated during interstitial ablation on elastographic depiction of in vitro thermal lesions. J Ultrasound Med. 2004;23(4):535–44; quiz 45-6

21. Korourian S, Klimberg S, Henry-Tillman R, Lindquist D, Jones M, Eng DC, et al. Assessment of proliferating cell nuclear antigen activity using digital image analysis in breast carcinoma following magnetic resonance-guided interstitial laser photocoagulation. Breast J. 2003;9(5):409–13.

22. van Esser S, van den Bosch MA, van Diest PJ, Mali WT, Borel Rinkes IH, van Hillegersberg R. Minimally invasive ablative therapies for invasive breast carcinomas: an overview of current literature. World J Surg. 2007;31(12):2284–92.

23. Fornage BD, Hwang RF. Current status of imaging-guided percutaneous ablation of breast cancer. AJR Am J Roentgenol. 2014;203(2):442–8.

24. Sabel MS. Nonsurgical ablation of breast cancer: future options for small breast tumors. Surg Oncol Clin N Am. 2014;23(3):593–608.

25. van Esser S, Veldhuis WB, van Hillegersberg R, van Diest PJ, Stapper G, ElOuamari M, et al. Accuracy of contrast-enhanced breast ultrasound for pre-operative tumor size assessment in patients diagnosed with invasive ductal carcinoma of the breast. Cancer Imaging. 2007;7:63–8.

26. Medina-Franco H, Soto-Germes S, Ulloa-Gomez JL, Romero-Trejo C, Uribe N, Ramirez-Alvarado CA, et al. Radiofrequency ablation of invasive breast carcinomas: a phase II trial. Ann Surg Oncol. 2008;15(6):1689–95.

27. Fleming MM, Holbrook AI, Newell MS. Update on image-guided percutaneous ablation of breast cancer. AJR Am J Roentgenol. 2017;208(2):267–74.

28. Ivarsson K, Myllymaki L, Jansner K, Stenram U, Tranberg KG. Resistance to tumour challenge after tumour laser thermotherapy is associated with a cellular immune response. Br J Cancer. 2005;93(4):435–40.

29. SchwartzbergBS, AbdelatifOM, LewinJ, et al. Multicenter clinical trial of percutaneous laser ablation for early stage primary breast cancer: results of 49 cases with radiographic and pathological correlation. San Antonio Breast Cancer Symposium website. Published 2015. www.sabcs.org/Portals/SABCS2016/San Antonio. Accessed 28 Sep 2016.

30. Mumtaz H, Barone GW, Ketel BL, Ozdemir A. Successful management of a nonmalignant esophageal perforation with a coated stent. Ann Thorac Surg. 2002;74(4):1233–5.

31. Manenti G, Perretta T, Gaspari E, Pistolese CA, Scarano L, Cossu E, et al. Percutaneous local ablation of unifocal subclinical breast cancer: clinical experience and preliminary results of cryotherapy. Eur Radiol. 2011;21(11):2344–53.

32. Basu S, Ravi B, Kant R. Interstitial laser hyperthermia, a new method in the management of fibroadenoma of the breast: A pilot study. Lasers Surg Med. 1999;25(2):148–52.

33. Dowlatshahi K, Wadhwani S, Alvarado R, Valadez C, Dieschbourg J. Interstitial laser therapy of breast fibroadenomas with 6 and 8 year follow-up. Breast J. 2010;16(1):73–6.

34. Mauri G, Sconfienza LM, Pescatori LC, Fedeli MP, Ali M, Di Leo G, et al. Technical success, technique efficacy and complications of minimally-invasive imaging-guided percutaneous ablation procedures of breast cancer: A systematic review and meta-analysis. Eur Radiol. 2017;27(8):3199–210.

35. Rageth CJ, O'Flynn EA, Comstock C, Kurtz C, Kubik R, Madjar H, et al. First International Consensus Conference on lesions of uncertain malignant potential in the breast (B3 lesions). Breast Cancer Res Treat. 2016;159(2):203–13.

11

Tian'an Jiang, Ping Liang, and Jie Yu

11.1 Introduction

Pancreatic cancer (PC) is the most lethal abdominal malignancy and one of leading causes of cancer-related death with a 5-year survival rate<10% for all stages [1]. Because most patients suffer from a primarily locally unresectable tumor or metastatic disease at the time of diagnosis, chemo- and radiotherapy so far have been the major treatment modalities but with limited survival benefit and severe toxicity reaction [2]. Minimally invasive ablation therapy has attracted great interest for the management of focal malignant disease during the past decade [3]. Potential advantages of ablation therapy include real-time imaging guidance, the ability to ablate tumor in patients who lose the surgical chance and reduced morbidity compared to surgery.

Several minimally invasive strategies including radiofrequency, high-intensity focused ultrasound (US), laser energy and cryoablation have been applied to pancreas in animal studies or limited clinical application [4–10]. Laser ablation (LA) energy is transmitted through an optic fiber

and the absorption of thermal energy within the tissue results in localized heating and cellular death. The main advantage of applying laser ablation system is the less trauma with the use of thin devices and more accurate thermal field control [4, 5, 11]. LA has been used in many therapies such as retroperitoneal lymph nodes, kidney, prostate, thyroid and risky liver tumors [12–17]. However, lagging behind other ablation techniques, LA achieved only limited experimental results in porcine pancreas and few case reports on endoscopic US-guided ablation of unresectable or recurrent pancreatic tumor [18–21].

LA uses a 21-G fine needle and allows for accurate thermal field control. The advantages of the small needle and precise thermal energy distribution theoretically could minimize the risk of off-target burning, which makes LA particularly suitable for treating tumors in difficult anatomical locations [11, 16, 22]. Using the endoscopic ultrasound guide (EUS-g) laser energy can be successfully transferred in target locations [19, 21, 23].

EUS was first established as a diagnostic method in gastrointestinal cancer staging. It helps in the staging of gastrointestinal cancers by offering high-resolution imaging and fine-needle biopsy of tumors, lymph nodes and pancreatic masses [24, 25]. In the recent decade, EUS was used not only as a noninvasive diagnostic tool but also as a therapeutic modality. Endovascular therapy for ablation of gastric varices and feeding

T. Jiang (✉)
Department of Ultrasound, First Affiliated Hospital,
College of Medicine, Zhejiang University,
Hangzhou, China
e-mail: tiananjiang@zju.edu.cn

P. Liang · J. Yu
Department of Interventional Ultrasound, Chinese
PLA General Hospital, Beijing, China

© Springer Nature Switzerland AG 2020
C. M. Pacella et al. (eds.), *Image-guided Laser Ablation*,
https://doi.org/10.1007/978-3-030-21748-8_11

vessels can be performed by EUS, because of the real-time visualization of flow in adjacent blood vessels using Doppler ultrasound. Besides, the application of EUS is wide, including bilioenteric and enteroenteric anastomosis in a minimally invasive manner, EUS-guided gastroenterostomy (EUS-GE) which has recently emerged as a feasible procedure to treat patients with gastric outlet obstruction [26], EUS-guided photodynamic therapy [27, 28] and EUS-g fine-needle injection (EUS-FNI) technique [29].

Currently, a preliminary study has shown that pancreatic tissue could be successfully destroyed by EUS-guided radiofrequency ablation [30]. EUS-RFA was performed in all six patients with pancreatic cancer located in the head or body of the pancreas successfully. In this study, no events such as pancreatitis or bleeding were found except that two patients experienced mild abdominal pain after the procedure. Complications reported in previous studies after EUS-RFA, however, might include abdominal pain, duodenal bleeding, jaundice, and duodenal stricture [26]. The aim of this chapter is to describe the technique and the results of LA in the treatment of PC.

11.2 Patients

Patients with unresectable clinically locally advanced PC and with limited metastasis (less than two metastatic organs outside the pancreas) not responsive to chemo- or radiotherapy may undergo LA treatment [31]. Exclusion criteria are grades 4 and 5 according to Eastern Cooperative Oncology Group (ECOG) score[32] and advanced heart or pulmonary disease (American Society of Anesthesiologists grade IV). All PCs must be diagnosed on the basis of pathological data obtained by targeted biopsy. Contrast enhanced abdominal magnetic resonance imaging (MRI)/computed tomography (CT) and real-time ultrasound (US) and CA 19–9 tumor markers should be obtained prior to LA. The LA technique, thanks to the use of thin devices, can be performed under the guidance MRI/CT/US.

11.3 Ablation Procedure

11.3.1 Percutaneous Approach

Pancreatic tumors may be treated using minimally invasive percutaneous ablation techniques when they are well detectable by imaging and result in a relatively safe and easy access pathway. Our group have performed eight cases of LA of PC by percutaneous US guidance with use of US scanner of 4–10 MHz frequency. Then color Doppler US was used to observe the blood flow around the puncture site. LA was performed by local anesthesia with 1% lidocaine applied to the skin, the subcutaneous tissue and the peritoneum. We used a multisource semiconductor diode laser system working in continuous mode with a wavelength of 1064 nm integrated with a latest generation ultrasound system (EchoLaser, Elesta, Calenzano (FI), Italy). The laser unit allows the use of multiple sources (up to four) both simultaneously and separately from each other even at different output powers. The insertion route was carefully determined by US to avoid the normal pancreas, bowel, vessels, pancreatic duct and bile ducts. One or two 21-G needles were inserted into PC with the tip of needle 10 mm away from the distal borderline of tumor and with the shaft of needle 5–10 mm from the tumor's lateral border. Then a 300-µm diameter plane-cut quartz optical bare fiber was advanced through the sheath of the needle which is then pulled back so as to expose the fiber in direct contact with the tumor tissue by 5 mm. The output power of laser was set at 5 W, and the energy set for 3 KJ. For larger tumors, the needle and fiber were repositioned or pulled back to ablate each part of the tumor, and additional energy was applied until the whole lesion became hyperechoic. The total delivered energy was automatically calculated by the equipment. The number of fibers used (from one to two) was related to the size of the PC at baseline and to the reciprocal anatomical relationships of the lesion with adjacent tissues. If two fibers were inserted simultaneously during LA to obtain a larger ablation zone, the distance between the fibers of no more than 10 mm was used. The correct needle position and the distance between the fibers were verified using the US image. Upon completion of the ablation procedure, the CEUS (contrast-enhanced US) scan was performed to confirm the technical effect (no increase in tumor).

11.3.2 Endoscopic Approach

Since the percutaneous approach is not always possible and it is difficult without the particular experience of the operator, it is possible to resort to endoscopic EUS-g ablation to debulking tumor mass. This is a better method for providing the best combination of precise localization, excellent visualization and real-time imaging guidance with minimal invasiveness [19–21, 33]. Many authors used curved linear array echoendoscope of different vendors.

After an 8-hour fast, patients undergo endoscopic maneuver under deep sedation with propofol. Some authors do not report the prophylactic administration of antibiotics [20], while others use it by administering antibiotics immediately before the procedure and for 3 days thereafter [21]. EUS-LA is performed orally by an experienced endoscopist to detect pancreatic lesions, and then use color Doppler ultrasonography to observe the blood flow around the puncture site. CEUS is performed both before and after each LA procedure, using an intravenous 5 mL of ultrasound contrast medium injection (SonoVue, Bracco, Milan, Italy) through an antecubital vein with a 20-gauge catheter followed by a 10-mL saline solution flush.

After determining the depth, a 22-G needle is inserted in the lesions. Once in the target site, the needle is gently pulled back so that the 300-μm optical fiber comes in direct contact with the tissue to be ablated. After retraction of the needle sheath, the bare flat fiber in direct contact for 5 mm with the tumor tissue is inserted in the center of the tumor away from the lower edge of the tumor for about 13–15 mm. The laser light generator is activated and the energy is transferred to the tumor tissue. The procedure can be performed several times in the same session using the pull-back maneuver and/or repositioning the applicator (sheath and fiber) parallel to the previous ablated area to proceed with other ablations in untreated sites. It is possible to repeat the maneuver also in the following days both to obtain a greater area of ablation and to ablate any residual vital tissue discovered using the CEUS [19–21]. The laser has been used both in animal models and in patients with different power settings from 2 W to 5 W with variable energy transfer from 800 to 1800 J per fiber in one or more sessions [5, 18–21, 34].

11.4 Results

In 2010, the first LA of pancreas study on eight healthy pigs was performed by means of EUS guidance. All applications (at 2 W and 3 W, with 500 J and 1000 J energy delivery) were directed toward the body and tail of the pancreas, using a transgastric approach. After 24 h, the pigs were sacrificed and the ablated lesions were excised for histopathologic evaluation [18]. The acquired data confirmed the results of previous in vivo experimental studies on other organs in animal models [35] and demonstrated an area of coagulative zone well delimited without signs of damage to the adjacent vital tissue and without signs of pancreatitis. Furthermore, a good correlation between the released energy and the extent of the ablated area has been shown.

Currently there are few clinical studies that report the initial results of the method with a still very limited number of patients treated with EUS approach [19–21]. They all showed the technique was safe for unresectable or recurrent PC patients.

In Jiang et al.'s study, EUS-guided LA (EUS-g LA) was performed on a 61-year-old man with pancreatic carcinoma, and CEUS showed nearly complete necrosis and shrinkage of the tumor 2 months after the ablation. The lesion located in the head of the pancreas with a maximum size of 5.3 cm was treated with several treatments and several sessions at different times and with different amounts of energy per treatment (up to total of 17.500 J). There were no serious procedure-related complications [20] (Fig. 11.1).

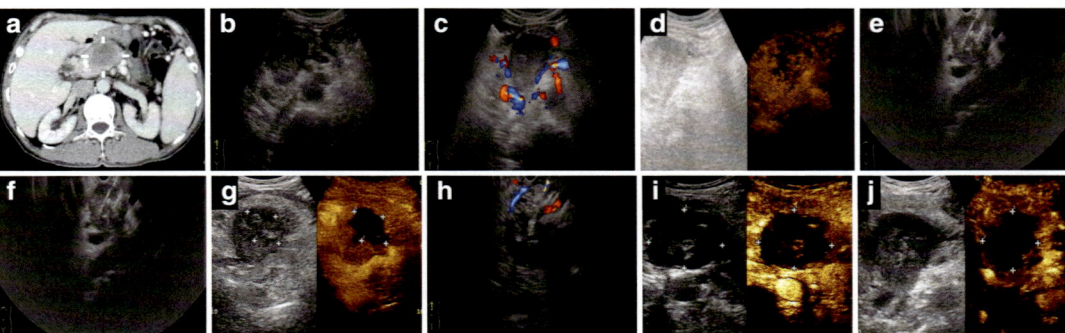

Fig. 11.1 A 61-year old male with pancreatic cancer. Preoperative computed tomography scan and contrast-enhanced ultrasound image showed a tumor measuring 5.3 × 4.6 cm in size in the pancreatic head (**a–d**) (*arrowheads*). Endoscopic ultrasonography real time guided laser fiber being inserted into the center of tumor away from the capsule wall (approximately 1.3 cm) (**e, f**). Two days later, contrast-enhanced ultrasound showed an abnormal residual near the left of the tumor (**g**). Then, after 6 days, another endoscopic ultrasonography guided laser ablation was performed for target tumor (**h**), and the follow-up contrast-enhanced ultrasound image showed the mass was completed necrotized without enhancement (**i**). And 2 months later after two ablations, contrast-enhanced ultrasound showed the tumor nearly complete necrosis and shrunk (**j**)

The prospective cohort single-center study by Di Matteo et al. reported the outcomes obtained in nine patients with stage IIb-III pancreatic ductal adenocarcinoma unresectable and unresponsive to chemo-radiotherapy. Most of the lesions were in the head of the pancreas (six patients). The mean lesions size was 35.4 mm (range 21–45 mm). The patients were divided into three groups and treated with a total delivered energy of 800, 1000 and 1200 J, at a low power setting (2, 3 and 4 W), respectively. Each patient was treated with a single application of one of these settings. The application time of power setting ranged from 200 to 600 s. All the procedures were performed under EUS guidance with color Doppler analysis to prevent injury of surrounding vessels and structures. In accordance with the guidelines of the American Society Gastrointestinal Endoscopy (ASGE)[36], no major complication was detected. Three patients developed thin pericapsular fluid collections during the following 7 days after the maneuver and they spontaneously disappeared within 30 days. Only two patients presented an increase in serum amylase level without the need to prolong hospital stay. The low power setting avoided damage to normal tissue adjacent to the tumor and avoided possible pancreatitis. In addition, the data of the study seem to attest that the power of 4 W/1000 J is the setting most suitable to obtain the largest volume of ablation. Median overall survival was 7.4 months (range 29–662 days). All patients died after disease progression. There is no information on the relationship between the areas of coagulative zone and the duration of survival that should be provided by further studies [21]. So even if small, the sample of cases available so far suggests that EUS-g LA might be a promising alternative to surgery in selected cases. However, it needs to be confirmed by more prospective studies with long-term follow-up in the future.

As for the percutaneous approach, our group has an initial experience. Between September 2016 and October 2018, according to the Strengthening the Reporting of Observational Studies in Epidemiology statement for observational studies [37], eight patients with locally advanced and metastatic PC were evaluated for inclusion by the multidisciplinary tumor board in a prospective study. The mean largest tumor diameter was 5.3 ± 1.1 cm (range, 4.2–6.9 cm). One lesion was located at the body of pancreas and three at tails and four at both bodies and tails. The median time from diagnosis to LA was 27 days (range, 9–53 days). Three patients were with locally advanced PC (stage III), three with liver metastases (stage IV) and two with both liver and retroperitoneal lymph node metastases

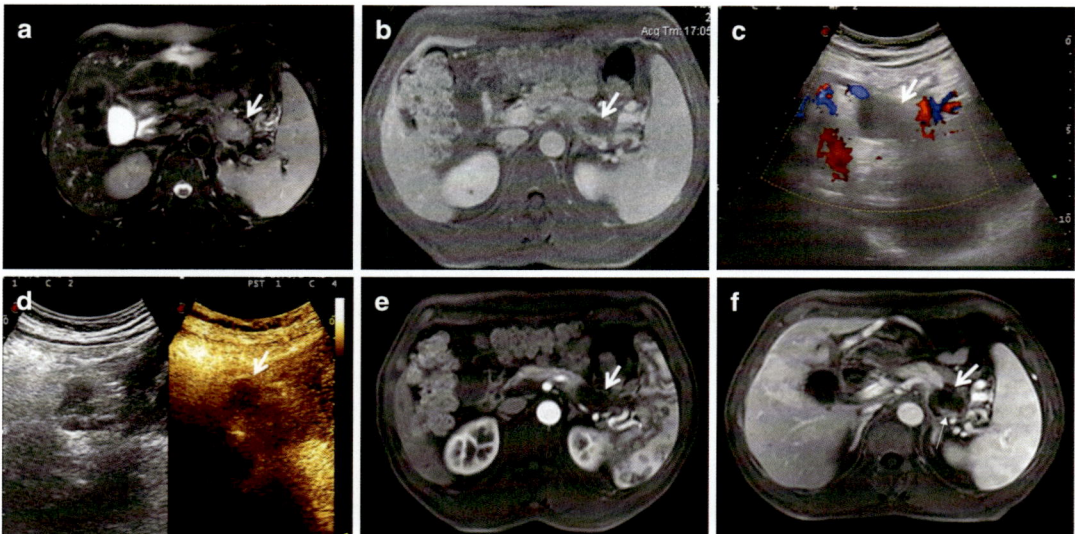

Fig. 11.2 Representative case of pancreatic cancer treated percutaneously. Transverse images in a 62-year-old man with a 4.9 × 3.2 cm cancer in pancreatic tail treated with percutaneous laser ablation. (**a**) Preablation T2 magnetic resonance imaging (MRI) scan shows the lesion is heterogeneous hyperintense (arrow). (**b**) Preablation contrast-enhanced MRI scan shows the lesion is heterogeneous hypointense (arrow). (**c**) Preablation ultrasound (US) scan shows one hypoechoic lesion (arrow) with poor blood supply on color Doppler flow imaging. (**d**) Preablation contrast-enhanced US scan shows the lesion is heterogeneous hypo-enhancement (arrow) in arterial phase. (**e**) On contrast-enhanced MRI scan obtained 3 days after ablation, no enhancement is seen in the ablation zone (arrow) and without obvious residual tumor in arterial phase. (**f**) On contrast-enhanced MRI scan obtained 3 days after ablation, no enhancement is seen in the ablation zone (arrow) and with a little residual tumor in late phase (fine arrow)

(stage IV). The total number of metastatic lesions for each stage IV patient was less than three and the size for each lesion was less than 2 cm. For these eight patients, the aim of LA was to decrease the tumor burden and manage the pain. No patient was lost to follow up. Technique success (successful fiber placement and laser delivery) was achieved in all patients. Fibers were placed ventrally in all the patients with supine position. The number of fibers used was one in two patients and two in six patients. A fiber pullback was performed in all the patients. The mean insertion number of needle was 2.6 ± 0.9 (range 2–4). Ablation power of all patients was 5 W and the mean ablation energy was 9.5 ± 1.8 KJ (range 7.6–12KJ). The metastases of liver and retroperitoneal lymph nodes were treated by LA during the PC ablation procedure. Additionally, in all cases, a contrast-enhanced US by means of a previous 5 mL of SonoVue injection followed by a 5-mL saline solution flush was performed before and after LA. The median post-procedural hospital stay was 5 days (range 4–9 days). Mean pancreas volume was 93.2 ± 20.4 mL (range 71.1–123.2 mL). Mean tumor volume was 16.1 ± 3.8 mL (range 14.5–23.1 mL) and ablation volume was 16.1 ± 3.8 mL (range 13.0–22.1 mL), which reached 89.1 ± 7.4% (range 80.2–98.0%) of tumor volume. Two patients received chemotherapy of eight cycles with gemcitabine after LA and four received five cycles. The neuroendocrine cancer patient and one stage IV patient refused to receive any therapy after LA. Four stage IV patients died at 6.5, 7.7, 9.4 and 12.5 months after LA because of hepatic encephalopathy (n = 1) and tumor progression (n = 3), respectively. The other four patients all survived during follow-up. After a median follow-up period of 9.7 months (range, 6–15 months), the median OS from diagnosis was 11 months (95% confidence interval [CI]: 7 months, 14 months) and the median OS from LA was 10 months

(95% CI:5 months, 13 months). All the patients completed the QOL questionnaires [38] and pain score scale (visual pain scores from 0 to 10) before LA. All completed the questionnaires at 4 weeks and every 3 months after LA. The QOL questionnaires revealed that after LA, patients experienced ameliorative physical function and pain degree compared to baseline at 1-month follow-up. No patients died within 90 days after LA. According to criteria of Society of Interventional Radiology (SIR) clinical practice guidelines [39, 40], no major complications including pancreatitis, bile leakage and biliary obstruction occurred. Gastrointestinal side effects such as nausea, abdominal pain and loss of appetite were observed in all the patients within 3 days after LA. Two patients developed pancreatic pseudocyst (2.4×2.3 cm and 2.0×1.8 cm, respectively) 3 days after LA with the symptom of mild pain, and the cysts were absorbed or decreased in 1 month after LA without any treatment. There was no significant increase in amylase and lipase levels and blood glucose level during 1 week after LA compared to baseline level ($P = 0.5$, $P = 0.8$ and $P = 0.06$, respectively).

11.5 Conclusion

As a novel technique, the results of LA for PC were only reported by a few experimental studies in porcine pancreatic tissue and case report of tumor ablation guided by endoscopic US or peroral pancreatoscopy. In human experience, LA was feasible and well tolerated in patients with pancreatic cancer. Theoretically, LA has some advantages for PC therapy. The major difficulties of PC ablation are the risks of inadvertent thermal injury for adjacent tissues and the impossibility of the complete ablation of all tumor bulk. Laser can create accurate, predictable, and reproducible ablation zones that induce minimal changes outside the targeted ablation zone. It uses a 21–22 gauge guidance needle as the ethanol ablation, which avoids the larger diameter of the radiofrequency or cryoablation needle puncture and reduces potential injury to gastrointestinal tract. And different from ethanol

ablation that produces liquid distribution non-uniformly in the tumor and the limited ablation area [41], LA can induce a controlled, well-defined ablation area by fine optical fibers. These characteristics may offer potential advantages over other ablative techniques for PC treatment. Percutaneous or EUS-guided LA for locally advanced and metastatic PC appears to be a safe and feasible focal therapy option with minimal invasion. The technique shows an encouraging pain control effect and could be a promising alternative to surgery in selected cases. However, more large-scale prospective studies with long-term follow-up are necessary to confirm this finding in the future.

References

1. Vincent A, Herman J, Schulick R, Hruban RH, Goggins M. Pancreatic cancer. Lancet. 2011;378(9791):607–20.
2. Tempero MA, Arnoletti JP, Behrman SW, Ben-Josef E, Benson AB 3rd, Casper ES, et al. Pancreatic adenocarcinoma, version 2.2012: featured updates to the NCCN guidelines. J Natl Compr Cancer Netw. 2012;10(6):703–13.
3. Gillams A, Goldberg N, Ahmed M, Bale R, Breen D, Callstrom M, et al. Thermal ablation of colorectal liver metastases: a position paper by an international panel of ablation experts, the interventional oncology sans Frontieres meeting 2013. Eur Radiol. 2015;25(12):3438–54.
4. Ahmed M, Brace CL, Lee FT Jr, Goldberg SN. Principles of and advances in percutaneous ablation. Radiology. 2011;258(2):351–69.
5. Di Matteo F, Martino M, Rea R, Pandolfi M, Panzera F, Stigliano E, et al. US-guided application of Nd:YAG laser in porcine pancreatic tissue: an ex vivo study and numerical simulation. Gastrointest Endosc. 2013;78(5):750–5.
6. Schena E, Majocchi L. Assessment of temperature measurement error and its correction during Nd:YAG laser ablation in porcine pancreas. Int J Hyperth. 2014;30(5):328–34.
7. Ungureanu B, Pirici D, Mărgăritescu C, S L, Pătraşcu S, Şurlin V, et al. Endoscopic ultrasound-guided radiofrequency ablation of the pancreas: an experimental study with pathological correlation. Endoscopic Ultrasound. 2016;4:330–5.
8. Luo XM, Niu LZ, Chen JB, Xu KC. Advances in cryoablation for pancreatic cancer. World J Gastroenterol. 2016;22(2):790–800.
9. Linecker M, Pfammatter T, Kambakamba P, DeOliveira ML. Ablation strategies for locally advanced pancreatic cancer. Dig Surg. 2016;33(4):351–9.

10. Duprè A, Melodelima D, Pflieger H, Chen Y, Vincenot J, Kocot A, et al. Thermal ablation of the pancreas with intraoperative high-intensity focused ultrasound: safety and efficacy in a porcine model. Pancreas. 2017;46(2):219–24.

11. Pacella CM, Francica G, Di Lascio FM, Arienti V, Antico E, Caspani B, et al. Long-term outcome of cirrhotic patients with early hepatocellular carcinoma treated with ultrasound-guided percutaneous laser ablation: a retrospective analysis. J Clin Oncol. 2009;27(16):2615–21.

12. Oto A, Sethi I, Karczmar G, McNichols R, Ivancevic MK, Stadler WM, et al. MR imaging-guided focal laser ablation for prostate cancer: phase I trial. Radiology. 2013;267(3):932–40.

13. Mou Y, Zhao Q, Zhong L, Chen F, Jiang T. Preliminary results of ultrasound-guided laser ablation for unresectable metastases to retroperitoneal and hepatic portal lymph nodes. World J Surg Oncol. 2016;14(1):165.

14. Sartori S, Mauri G, Tombesi P, Di Vece F, Bianchi L, Pacella CM. Ultrasound-guided percutaneous laser ablation is safe and effective in the treatment of small renal tumors in patients at increased bleeding risk. Int J Hyperth. 2018;35(1):19–25.

15. Zhou W, Jiang S, Zhan W, Zhou J, Xu S, Zhang L. Ultrasound-guided percutaneous laser ablation of unifocal T1N0M0 papillary thyroid microcarcinoma: preliminary results. Eur Radiol. 2017;27(7):2934–40.

16. Francica G, Petrolati A, Di Stasio E, Pacella S, Stasi R, Pacella CM. Effectiveness, safety, and local progression after percutaneous laser ablation for hepatocellular carcinoma nodules up to 4 cm are not affected by tumor location. AJR Am J Roentgenol. 2012;199(6):1393–401.

17. Pacella CM, Bizzarri G, Francica G, Bianchini A, De Nuntis S, Pacella S, et al. Percutaneous laser ablation in the treatment of hepatocellular carcinoma with small tumors: analysis of factors affecting the achievement of tumor necrosis. J Vasc Interv Radiol. 2005;16(11):1447–57.

18. Di Matteo F, Martino M, Rea R, Pandolfi M, Rabitti C, Masselli GM, et al. EUS-guided Nd:YAG laser ablation of normal pancreatic tissue: a pilot study in a pig model. Gastrointest Endosc. 2010;72(2):358–63.

19. Di Matteo F, Picconi F, Martino M, Pandolfi M, Pacella CM, Schena E, et al. Endoscopic ultrasound-guided Nd:YAG laser ablation of recurrent pancreatic neuroendocrine tumor: a promising revolution? Endoscopy. 2014;46(Suppl 1 UCTN):E380–1.

20. Jiang T, Deng Z, Li J, Tian G. Pancreatic cancer: does it work if EUS and laser ablation get married? Endosc Ultrasound. 2018;7(3):207–9.

21. Di Matteo FM, Saccomandi P, Martino M, Pandolfi M, Pizzicannella M, Balassone V, et al. Feasibility of EUS-guided Nd:YAG laser ablation of unresectable pancreatic adenocarcinoma. Gastrointest Endosc. 2018;88(1):168–74 e1.

22. Jiang T, Deng Z, Tian G, Chen F, Bao H, Li J, et al. Percutaneous laser ablation: a new contribution to unresectable high-risk metastatic retroperitoneal lesions? Oncotarget. 2017;8(2):2413–22.

23. Di Matteo F, Grasso R, Pacella CM, Martino M, Pandolfi M, Rea R, et al. EUS-guided Nd:YAG laser ablation of a hepatocellular carcinoma in the caudate lobe. Gastrointest Endosc. 2011;73(3):632–6.

24. Camellini L, Carlinfante G, Azzolini F, Iori V, Cavina M, Sereni G, et al. A randomized clinical trial comparing 22G and 25G needles in endoscopic ultrasound-guided fine-needle aspiration of solid lesions. Endoscopy. 2011;43(8):709–15.

25. Tian G, Bao H, Li J, Jiang T. Systematic review and meta-analysis of diagnostic accuracy of endoscopic ultrasound (EUS)-guided fine-needle aspiration (FNA) using 22-gauge and 25-gauge needles for pancreatic masses. Med Sci Monit. 2018;24:8333–41.

26. Sreenarasimhaiah J. Interventional endoscopic ultrasound: the next frontier in gastrointestinal endoscopy. Am J Med Sci. 2009;338(4):319–24.

27. Chan HH, Nishioka NS, Mino M, Lauwers GY, Puricelli WP, Collier KN, et al. EUS-guided photodynamic therapy of the pancreas: a pilot study. Gastrointest Endosc. 2004;59(1):95–9.

28. Yusuf TE, Matthes K, Brugge WR. EUS-guided photodynamic therapy with verteporfin for ablation of normal pancreatic tissue: a pilot study in a porcine model (with video). Gastrointest Endosc. 2008;67(6):957–61.

29. Irisawa A, Takagi T, Kanazawa M, Ogata T, Sato Y, Takenoshita S, et al. Endoscopic ultrasound-guided fine-needle injection of immature dendritic cells into advanced pancreatic cancer refractory to gemcitabine: a pilot study. Pancreas. 2007;35(2):189–90.

30. Carrara S, Arcidiacono PG, Albarello L, Addis A, Enderle MD, Boemo C, et al. Endoscopic ultrasound-guided application of a new hybrid cryotherm probe in porcine pancreas: a preliminary study. Endoscopy. 2008;40(4):321–6.

31. Wolfgang CL, Herman JM, Laheru DA, Klein AP, Erdek MA, Fishman EK, et al. Recent progress in pancreatic cancer. CA Cancer J Clin. 2013;63(5):318–48.

32. Oken MM, Creech RH, Tormey DC, Horton J, Davis TE, McFadden ET, et al. Toxicity and response criteria of the Eastern Cooperative Oncology Group. Am J Clin Oncol. 1982;5(6):649–55.

33. Rustagi T, Chhoda A. Endoscopic radiofrequency ablation of the pancreas. Dig Dis Sci. 2017;62(4):843–50.

34. Schena E, Saccomandi P, Giurazza F, Caponero MA, Mortato L, Di Matteo FM, et al. Experimental assessment of CT-based thermometry during laser ablation of porcine pancreas. Phys Med Biol. 2013;58(16):5705–16.

35. Pacella CM, Rossi Z, Bizzarri G, Papiini E, Marinozzi V, Paliotta D, et al. Ultrasound-guided percutaneous laser ablation of liver tissue in a rabbit model. Eur Radiol. 1993;3:26–32.

36. Cotton PB, Eisen GM, Aabakken L, Baron TH, Hutter MM, Jacobson BC, et al. A lexicon for endoscopic adverse events: report of an ASGE workshop. Gastrointest Endosc. 2010;71(3):446–54.

37. von Elm E, Altman DG, Egger M, Pocock SJ, Gotzsche PC, Vandenbroucke JP, et al. The strengthening the reporting of observational studies in epidemiology (STROBE) statement: guidelines for reportingobservationalstudies.Lancet.2007;370(9596): 1453–7.

38. Aaronson NK, Ahmedzai S, Bergman B, Bullinger M, Cull A, Duez NJ, et al. The European Organization for Research and Treatment of Cancer QLQ-C30: a quality-of-life instrument for use in international clinical trials in oncology. J Natl Cancer Inst. 1993;85(5):365–76.

39. Sacks D, McClenny TE, Cardella JF, Lewis CA. Society of Interventional Radiology clinical practice guidelines. J Vasc Interv Radiol. 2003;14(9Pt 2):S199–202.

40. Ahmed M, Solbiati L, Brace CL, Breen DJ, Callstrom MR, Charboneau JW, et al. Image-guided tumor ablation: standardization of terminology and reporting criteria—a 10-year update. Radiology. 2014;273(1):241–60.

41. Ofosu A, Ramai D, Adler DG. Endoscopic ultrasound-guided ablation of pancreatic cystic neoplasms: ready for prime time? Ann Gastroenterol. 2019;32(1):39–45.

Lung Tumors Laser Ablation

12

2

Tian'an Jiang and Qiyu Zhao

12.1 Introduction

Lung cancer is one of the most common malignant tumors in the world. It is also the second most common cancer disagnoses by gender, after prostate cancer for men and beast cancer for women. Recent statistical data shows there were 1.8 million new cases and 1.6 million deaths globally in 2012. Among these new cases, a large portion of the increase occurs in developing countries [1–3]. Environmental exposures, behavior and genetic factors contribute mainly to tumor development. Additionally, lung is also the most common site of malignant metastases.

Surgery is the recommended treatment for patients with stage I–II non-small-cell lung cancer (NSCLC) and 5-year survival is over 56% [4, 5], but only about one-third of the patients were suitable for radical resection, and nearly 50% of the I-IIIA patients had recurrence within 5 years after resection. High-dose stereotactic body radiation therapy was also recommended for early stage NSCLC if surgical resection is not an option [6,

7]; however, it needs sophisticated planning and delivery technology. For patients with stage IB–IIIA disease, chemotherapy could benefit the survival rate [8, 9]. Surgical resection is determined by the tumor location and resectablility. Treatment for locally advanced NSCLC (stages III and IV) not suitable for surgical resection usually can take advantage of a combined thoracic radiotherapy with concurrent chemotherapy [10–13].

As most lung cancers are unresectable and benefits from radiotherapy and chemotherapy are limited, many new local treatments have emerged, including thermal ablation. Tumor thermal ablation is a minimally invasive procedure that delivering heat to tumor cells induce irreversible damage and coagulative necrosis. Thermal ablation methods include microwave ablation (MWA), radiofrequency ablation (RFA), cryoablation and laser ablation (LA). This treatment options have been proven to be safe and effective. Laser ablation is one of the treatment that not commonly used but many recent studies have demonstrated that image-guided laser ablation could benefit patients with primary lung cancer or unresectable pulmonary metastases [14–18].

12.2 Technique and Devices

Imaging guidance techniques for lung tumor laser ablation include CT, MRI and ultrasound. CT is the most commonly used. With T1-weighted

T. Jiang (✉)
Department of Ultrasound, First Affiliated Hospital, College of Medicine, Zhejiang University, Hangzhou, China
e-mail: tiananjiang@zju.edu.cn

Q. Zhao
Department of Ultrasound, The First Affiliated Hospital, College of Medicine, Zhejiang University, Hangzhou, China

© Springer Nature Switzerland AG 2020
C. M. Pacella et al. (eds.), *Image-guided Laser Ablation*,
https://doi.org/10.1007/978-3-030-21748-8_12

Fig. 12.1 A 64-year-old man with lung metastasis from sigmoid colon cancer. Axial unenhanced CT images revealed laser fibers ablating the tumor 1 cm outside the lesion (**a**) Before ablation; (**b**) After ablation (yellow arrows); (**c**) Axial CT image after treatment shows retraction of needles from the treatment site (yellow arrow); (**d**) Axial CT documents clear fibrosis and cavitation at the site of ablative treatment to confirm adequate ablation of the lesion (yellow arrow)

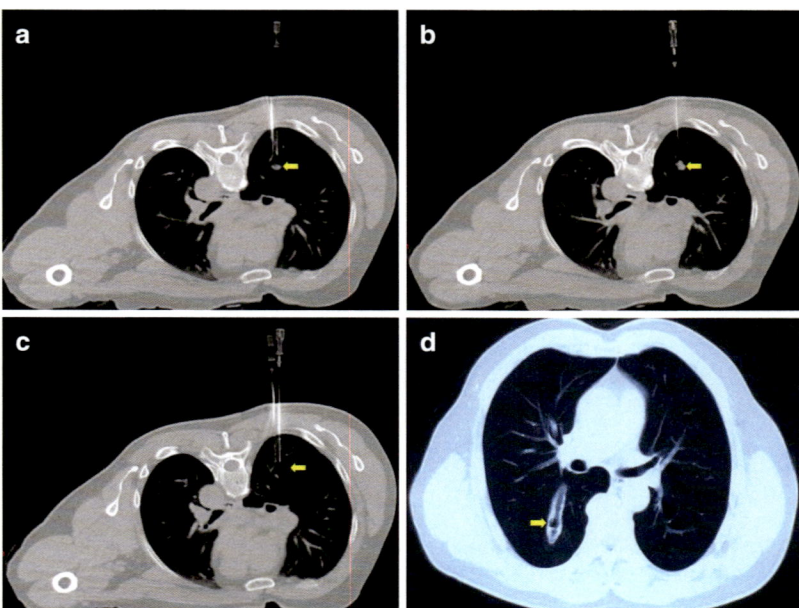

thermal sequences, changes in intratumoral temperature can be monitored by MRI during the procedure [19]. For tumors near or adherent to the chest wall, ultrasound guidance can be used if the tumor could be visualized and the whole picture could be observed with ultrasound [20].

Laser fiber is introduced into the lung by 21-gauge Chiba needle, which is thinner than RFA or MWA, so the LA manifests fewer side effects such as pneumothorax [14, 15, 18]. Local anesthesia with lidocaine 1% or mepivacaine hydrochloride 0.5% is used as well as intravenous injection of sedative and analgesic medication [21]. Under CT/MRI/US guidance, the interventional radiologist uses a 21-gauge Chiba needle (Top, Tokyo, Japan) into the lesion. After removing the mandrel from the needle, the laser fiber is inserted into the sheath, making sure that the bare fiber is out of about 0.5 cm. If the tumor size is not more than 1 cm, one or two laser fibers are used to ablate it. But for the tumor larger in size, three or four laser fibers are applied in parallel or crossed positions, each of which has output power of 3–5 W for 1800 J using a multisource semiconductor diode laser (EchoLaser, Elesta Srl, Florence, Italy) operating a wavelength of 1064 nm. The needle pullback technique in treating larger liver tumor

can also be used in large tumor of lung [14, 18]. Immediately after ablation, CT or MR scan will be performed to evaluate the ablation area. If there is residual vital tissue left unablated, an additional ablation maneuver can be carried out. Figures 12.1, 12.2, 12.3, 12.4, 12.5 and 12.6 are representative and significant examples of primary and secondary tumors treated by laser technique using one or more light sources, taking into account the site, the morphology and the size of the lesions. The legend of each case can help the reader to understand the laser methodology used.

12.3 Results

12.3.1 Lung Metastases Ablation

Lung is a common site of malignant metastases where 15% of colorectal carcinoma patients and 30–50% of other cancer patients develop pulmonary metastases [22]. The standard treatment is still metastasectomy that offers best disease-free survival [23]; however, only 20–30% of patients are suitable for surgical resection [24]; therefore, other treatments that can provide local tumor control and benefit survival have been increasingly

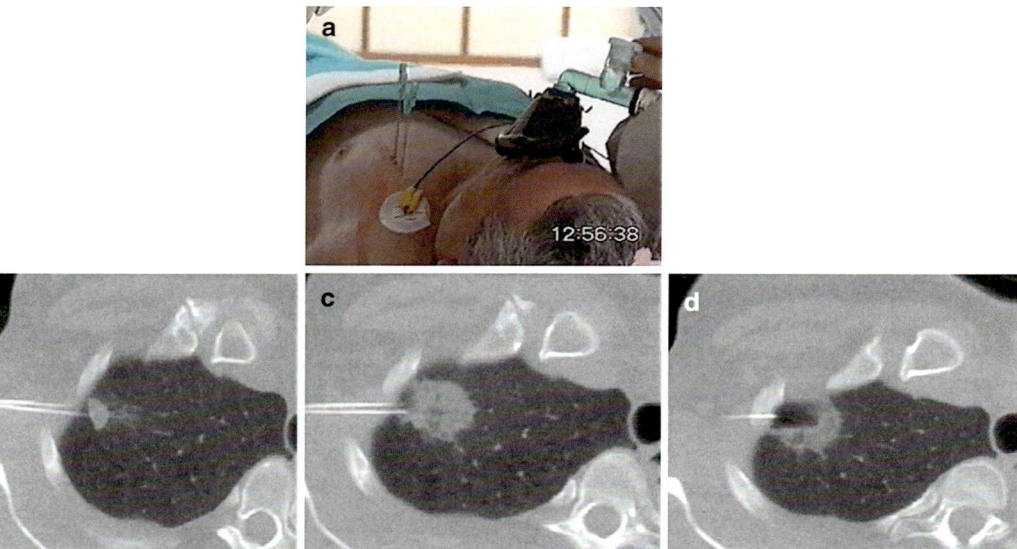

Fig. 12.2 Representative case of 65-year-old man with NSCLC with an axial diameter of 2.3 cm in the right upper lobe treated with LA. (**a**) Photo of the patient in the supine position inside the gantry of the CT device. The two needles used for the ablation maneuvers are clearly visible. (**b**) Axial CT image obtained before ablation shows the lesion in which two 21-gauge needles have been correctly positioned. (**c**) Axial CT image immediately after the end of treatment after fiber retraction shows a volumetric increase of the lesion surrounded by modest ground glass due to hyperemia and edema. (**d**)Axial CT image shows an area of cavitation within the lesion due to vaporization for coagulative necrosis (Courtesy of R. Regine, A. Cardarelli Hospital, Naples, Italy)

adopted. Image-guided tumor ablation enables direct destruction of solid neoplasms and allows for the control by using thermal energy. The advantages of tumor ablation in comparison with surgery include less damage of lung tissue, repeatability, less breathing impairment [25]. Some doctors using an miniaturized internally cooled applicator system diameter 5.5-French [26] connected to a 1064 nm Nd: YAG laser generator equipped with optional beam splitters [27] treated prospectively 108 lung metastatic nodules in 64 patients and achieved complete ablation in 31 out of 64 patients with 136 interventional procedures. The laser source setting can be used simultaneously or changed for each individual diffuser fibers. Local tumor control was 78% (85 of 108 tumors). Among the 31 patients (mean target diameter of 2.1 cm) who were treated completely or have undergone definitive ablative therapy, the 1-, 2-, 3-, 4- and 5-year survival rates after ablative therapy were 81, 59, 44, 44 and

27%, respectively. The median progression-free interval was 7.4 months. Pneumothorax in which periprocedural drainage was required occurred in 5% of all cases [17]. A retrospective study with 109 colorectal lung metastases patients treated by the thermal ablation showed that LA, RFA and MWA could be used as therapeutic options for lung metastases. The local tumor control was higher (88.3%) with MWA than RFA (69.2%) and LA (68.0%). No significant differences were detected in local progression and survival rates [28]. Studies have shown that three-year overall survival rate of RFA treating pulmonary metastases was nearly 50% against that (60%) with pulmonary metastasectomy [29]. Data from the two studies mentioned above correlate favorably both with survival rates after radiofrequency ablation and those of patients undergoing surgical resection for pulmonary metastases [30, 31]. However, RFA has a higher impedance in the lung, which means poor energy spreading,

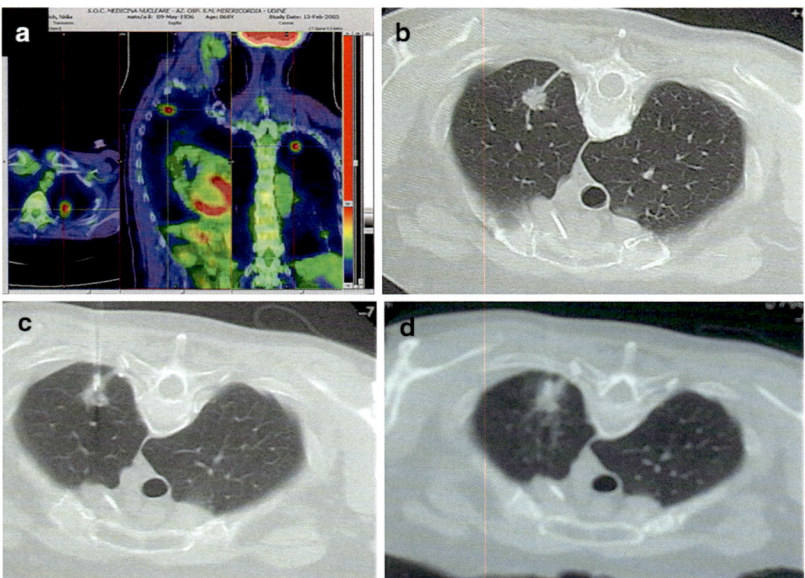

Fig. 12.3 Representative case of 55-year-old man with NSCLC located on the right upper lobe with an axial diameter of 2.5 cm. (**a**) Axial, sagittal and coronal positron tomographic image (CT-PET) clearly shows the intense metabolic activity in the lesion. (**b**) Axial CT image confirms the lesion in the posterior aspect of the right upper lobe. (**c**) Axial CT image shows two needles positioned correctly in the lesion before treatment with LA. (**d**) Axial CT obtained immediately after ablation. A modest swelling is visible with modest irregularity of the margins of the induced coagulation zone. The tumor was treated by delivering laser energy equal to 3600 J per needle (Courtesy of M. Sponza, Angiographic Diagnostics and Interventional Radiology, Integrated University Health Hospital of Udine, Italy)

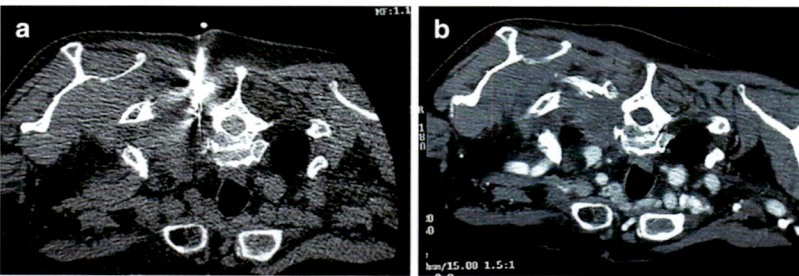

Fig. 12.4 Representative case of NSCLC nodule of 3.9 cm in maximum diameter located at the top of the lung in a 76-year-old patient. Pancoast's syndrome in patient with shoulder pain, arm pain and weakness in the hand. The first signs of ipsilateral Horner's syndrome were also present. Two applicators (**a**) spaced apart of 1.0 cm were placed and two treatments were performed using a pullback technique in the same session. A total of 7200 Js (1800 J per fiber) were deployed on the entire neoplastic tissue. (**b**) Axial CT image after laser treatment shows the nodule is avascular after administration of contrast medium. The patient had a marked improvement in symptoms for a duration of about 3 months. The case is a good example of how it is possible to obtain with a smaller number of sources (in this case, two) large areas of ablation using the pullback technique to deploy in the tumor an amount of energy equal to what would have occurred inserting four applicators in a square configuration spaced by 1.0 cm each from the other (Courtesy of R. Regine, A. Cardarelli Hospital, Naples, Italy)

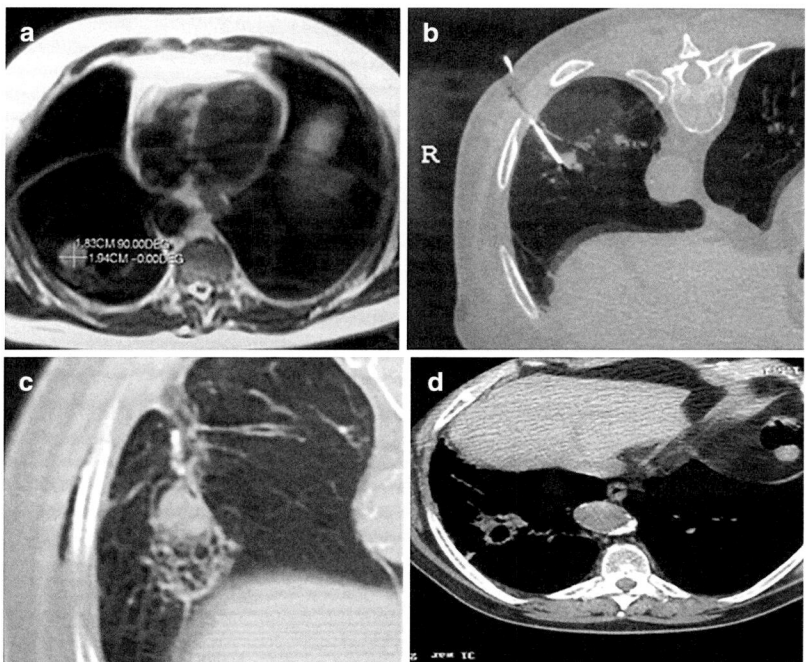

Fig. 12.5 55-year-old man with solitary pulmonary metastasis from colorectal carcinoma in right inferior lobe treated by LA. (**a**) Axial CT image obtained before laser ablation shows lung metastasis with axial diameter of 1.9 cm located in posterior aspect of inferior right lobe. (**b**) Axial CT image shows a thin needle within lesion. (**c**) Axial CT image obtained 12 h after ablation shows an ablation zone larger than basal lesion with a zone of ground-glass opacification surrounding lesion. (**d**) Axial CT image 12 months after ablation shows residual scarring in ablation bed with cavitation denoting complete eradication of lesion. 3600 J deployed using one applicator and pullback technique (Courtesy of R. Regine, A. Cardarelli Hospital, Naples, Italy)

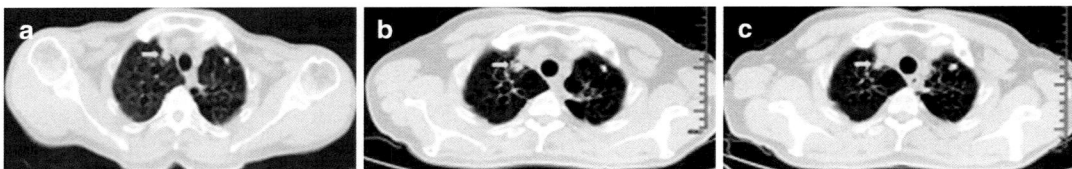

Fig. 12.6 Representative case of tumor adjacent to large blood vessels. (**a**) The axial CT scan shows before LA the lesion of 15.4 × 10.7 mm in diameter very close to the blood vessels of the neck (yellow arrow). The CT (**b**) and (**c**) images obtained 2 and 4 months after the LA show stationarity of the lesion (yellow arrows) without variations in size and morphological appearance, probably due to the absence of tumor vitality. No damage to the structures of the contiguous vessels is noticed

whereas LA with less impedance problems and lower cooling effects induces larger ablation volumes and more predictable coagulation zone than the RF due to the less influence of electrical conductivity in heat deposition [32]. The greatest advantage of LA is being able to perform under real-time guidance of MRI which allows monitoring increasing temperature in the ablated area, permitting evaluation of coagulation necrosis [21, 33].

LA has more advantages compared to other methods including the lower risk of bleeding, infection or injuries of adjacent organs, which means LA is able to destroy tumor directly while reducing the collateral damage to surrounding structures. Thus, LA is advisable for tumors adjacent to vital regions [16], like what happens in other organs that have particularly vulnerable vital structures such as the liver [34] and pancreas [35, 36]. The most common complications for thermal ablation are pneumothorax, bleeding, pleural effusion and subcutaneous emphysema. Pneumothorax occurred in 9.7% of lesions treated with LA, much less than that of MWA (30%) and RFA (17.3%). Subcutaneous emphysema also had a statistically significantly lower rate of occurrence after LA [28]. These complications are even rarer when using thin applicators with a caliper below the millimeter. Based on the data so far known in the literature on 28 patients with 33 nodules, of which 19 primary lung tumors and 15 metastatic nodules, treated with these thin devices and low wattage laser light, there were local side effects easily managed only in two cases (a slight self-limiting hemoptysis and a pleural empyema) and a single case of minimal pneumothorax in which no treatment was necessary. Only one case of small pneumothorax equal to 0.3% of the whole series in a patient suffering from severe pulmonary dysfunction with diffuse pulmonary bullae required chest drainage [14, 15, 18].

The Cardiovascular and Interventional Radiological Society of Europe (CIRSE) guidelines 2012 state that there is no specifically defined number of lesions for metastases palliative ablation [37]; however, most centers treat patients with five or fewer metastases. The guideline in China states that the metastases foci should be limited to ≤3 unilateral lung lesions (bilateral ≤5) for multiple metastases, with maximum diameters of ≤3 cm, or ≤5 cm for a unilateral single metastasis with no metastasis at any other site [38]. Multiple laser fibers were used parallelly for larger lesions, and the combination required less energy for focal ablation. For patients with bilateral pulmonary metastatic disease, bilateral simultaneous ablation is not rec-

ommended [39]. Some researchers believe that when thermal energy input is excessive, it might lead to malignant tumor recurrence and rapid expansion [39–41]. Therefore, in order to inactivate tumor, lower wattage and lower energy were used to produce better prognosis.

Contraindications for treatment include underlying interstitial disease, such as pulmonary fibrosis that may result in severe pulmonary failure and even death. Patients with severe respiratory disease, severe bleeding tendency, poorly controlled ipsilateral pleural malignant effusions, severe liver, kidney, heart, lung function insufficiency, severe anemia, severe dehydration or systemic infections, high fever that cannot be corrected or improved in the short term and a life expectancy estimated at <1 year are not considered good candidates for treatment [38, 42, 43]. Pneumothorax and pleural effusion are more common than parenchymal bleeding and hemoptysis [16].

12.3.2 Primary Lung Tumor Ablation

Worldwide, lung cancer is the most commonly diagnosed cancer (11.6% of the total cases) and the leading cause of cancer death (18.4% of the total cancer deaths) [44]. Due to the complexity of tumorigenesis, development and pathological pattern, the treatments of primary lung cancer now in use gain unsatisfied effectiveness. No matter what pathological type is, NSCLC or Small Cell Lung Cancer (SCLC), the main treatments are surgical resection, typically by lobectomy, radiotherapy, chemotherapy and targeted therapy [4]. Patients who come to our observation in conditions of advanced disease lose the opportunity to be treated with the available therapies even in the case of simple palliation. In other words, minimally invasive ablation techniques can obtain good local control and progression-free survival in patients with treatment-naïve T1 lung tumors, including patients with metachronous and synchronous tumors [45].

Hence, new way for palliative care that is safe, minimal invasive and stable has to be found. And new local lung tumor therapy comes, including resection under thoracoscopy, thermal ablation and cryoablation, which is made possible by technical advancements in computed tomography (CT) and ultrasound technology [46]. Thermal ablation modalities consisting of radiofrequency (RF), microwave and laser have the advantage of the selective damage to targeted tissue so that it can preserve the maximum of normal lung tissues in patients with poor lung function [47]. Radiofrequency ablation (RFA) and microwave ablation (MWA) have been considered as useful treatment options for patients with lung cancer who are not able to receive surgery [48]. Especially, an article about 566 patients showed that RFA illustrated a 53.7% 3-year, and a 44.1% 4-year control rate of lung metastatic disease [49]. Although large series researches suggested that laser ablation (LA), also called laser interstitial thermotherapy (LITT), has high efficacy of ablation compared to surgical resection in liver tumors, it is not widely used in primary lung tumors to date [16, 21, 50].

RFA uses electromagnetic energy deposition, utilizing energy sources typically from 375 to 500 KHz (less than 30 MHz) while MWA encompasses energy sources of a range from 30 MHz to 30 GHz [37, 51]. Laser ablation (LA) is performed by utilizing neodymium–yttrium aluminium garnet (Nd:YAG) laser fiber [52]. In contrast to RFA and MWA, LA has the advantages of lower cooling effect, absence of impedance problem, feasible induction of accurate ablated area, larger volumes and thermometry, yet it has the disadvantages of tissue carbonization [21]. And the laser fiber may have the smallest size so that the incidence of pneumothorax may decrease. Still, the most meaningful advantage of laser ablation is the real-time monitoring under MRI guidance [53].

Most often, laser is used in adjuvant therapeutic combinations under video-assisted thoracoscopic surgery, bronchoscope or CT: pre-treatment Nd:YAG-laser enables rapid removal of obstruction, symptom control and reduction of bleeding in mechanical removal [11, 54]. The reports reveal that temperature development during laser ablation is influenced by ventilation and

perfusion-mediated tissue cooling, and the same temperature reaches in both tumor tissue and normal one. They also proved that the use of two laser fibers increases the achieved temperatures and the coagulation size correlates with temperature positively [55–57].

Maybe one day, laser ablation can become a candidate for primary pulmonary malignancy treatment. Before that, further researches and more clinical trials are needed. In a word, current studies indicate that CT/MR/US-guided LA could be promising for the treatment of lung tumors. Furthermore, there are still the needs for more large-scale prospective studies to convince the use of multi-needle LA in large tumors in the future.

References

1. de Groot PM, Wu CC, Carter BW, Munden RF. The epidemiology of lung cancer. Trans Lung Cancer Res. 2018;7(3):220–33.
2. Siegel RL, Miller KD, Jemal A. Cancer statistics, 2018. CA Cancer J Clin. 2018;68(1):7–30.
3. Dela Cruz CS, Tanoue LT, Matthay RA. Lung cancer: epidemiology, etiology, and prevention. Clin Chest Med. 2011;32(4):605–44.
4. Vansteenkiste J, Crino L, Dooms C, Douillard JY, Faivre-Finn C, Lim E, et al. 2nd ESMO Consensus Conference on Lung Cancer: early-stage non-small-cell lung cancer consensus on diagnosis, treatment and follow-up. Ann Oncol. 2014;25(8): 1462–74.
5. Goldstraw P, Chansky K, Crowley J, Rami-Porta R, Asamura H, Eberhardt WE, et al. The IASLC lung cancer staging project: proposals for revision of the TNM stage groupings in the forthcoming (eighth) edition of the TNM classification for lung cancer. J Thorac Oncol. 2016;11(1):39–51.
6. Timmerman R, Paulus R, Galvin J, Michalski J, Straube W, Bradley J, et al. Stereotactic body radiation therapy for inoperable early stage lung cancer. JAMA. 2010;303(11):1070–6.
7. Fakiris AJ, McGarry RC, Yiannoutsos CT, Papiez L, Williams M, Henderson MA, et al. Stereotactic body radiation therapy for early-stage non-small-cell lung carcinoma: four-year results of a prospective phase II study. Int J Radiat Oncol Biol Phys. 2009;75(3):677–82.
8. Pignon JP, Tribodet H, Scagliotti GV, Douillard JY, Shepherd FA, Stephens RJ, et al. Lung adjuvant cisplatin evaluation: a pooled analysis by the LACE Collaborative Group. J Clin Oncol. 2008;26(21):3552–9.

9. NSCLC Meta-analysis Collaborative Group. Preoperative chemotherapy for non-small-cell lung cancer:a systematic review and meta-analysis of individualparticipant data. Lancet. 2014;383:1561–71.

10. Curran WJ Jr, Paulus R, Langer CJ, Komaki R, Lee JS, Hauser S, et al. Sequential vs. concurrent chemoradiation for stage III non-small cell lung cancer: randomized phase III trial RTOG 9410. J Natl Cancer Inst. 2011;103(19):1452–60.

11. Auperin A, Le Pechoux C, Rolland E, Curran WJ, Furuse K, Fournel P, et al. Meta-analysis of concomitant versus sequential radiochemotherapy in locally advanced non-small-cell lung cancer. J Clin Oncol. 2010;28(13):2181–90.

12. Govindan R, Page N, Morgensztern D, Read W, Tierney R, Vlahiotis A, et al. Changing epidemiology of small-cell lung cancer in the United States over the last 30 years: analysis of the surveillance, epidemiologic, and end results database. J Clin Oncol. 2006;24(28):4539–44.

13. Lemjabbar-Alaoui H, Hassan OU, Yang YW, Buchanan P. Lung cancer: Biology and treatment options. Biochim Biophys Acta. 2015;1856(2):189–210.

14. Sponza M, Aprile G, Gasparini D, Iaiza E, De Pauli F, Giovannoni M, et al. Percutaneous laser-induced thermoablation (LIT) of non-resectable lung metastases and primary lung tumors: A preliminary evaluation of technical aspects and local efficiency. ASCO Annual Meeting Proceedings (Post-Meeting Edition). J Clin Oncol. 2006;24:18S.

15. Regine R, Stavolo C, Maglione F. Laser thermoablation of smal pulmonary tumors : immediate and long-term follow-up CT features. In: C 23; First World Congress of ThoracicImaging and Diagnosis in Chest Disease. NaplesItaly: Pozzuoli; 2005.

16. Weigel C, Rosenberg C, Langner S, Frohlich CP, Hosten N. Laser ablation of lung metastases: results according to diameter and location. Eur Radiol. 2006;16(8):1769–78.

17. Rosenberg C, Puls R, Hegenscheid K, Kuehn J, Bollman T, Westerholt A, et al. Laser ablation of metastatic lesions of the lung: long-term outcome. AJR Am J Roentgenol. 2009;192(3):785–92.

18. Zhao Q, Tian G, Chen F, Zhong L, Jiang T. CT-guided percutaneous laser ablation of metastatic lung cancer: three cases report and literature review. Oncotarget. 2017;8(2):2187–96.

19. Vogl TJ, Fieguth HG, Eichler K, Straub R, Lehnert T, Zangos S, et al. Laser-induced thermotherapy of lung metastases and primary lung tumors. Radiologe. 2004;44(7):693–9.

20. Liu B, Ye X, Fan W, Li X, Feng W, Lu Q, et al. Expert Consensus for Image-guided Radiofrequency Ablation of Pulmonary Tumors (2018 Version). Zhongguo Fei Ai Za Zhi. 2018;21(2):76–88.

21. Vogl TJ, Naguib NN, Lehnert T, Nour-Eldin NE. Radiofrequency, microwave and laser ablation of pulmonary neoplasms: clinical studies and technical considerations--review article. Eur J Radiol. 2011;77(2):346–57.

22. Inoue M, Kotake Y, Nakagawa K, Fujiwara K, Fukuhara K, Yasumitsu T. Surgery for pulmonary metastases from colorectal carcinoma. Ann Thorac Surg. 2000;70(2):380–3.

23. RobinsonLA, RuckdeschelJC, WagnerH, Jr., StevensCW, American College of Chest P. Treatment of non-small cell lung cancer-stage IIIA: ACCP evidence-based clinical practice guidelines (2nd edition). Chest2007;132(3 Suppl):243S–265S.

24. Mazzone P. Preoperative evaluation of the lung resection candidate. Cleve Clin J Med. 2012;79(Electronic Suppl 1):eS17–22.

25. Hiraki T, Gobara H, Iguchi T, Fujiwara H, Matsui Y, Kanazawa S. Radiofrequency ablation as treatment for pulmonary metastasis of colorectal cancer. World J Gastroenterol. 2014;20(4):988–96.

26. Hosten N, Stier A, Weigel C, Kirsch M, Puls R, Nerger U, et al. Laser-induced thermotherapy (LITT) of lung metastases: description of a miniaturized applicator, optimization, and initial treatment of patients. Rofo. 2003;175(3):393–400.

27. Roggan A, Mesecke-von Rheinbaben I, Knappe V, Vogl T, Mack MG, Germer C, et al. Applicator development and irradiation planning in laser-induced thermotherapy (LITT). Biomed Tech (Berl). 1997;42(Suppl):332–3.

28. Vogl TJ, Eckert R, Naguib NN, Beeres M, Gruber-Rouh T, Nour-Eldin NA. Thermal Ablation of Colorectal Lung Metastases: Retrospective Comparison Among Laser-Induced Thermotherapy, Radiofrequency Ablation, and Microwave Ablation. AJR Am J Roentgenol. 2016;207(6):1340–9.

29. Kim HJ, Kye BH, Lee JI, Lee SC, Lee YS, Lee IK, et al. Surgical resection for lung metastases from colorectal cancer. J Kor Soc Coloproctol. 2010;26:354–8.

30. Pfannschmidt J, Muley T, Hoffmann H, Dienemann H. Prognostic factors and survival after complete resection of pulmonary metastases from colorectal carcinoma: experiences in 167 patients. J Thorac Cardiovasc Surg. 2003;126(3):732–9.

31. Yamakado K, Hase S, Matsuoka T, Tanigawa N, Nakatsuka A, Takaki H, et al. Radiofrequency ablation for the treatment of unresectable lung metastases in patients with colorectal cancer: a multicenter study in Japan. J Vasc Interv Radiol. 2007;18(3):393–8.

32. Knappe V, Mols A. Laser therapy of the lung: biophysical background. Radiologe. 2004;44(7):677–83.

33. Haemmerich D, Lee FT Jr. Multiple applicator approaches for radiofrequency and microwave ablation. Int J Hyperth. 2005;21(2):93–106.

34. Francica G, Petrolati A, Di Stasio E, Pacella S, Stasi R, Pacella CM. Effectiveness, safety, and local progression after percutaneous laser ablation for hepatocellular carcinoma nodules up to 4 cm are not affected by tumor location. AJR Am J Roentgenol. 2012;199(6):1393–401.

35. Di Matteo F, Picconi F, Martino M, Pandolfi M, Pacella CM, Schena E, et al. Endoscopic ultrasound-guided Nd:YAG laser ablation of recurrent pancre-

atic neuroendocrine tumor: a promising revolution? Endoscopy. 2014;46(Suppl 1 UCTN):E380–1.

36. Di Matteo FM, Saccomandi P, Martino M, Pandolfi M, Pizzicannella M, Balassone V, et al. Feasibility of EUS-guided Nd:YAG laser ablation of unresectable pancreatic adenocarcinoma. Gastrointest Endosc. 2018;88(1):168–74 e1.

37. Pereira PL, Masala S. Cardiovascular, Interventional Radiological Society of E. Standards of practice: guidelines for thermal ablation of primary and secondary lung tumors. Cardiovasc Intervent Radiol. 2012;35(2):247–54.

38. Ye X, Fan WJ, Chen JH, Feng WJ, Gu S, Han Y, et al. Chinese expert consensus workshop report: Guidelines for thermal ablation of primary and metastatic lung tumors. Thoracic Cancer. 2015;6:112–21.

39. Dong S, Kong J, Kong F, Kong J, Gao J, Ke S, et al. Insufficient radiofrequency ablation promotes epithelial-mesenchymal transition of hepatocellular carcinoma cells through Akt and ERK signaling pathways. J Transl Med. 2013;11:273.

40. Brunello F, Carucci P, Gaia S, Rolle E, Brunocilla PR, Castiglione A, et al. Local tumor progression of hepatocellular carcinoma after microwave percutaneous ablation: a preliminary report. Gastroenterology Res. 2012;5(1):28–32.

41. Ohno T, Kawano K, Yokoyama H, Tahara K, Sasaki A, Aramaki M, et al. Microwave coagulation therapy accelerates growth of cancer in rat liver. J Hepatol. 2002;36(6):774–9.

42. Dupuy DE, Mayo-Smith WW, Abbott GF, DiPetrillo T. Clinical applications of radio-frequency tumor ablation in the thorax. Radiographics. 2002;22 Spec No:S259–69.

43. McTaggart RA, Dupuy DE, Dipetrillo T. Image guided ablation in the thorax. In: Geschwind J-FH SM, editor. Interventional oncology: principles and practice. New York, NY: Cambridge University Press; 2008. p. 440–74.

44. Bray F, Ferlay J, Soerjomataram I, Siegel RL, Torre LA, Jemal A. Global cancer statistics 2018: GLOBOCAN estimates of incidence and mortality worldwide for 36 cancers in 185 countries. CA Cancer J Clin. 2018;68(6):394–424.

45. Ridge CA, Silk M, Petre EN, Erinjeri JP, Alago W, Downey RJ, et al. Radiofrequency ablation of T1 lung carcinoma: comparison of outcomes for first primary, metachronous, and synchronous lung tumors. J Vasc Interv Radiol. 2014;25(7):989–96.

46. Dempsey PJ, Ridge CA, Solomon SB. Advances in interventional oncology: lung cancer. Cancer J. 2016;22(6):393–400.

47. Vogl TJ, Helmberger TK, Mack MG, Reiser MFE. Percutaneous tumor ablation in medical radiology. Berlin: Springer-Verlag; 2008.

48. Donington J, Ferguson M, Mazzone P, Handy J Jr, Schuchert M, Fernando H, et al. American College of Chest Physicians and Society of Thoracic Surgeons consensus statement for evaluation and management for high-risk patients with stage I non-small cell lung cancer. Chest. 2012;142(6):1620–35.

49. de Baere T, Auperin A, Deschamps F, Chevallier P, Gaubert Y, Boige V, et al. Radiofrequency ablation is a valid treatment option for lung metastases: experience in 566 patients with 1037 metastases. Ann Oncol. 2015;26(5):987–91.

50. Vogl TJ, Straub R, Eichler K, Sollner O, Mack MG. Colorectal carcinoma metastases in liver: laser-induced interstitial thermotherapy--local tumor control rate and survival data. Radiology. 2004;230(2):450–8.

51. Goldberg SN, Grassi CJ, Cardella JF, Charboneau JW, Dodd GD 3rd, Dupuy DE, et al. Image-guided tumor ablation: standardization of terminology and reporting criteria. J Vasc Interv Radiol. 2005;16(6): 765–78.

52. Dupuy DE. Image-guided thermal ablation of lung malignancies. Radiology. 2011;260(3):633–55.

53. Okuma T, Matsuoka T, Tutumi S, Nakmura K, Inoue Y. Air embolism during needle placement for CT-guided radiofrequency ablation of an unresectable metastatic lung lesion. J Vasc Interv Radiol. 2007;18(12):1592–4.

54. Bolliger CT. Multimodality treatment of advanced pulmonary malignancies. In: Interventional bronchoscopy, vol. 30. Basel: Karger Publishers; 2000. p. 187–96.

55. Vietze A, Koch F, Laskowski U, Linder A, Hosten N. Measurement of ventilation- and perfusion-mediated cooling during laser ablation in ex vivo human lung tumors. Eur J Radiol. 2011;80(2): 569–72.

56. Hoffmann CO, Rosenberg C, Linder A, Hosten N. Residual tumor after laser ablation of human non-small-cell lung cancer demonstrated by ex vivo staining: correlation with invasive temperature measurements. MAGMA. 2012;25(1):63–74.

57. Koch F, Vietze A, Laskowski U, Ritter C, Linder A, Hosten N. Ex-vivo human lung tumor model: use for temperature measurements during thermal ablation of NSCLC. In: RöFo-Fortschritte auf dem Gebiet der Röntgenstrahlen und der bildgebenden Verfahren, vol. 183, No. 03. New York: Georg Thieme; 2011. p. 251–9.

Benign Prostatic Hyperplasia and Prostate Cancer Laser Ablation

Claudio Maurizio Pacella, Giovanni Mauri, Guglielmo Manenti, Tommaso Perretta, and Gianluigi Patelli

13.1 Benign Prostatic Hyperplasia

13.1.1 Background

The search for new minimally invasive therapies (MIT) for the treatment of bothersome symptoms of the lower urinary tract from benign prostatic hyperplasia (LUTS/BPH) arises from the need to offer an effective and long-lasting alternative cure to many patients who do not tolerate adverse events of medical care and that do not experience the improvements expected from their use, while they often suffer from complications related to the prolonged use of these expensive drugs. In addition, patients, particularly those with mild-to-moderate symptoms, choose to observe symptom development or follow medical care over time. These medical strategies with alpha-blockers or 5-alpha-reductase inhibitors or their combination often do not give good results and a part of them eventually require more invasive surgical treatments [1, 2]. Finally, in the population that suffers from these disorders there are some individuals who do not want to run the risks of potential complications related to invasive surgical procedures [3].

Bladder outlet obstruction (BOO) is a common condition affecting with different severity 70% of the male population between 60 and 69 years and 80% of those aged 80 years or older [4]. In this population approximately 70% of men with LUTS/BPH exhibit coexisting erectile dysfunction (ED) whose prevalence ranges from 35% to 95% and increases with the severity of LUTS [5]. The aim of any therapy is to reduce benign prostatic obstruction (BPO) and at the same time minimize complications and adverse events related to simple (open) prostatectomy, when applied to large adenoma, and transurethral resection of the prostate (TURP) [3, 6]. This latter is associated with a small but significant risk, with a 30-day mortality of 0.3% and a variety of morbidities including transurethral resection syndrome (1%) which is related to the absorption of irrigating fluid leading to confusion and collapse, hemorrhage during the operation (transfusion rate of 5%), and subsequent urinary tract infection [7, 8]. On the other hand, transurethral therapies that use lasers such as holmium laser and current GreenLight laser-photo-selective

C. M. Pacella (✉)
Department of Diagnostic Imaging and Interventional Radiology, Regina Apostolorum Hospital, Albano Laziale, Rome, Italy

G. Mauri
Division of Interventional Radiology, European Institute of Oncology, IRCCS, Milan, Italy

G. Manenti · T. Perretta
Department of Diagnostic Imaging and Interventional Radiology, Tor Vergata University, Rome, Italy

G. Patelli
Department of Diagnostic and Interventional Radiology, Pesenti-Fenaroli Hospital-ASST Bergamoest, Alzano Lombardo, Italy

© Springer Nature Switzerland AG 2020
C. M. Pacella et al. (eds.), *Image-guided Laser Ablation*,
https://doi.org/10.1007/978-3-030-21748-8_13

vaporization (PVP), offered as alternatives to TURP, have some not negligible limits. In particular, there have not been long-term comparative data nor direct comparisons and for now they cannot be a suitable technique for the general urologist [9, 10].

The flourishing of minimally invasive surgical therapies (MIST) arises also from the need to offer options personalized based on patients and pathological factors [11]. The available armamentarium of these therapies today includes thermal therapies such as conductive transurethral needle ablation of the prostate (TUNA) [12, 13], transurethral microwave thermotherapy (TUMT) [14], mechanical therapies such as prostatic urethral lift (PUL) [15, 16], intraoperative stents [17], intraoperative injection [18–21], and many other emerging therapies such as convective radiofrequency thermal therapy (CRTT) [22], prostatic artery embolization (PAE) [23, 24], aquablation [25, 26], and histotripsy [27]. Some of these are in decline, others remain experimental, and others seem to provide promising results.

13.1.2 Historical Notes

About minimally invasive therapies that used laser energy, the first report, originally described in 1984, on the treatment with Nd:YAG laser of the prostate tissue involved the ablation of the residual tissue after the TURP debulking of a localized prostate carcinoma [28]. One year later, the first clinical experience with ten patients with prostate cancer was reported using an end-fire Nd:YAG laser in a contact modality [29]. Soon after, promising results of experimental studies on dog prostate were reported using a noncontact laser under US guidance in real time (TULIP) [30–32]. The problems analyzed by these studies consider both the improvement of the clinical symptomatology and the rate of flow [33]. The goal of interstitial treatment, according to the authors, was to induce intraprostatic coagulation. The absorption of the coagulated tissue decompresses the intraprostatic part of the urethra with consequent improvement of the LUTS [34]. In most of these works the approach was transure-

thral and only in some cases perineal [35–37]. In detail, in the most cited work, maneuvers were performed in the majority of cases transurethrally under direct vision of a cystoscope or percutaneously from the perineum under transrectal ultrasound guidance. As the urethra remains intact, in this latter case with percutaneous approach, no sloughing of tissue takes place. The treatment regimen consisted of doing a few punctures with constant power (10 W) for defined periods or more short punctures at powers from 20 W to 7 W in three separate steps. On average, 6.2 (2–15) fiber placement was done with 21,700 (2400–48,000) J of energy applied. The caliber of the applicators used was 1.9 mm. Significant complications were rare; most patients suffered from transient irritative symptoms, with 4% of patients suffering from strictures and 7% retrograde ejaculation. 9.6% of patients required retreatment during 12 months of follow-up. Twelve out of hundred twenty-seven patients with prostate smaller than 60 cc and with a pronounced median bar were additionally treated with transurethral incision of the bladder neck or prostate (TUIP) using a bare laser fiber in tissue contact at a 40 W power setting [34]. Finally, only in some cases the postoperative evaluation of the coagulation area was performed with magnetic resonance imaging (MRI) able of depicting the effects induced by laser therapy in various tissues [35]. From what has been said, it must be deduced that these interesting experiences show a very complex technique that is not easy to practice and requires a long learning period and have non-negligible complications. This approach deserves attention but must be simplified.

Hence in the feasibility study recently published the authors adopt the perineal approach for the percutaneous treatment of BPH patients using multi-fiber laser technology. Thanks to the experience gained in the debulking of benign thyroid nodules [38], the authors applied the same strategy for the debulking of the prostatic lobes, improving the symptomatology of patients affected by LUTS/BPH. The characteristics of the technology with thin introducers (less than 1 mm) make the transperineal approach safe and relatively easy.

13.1.3 Treatment Strategy

The inclusion criteria are as follows [39]: briefly (a) if male subject >50 years of age who have symptomatic BPH; (b) International Prostate Symptom Score (IPSS) score ≥13; (c) prostate volume ≥30 mL on transrectal ultrasonographic (TRUS) images; (d) peak urinary flow rate (Qmax): ≥5 to ≤15 mL/s; and (e) post-void residual (PVR) ≥50 mL. Exclusion criteria were as follows: (a) urethral stricture; (b) previous prostate bladder neck, or urethral surgery; (c) prostate cancer or patients who had a prostate-specific antigen (PSA) value greater than 4 ng/mL; and (d) patients with known neurological disorders, e.g., multiple sclerosis, Parkinson's disease, or known history of spinal cord injury. The use of anticoagulants or indwelling urinary catheters for urinary retention was not a criterion for exclusion. There are no morphological contraindications for use of this thermal therapy procedure in subjects with an intravesical median lobe or hyperplasia of the central zone. Preoperative evaluation included assessment of the following parameters: IPSS, quality-of-life score (QoL), Q_{max}, PVR, ultrasound examination of the prostate, and PSA blood testing. Obviously, all patients signed a dedicated informed consent.

The primary end points of this study were technical success, safety of transperineal percutaneous laser ablation (TPLA), and change in IPSS. The technical success was defined following the standard terminology adopted for tumor ablation [40]. Secondary end points were Qol, Qmax, PVR, and prostatic volume at the end of follow-up. Secondary judgment criteria included operative parameters including laser data (duration, joules, number of fibers used), adverse events during the procedure and within 24 h after the maneuver (periprocedural period), hospital stay, and duration of the catheterization. A postoperative visit was scheduled at 6, 12, and 24 months for evaluation of efficacy and delayed complications. The definition of complications was consistent with the standardized terminology and reporting criteria for image-guided tumor ablation proposed by other authors [41] and with the classification of surgical complications according to the modified Clavien system [3].

13.1.4 Technique

The patient is positioned in the radiological intervention suite in a urological position. A three-way Foley 18-F catheter is inserted with continuous irrigation of a saline solution during and after the maneuver. The technique has already been explicitly explained elsewhere in the first feasibility study [39]. In practice it consists of positioning under ultrasound guidance up to four applicators (one to two per lobe) consisting of a 21-gauge Chiba needle as introducer in whose lumen is inserted a bare optical fiber of quartz of 300 µm until it protrudes by 10 mm from the tip of the thin introducer. In the case of volumes less than or equal to 40 mL, a single applicator per lobe can be inserted while in the case of a prostate with a volume greater than 40 mL two applicators per lobe are used. It should be emphasized that since the technique allows to customize the treatment based on the volume of the lobes, in the case of volumetric asymmetry of the lobes it is possible to position a number of different introducers within the two lobes. In other words, it is possible to insert three introducers in the largest lobe and only one in the smallest lobe or even none if not necessary. The tip of the fiber should be placed 8–10 mm away from the outer wall of the urethra, 15 mm from the bottom of the bladder, and 10 mm from the outer edge of the prostate capsule. The position of the applicators must be carefully controlled using a biplanar ultrasound. In the case of two applicators, these must be positioned one after the other at a mutual distance of 8–10 mm. More generally, applicators must be positioned along a path that is as parallel as possible to the longitudinal plane of the prostate (Figs. 13.1 and 13.2). The access route is transperineal, hence the acronym TPLA which stands for transperineal laser ablation and underlines the extra-urethral approach to induced laser ablation. Each treatment is performed with patient under conscious sedation by IV of midazolam (2–3 mg) and with local anesthesia of the superficial tissues of the perineal region and prostate anesthesia by transrectal prostatic block or transperineally—to reduce

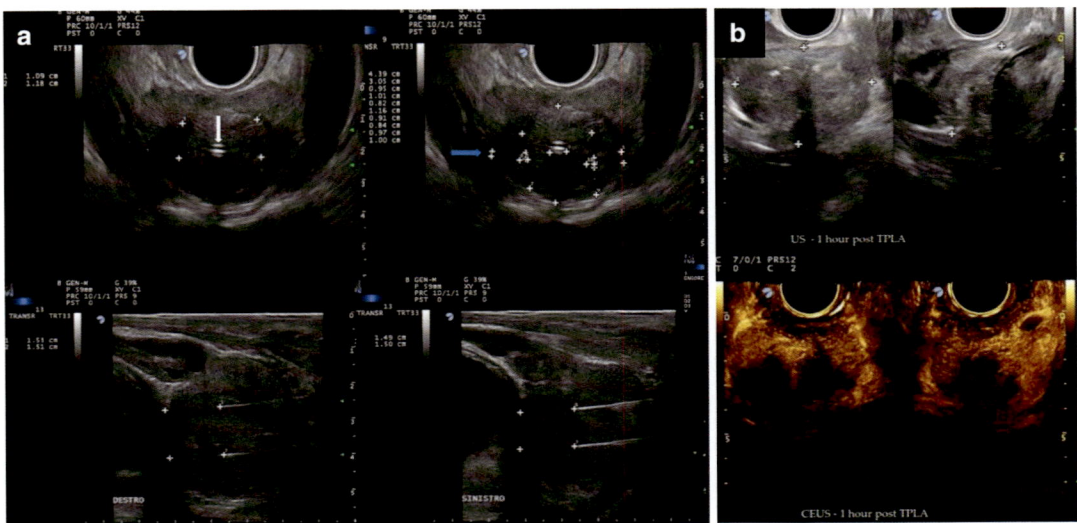

Fig. 13.1 Representative case of 61-year-old patient with a prostatic hyperplasia of 48 mL at baseline. (**a**). At the top axial TRUS images show the preliminary study to correctly position the heat sources at the safe distance from the urethral canal *(white arrow)* and from the capsule *(blue arrow)* before the treatment of LA. At the bottom the longitudinal TRUS images show the thin devices rightly spaced about 10 mm from each other at the correct distance from the prostatic capsule. (**b**). At the top from left to right the axial and longitudinal images of the gland 1 h after the treatment of LA. At the bottom, during the US study with ecocontrast, there are two areas of lack of enhancement due to the absence of vascularization in the coagulation zones

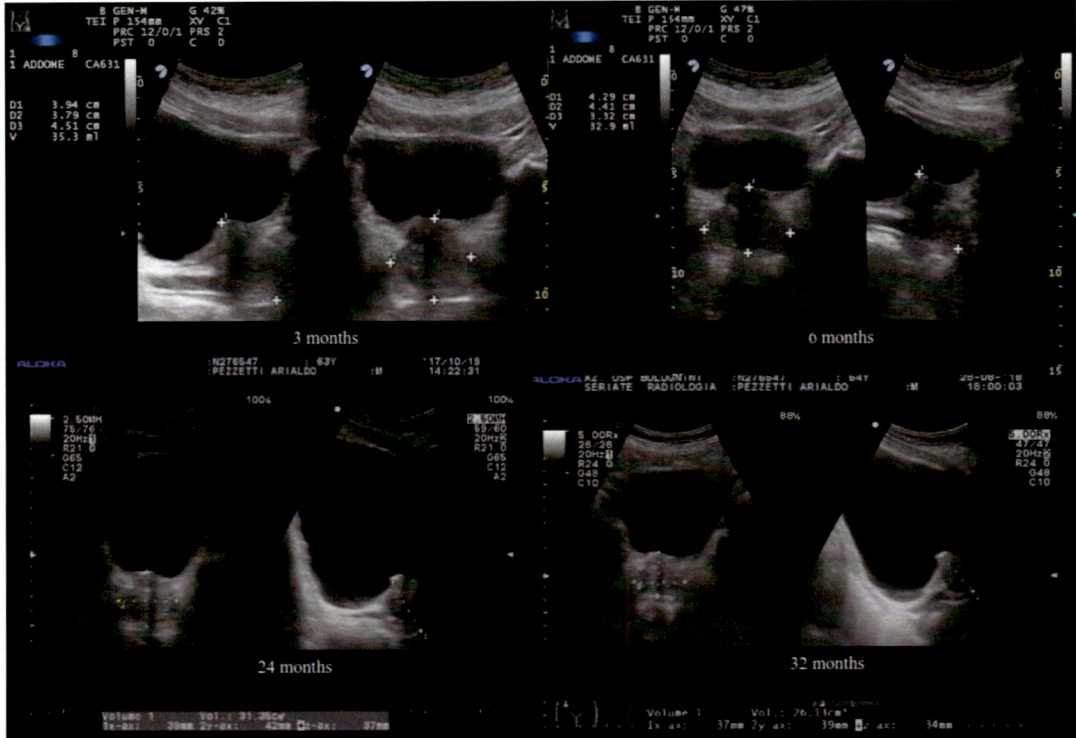

Fig. 13.2 Changes in prostate volume of the patient shown in Fig. 13.1 at 3, 6, 24, and 32 months after TPLA. To confirm the excellent durability of the laser ablation technique, all US axial and longitudinal images clearly show the progressive and marked reduction in prostate volume over time. The volumetric data confirm the persistence over time of the improvements induced by the percutaneous ablation maneuver

with this last choice the risk of infections—with lidocaine solution 2% (20 mL). This last maneuver has not always been followed by some operators who have started using this method to treat patients with LUTS/BPH in the light of the fact that the patients tolerate the maneuver well even without the anesthesia of the transrectal prostatic block.

As already mentioned above we have adopted a low-power laser and therefore each treatment is performed at a fixed power of 3 W changing the illumination time case by case according to prostate size. Depending on the size of the prostate, one to two consecutive illuminations are performed with a "pullback" technique during the same treatment session. The treatment ends when 1800 joules are reached for a single lighting or 3600 joules for two illuminations after the pullback. So the time needed to release these energies amounts to 600–1200 s. It is necessary to underline that, whatever the given condition, it is necessary to administer at least 1400 joules per single fiber per treatment to obtain a significant coagulation zone. At the end of the treatment based on the patient's clinical condition, anti-edema and anti-inflammatory drugs may be administered. After an observation period of about 1 h, the patient undergoes transrectal ultrasonography with the administration of an echo-amplifier contrast agent to evaluate the extent of the coagulation zone. For this specific problem we think in the future to use MRI imaging to get more detailed information on the effective extension of the ablated area as the use of ultrasound contrast gives us a rough information about the actual area of coagulation. The patient is kept in the hospital for 1–2 days and the catheter, in the absence of adverse events, was removed within 1 or 2 weeks after the procedure, taking into account the clinical condition of the patient, especially those with a history of long urinary retention and who have been holding urinary catheters permanently for a long time before treatment (see also paragraph 13.1.5 immediately following). The transperineal laser ablation is performed by the interventional radiology and urology team using the combined EchoLaser system (Elesta s.r.l. 50,041, Calenzano (FI), Italy).

13.1.5 Results

The following are the preliminary clinical data of the feasibility study on the first 18 patients treated with TPLA, while the medium-term results are ongoing evaluated on 81 patients with a mean follow-up of 16 months (range 3–45). At 3 months from treatment the mean IPSS score improved from 21.9 ± 6.2 to 10.7 ± 4.7, $p < 0.001$. Mean pre- and 3 months posttreatment QoL scores were 4.7 ± 0.6 and 2.1 ± 1.2, $p < 0.001$. Mean pre- and posttreatment Qmax (ml/s) scores were 7.6 ± 2.7 and 13.3 ± 76.2, $p < 0.001$. Mean pre- and posttreatment PVR (mL) scores were 199.9 ± 147.3 to 81.5 ± 97.8, $p < 0.001$. At 3 months from treatment the mean prostatic volume improved from 69.8 ± 39.9 to $54.8 \pm 29.8 \pm 29.8$, $p < 0.001$. Therefore, the improvements in percentage for the IPSS, QoL, Qmax, and prostatic volume were 47.0 ± 29.3, 54.5 ± 28.9, 82.5 ± 69.3, and 18.8 ± 17.1, respectively.

Procedural outcomes were (a) ablation time(s) 15.9 ± 3.9, (b) procedural time (min) 43.3 ± 8.7, (c) hospitalization time (days) 1.5 ± 0.4, and (d) catheterization time (days) 17.3 ± 10.0. The average volume of the ablated area was equal to 10.3 ± 3.6. So, the changes with the TPLA in IPSS, Qol, Qmax, and PVR scores were -11.2 points, -2.6 points, $+5.7$ mL/s, and -137.0 cc, respectively (Table 13.1).

These data demonstrate a significant improvement in all parameters at 3 months from treatment compared to baseline values. Only the reduction in prostate volume seems less significant than all other values, although statistically significant. The reactive process at the ablative insult occurs slowly with consequent slow reduction of the volume of the adenoma. In other words, TPLA is not an immediate ablative technique. Thus, the shrinking process is slow but progressive over time (Figs. 13.3 and 13.4). It is important that the volumetric improvement, accompanied by the improvement of all the other parameters, persists over time, proving a valid durability of the technique (Table 13.2). The long period of catheterization must be ascribed to the fact that in the feasibility study, the most complex patients unsuitable for surgery were carriers of bladder catheters for a long time before treatment with TPLA. In other words, many, if

Table 13.1 Data of the scores of the various technologies reported in the literature

Parameter	TPLA	Aquablation	CRTT	HoLEP[a]	TuVEP	PVP	TURP[a]	TURP[b]
IPSS	−11.2 pts	−16.6 pts	−11.5 pts	−21.2 pts	−18.7 pts	−13.2 pts	−10,3 pts	−15.4
QoL	−2.6 pts	−2.7 pts	−2.1 pts	−3.0 pts	−3,3 pts	–	−2.8 pts	−3.3
Qmax	+5.7 mL/s	+10.8 mL/s	+6.4 mL/s	+15.8 mL/s	+22.4 mL/s	+6.1 mL/s	+10.6 mL/s	+8.9 mL/s
PVR	−118.4 cc	−72 cc	−10.6 cc	−113.5	−162 cc	−76 cc	−126.7 cc	−64.0 cc

TPLA Transperineal percutaneous laser ablation, *CRTT* convective radiofrequency thermal therapy, *HoLEP* holmium laser, *TuVEP* thulium laser vapo-enucleation, *PVP* GreenLight laser photo-selective vaporization, *TURP* transurethral resection, *IPSS* International Prostate Symptoms Score, *QoL* quality of life, *Qmax* peak urinary flow, *PVR* post-void residual urine volume, *pts.* points
[a]Ref. [40]
[b]Ref. [42]

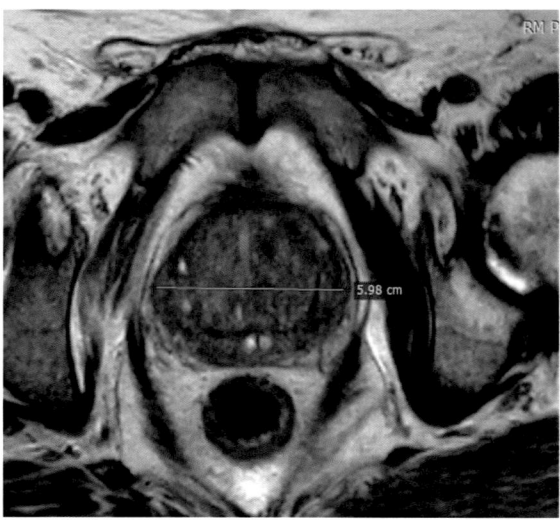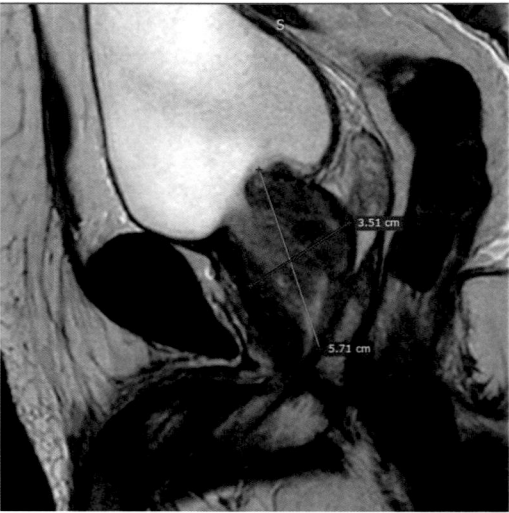

Fig. 13.3 Axial and sagittal T2-weighted MR images (TR/TE 5660/104; FA 160°) obtained before percutaneous transperineal laser ablation in an 81-year-old man with benign prostatic hyperplasia (BPH) and LUTS with a maximum transverse diameter of 5.98 cm and maximum sagittal diameter of 3.51 cm (prostate volume 119.6 mL)

not the majority, of this initial group of patients have kept, for their particular clinical conditions, the indwelling catheter for long periods of time before the ablation maneuver and therefore with strongly hypotonic bladder walls that obviously take a long time to get back to having a good wall contraction and efficient emptying. This drawback forces the operator to maintain the catheter in the bladder for longer at the patient's request, which senses burning and/or difficulty in urination in the absence of a catheter. However, some researchers believed that this therapeutic strategy was unnecessary and excessively conservative and suggested removing the catheter at the end of the procedure. According to these authors the modalities of the maneuver do not justify this therapeutic choice. To confirm this hypothesis, there are excellent results recently reported by some operators who removed the catheter at the end of the ablative maneuver in many of their patients without the latter complaining of adverse effects.

In our view, with TPLA in expert hands it is relatively easy to perform and control the various phases of the maneuver. The constant monitoring in real time of the treatment thanks to the low density of applied energy allows to avoid damages to the adjacent structures. By using the transperineal route, the bare laser flexible fibers can be placed directly within prostatic tissue keeping a safe distance from urethra and from bladder floor. Thus it is possible to induce a true debulking of prostatic lobes with a subsequent reduction in volume over time with no block to the urethral cavity and/or damage to urethral wall. In addition, this laser treat-

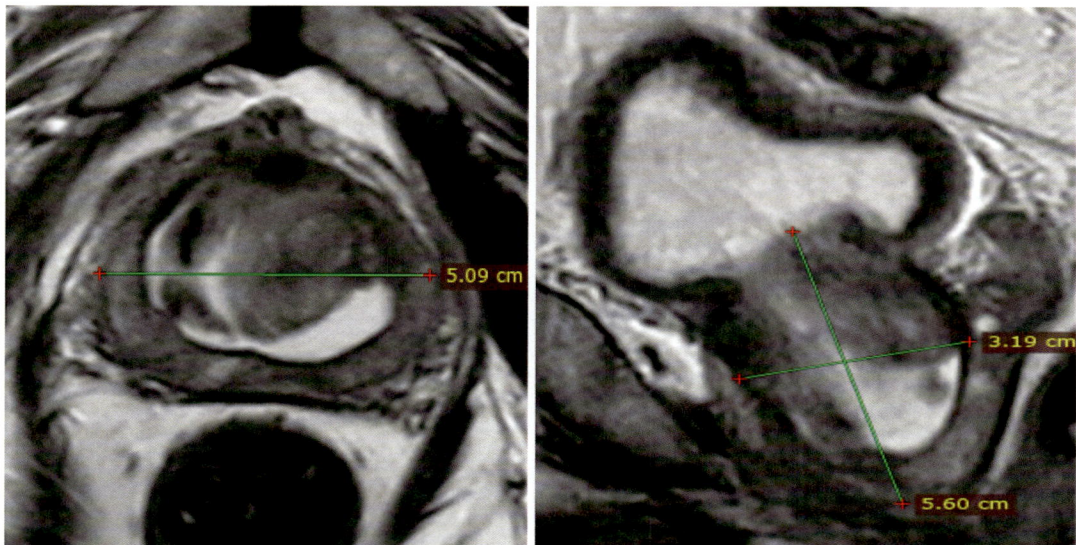

Fig. 13.4 Axial and sagittal T2-weighted MR images (TR/TE, 5660/104; flip angle 160°) at 1-month follow-up show a slight volume reduction (prostate volume 94.6 mL) but huge adenoma coagulative necrosis

Table 13.2 Changes over time of the 61-year-old patient's clinical parameters with a prostate volume of 48 mL at baseline shown in Figs. 13.1 and 13.2

P.A. (61 years)	Pretreatment	6 months	12 months	24 months	32 months
Prostatic volume	48 mL	35 mL	32 mL	31 mL	26 mL
Post-voiding residue	180	83	70 mL	100	88 mL
Qmax	8	13	15	14	9
IPSS score	32	3	4	4	1
QoL score	6	1	0	0	0

ment can be performed under conscious sedation and with local anesthesia during inpatient regimen.

13.1.6 Comparison of Technologies

Given that a comparison of data of the feasibility study mentioned above with those available in the literature cannot provide us with reliable conclusions, a knowledge of the most salient data of the various technologies operating in the clinical arena can enlighten us on their actual role and help us to choose the most suitable for a personalized treatment of patients who require our curative intervention. Some considerations are possible. The values of scores of TPLA at 3 months compare favorably with data reported with emerging technologies such as aquablation [26] and convective radiofrequency thermal therapy (CRTT) [22]. Comparisons are equally favorable with other methods such as HoLEP, PVP [42–44], and

thulium laser vapo-enucleation (ThuVEP) [45]. In the double-blind randomized controlled trial of Gilling, the IPSS, Qol, Qmax, and PVR scores of the TURP at 3 months were −15.4 points, −3.3 points, + 8.9 mL/s, and −64.0 cc [46]. The scores at 3 months of the IPSS, QoL, and post-void residual volume reported by Whelan in his prospective study were −13.2 points, +6.1 mL/s, and −76.0 cc for the PVP, and −13.9 points, +7.0 mLs, and −25 cc for the TURP [47] (see Table 13.1).

No severe complications were reported for TPLA. So far, the most frequent complaint reported by patients has been the sensation of irritating emptying for the reasons described above, which lasted for a period of about 14–15 days. With the precaution of continuously irrigating with cold saline solution the Foley catheter the times of this disorder have halved. No cases of intraoperative hemorrhage requiring transfusions, gross hematuria posttreatment, acute urinary retention, incontinence, acute urinary tract infection, urethral stricture, bladder neck contracture, bladder neck stenosis, surgical intervention for bleeding, capsular perforation, and erectile dysfunction have been reported. Over the years all the complications listed above have been reported with different incidences in the different methodologies. The various known complications occur in all techniques, but for grade 2–5 Clavien-Dindo event the trend in results is in favor of laser techniques compared to more strict surgical techniques such as TURP or simple (open) prostatectomy [7, 22, 43, 44, 46–51]. The preservation of sexual function is a key determinant in the surgical pathway for patients with LUTS secondary to BPH, especially in younger men. It is noteworthy that patients treated with HoLEP or TURP had a retrograde ejaculation in over 70% [7, 52] of cases and incontinence rate approximately 1–2% [53].

Finally, a brief mention deserves the technique of embolization of the prostatic artery (PAE) [54]. This technique has had a continuous evolution over the years and many single-arm studies have shown its efficacy and safety; however the amount of RCT data are limited and the few published comparisons with the TURP do not provide conclusive data [55, 56]. There are no studies that demonstrate the durability of the improvements induced by the PAE. It can be said that the technique appears to be complex, long, and relatively expensive, and requires the work of experienced interventional radiologists. In addition, it requires further technological advances, such as the type and size of the embolic material, and the development of an optimal technique to prevent the embolic flow to nontarget organs through PA anastomoses. In conclusion, the TPLA technique has good clinical results favorably comparable both with the more established techniques such as PVP, HoLEP, and TURP and with emerging techniques such as aquablation and CRTT in the absence of serious complications.

13.1.7 Final Considerations

Urologists around the world are constantly looking for the "gold standard" treatment for BPH. Recently, there has been a wave of new techniques such as holmium laser transurethral of the prostate (HoLEP) or thulium laser enucleation of the prostate (ThuLEP) that are replacing the GreenLight laser photo-selective vapo-enucleation (PVP) of the prostate and the bipolar TURP and its various modifications. These techniques based on various types of lasers have made great strides in their development from evaporation to enucleation techniques and various combinations. Urologists are constantly striving to acquire new skills to perform prostatectomy by laser enucleation rather than resorting to traditional TURP. The morcellation machines and their accessories helped the surgeons to achieve enucleation even in large prostates. Therefore every innovation in this field must be compared with the current operating trends.

The rise in MIT procedures represents a paradigm shift in the treatment of BPH. The aim of achieving a personalized medicine approach has led to the use of these "middle-ground" therapies that lie between medical therapy and invasive surgical intervention. The MIT group is varied and continually growing in its range of options based on patient and pathological factors. As the evidence for their utility is gathered, many of the MIT options remain experimental or without a robust evidence base. MIT should be used in a select patient group, particularly those that place importance on preserved sexual and continence function rather than urinary improvement. More mature data will help to identify the role of MIT in the evolving treatment pathway of BPH. In our view, our technique could be used profitably in younger patients even before medical treatment and in older patients who have significant comorbidities. It should be offered to patients with intermediate age in case of refusal of traditional surgery. In any case, among the possible customized choices, TPLA could have a crucial role.

13.2 Prostate Cancer

13.2.1 Epidemiology and History

Prostate cancer (PCa) is the most commonly diagnosed cancer and the second cause of cancer-related deaths for men in 2017 [57]. Prevalence in an autopsy study showed a PCa prevalence of 5% in persons at age <30 years, increasing to 59% by age >79 years [58]. Thanks to screening with PSA, development of new prostate biopsy protocols, and widespread use of magnetic resonance imaging for diagnostic purposes (multiparametric MRI and PIRADS scoring system), we have witnessed an increase in the accuracy of detection and localization [59]. As a result, today an ever-increasing number of small and low-grade cancer foci (index lesion as clinically relevant disease) are discovered in healthy young men. Radical treatments for prostate cancer such as surgery and radiotherapy involve the entire gland and are associated with urinary and sexual dysfunction. Therefore, for patients with very small, localized, and low-grade tumors, meaning grade group I (Gleason score ≤6—only individual discrete well-formed glands) and II (Gleason score 3 + 4—predominantly well-formed glands with a lesser component of poorly formed/fused/cribriform glands) [60], these treatments represent unnecessary overtreatment with undesirable secondary effects on their quality of life [61].

Today, 94% of low-risk cancers are treated with radical treatment [62]. In 2009, the European Randomized Study of Screening for Prostate Cancer (ERSPC) confirmed a substantial PCa mortality reduction due to PSA testing, with a substantially increased absolute effect at 13 years compared to findings after 9 and 11 years. So, a gain of survival of 27% among screened men aged 55–69 was demonstrated, with an average follow-up of 9 years after diagnosis. But this gain of survival was associated with a high rate of overdiagnosis and overtreatment [63]. Overdiagnosis occurs in approximately 40% of the screen-detected cases resulting in a high risk of overtreatment with unavoidable adverse effects. More generally, it should be remembered that for every individual saved, the number of people who receive a diagnosis of prostate cancer and therefore an irrelevant treatment on the duration of life, which negatively affects the quality of life itself, is not negligible. For example, the ERSPC study estimated that, for every life saved thanks to the early diagnosis of prostate cancer by the PSA, another 26 men discover that they have cancer and are therefore treated, suffering the undesirable effects of the therapies, for a disease, accidentally discovered through screening, which did not have time to manifest during their lifetime [63].

Prostate cancer does not induce symptoms in the early stages. Only in the later stages with a more advanced disease symptoms may be present. The PCa risk classification is based on a combination of digital rectal (DRE), PSA, and Gleason biopsy results. Gleason score is a parameter for aggression or tumor assessment. Gleason 3 is the lightest form and Gleason 5 is the most aggressive. The Gleason score is determined by adding the two most common variants. Low-risk tumors are not palpable or involve only half of a lobe or less, with a PSA of <10 ng/mL and a Gleason score of 3 + 3 = 6. Above all, these tumors have been found as a result of PSA test. When the tumors are palpable on the DRE, the Gleason score is higher or the PSA is >10 ng/mL, so a tumor is at intermediate or high risk (see Tables 13.3 and 13.4).

Table 13.3 Overview of the prostate cancer risk stratification

Low-risk	Intermediate-risk	High-risk	
PSA <10 ng/mL and GS <7 (ISUP grade 1)	PSA 10–20 ng/mL or GS 7 (ISUP grade2/3)	PSA >20 ng/mL or GS >7 (ISUP grade 4/5)	Any PSA any GS Any ISUP grade
Localized			**Locally advanced**

PSA Prostate-specific antigen, *GS* Gleason score, *ISUP* International Society of Urological Pathology (ISUP) Grading of Prostate Cancer

Table 13.4 Comparison ISUP *vs.* Gleason score

Risk group	ISUP grade group	Gleason score
Low	Grade group 1	Gleason score ≤6
Intermediate favorable	Grade group 2	Gleason score 7 (3 + 4)
Intermediate unfavorable	Grade group 3	Gleason score 7 (4 + 3)
High	Grade group 4	Gleason score 8
High	Grade group 5	Gleason score 9–10

ISUP International Society of Urological Pathology (ISUP) Grading of Prostate Cancer, *GS* Gleason score

13.2.2 Treatment Options

Radical treatment options with curative intent are surgery or radiotherapy and are indicated for intermediate- and high-risk tumors. According to the guidelines, the validated radical therapies are radical prostatectomy (RP) and radiotherapy as external beam radiotherapy and internal radiotherapy (brachytherapy) [58]. All radical treatments have side effects. When nerves are damaged during RP, the side effects induce incontinence and erectile dysfunction. Radiation therapy can also lead to late side effects, such as the effects of radiation that occur after years. The indication for a radical treatment in a larger disease with a higher risk is clear. When a small component of Gleason 4 is detected with the biopsy examination a radical treatment is formally indicated according to the guidelines. The side effects of radical treatment in these cases can be drastic.

Radical treatment in low-risk patients, as we have repeatedly stressed, involves overtreatment as many PCa, as the clinical history of these patients has revealed to us, will not develop clinically significant cancers. Therefore, active surveillance (AS) was introduced. AS is a regimen of regular PSA checks and prostate biopsies. The intent of this approach is to detect the progression of the disease and discover it in this way at an early stage where radical treatment could still be an option

for the good results that can be achieved with this choice. During the period of AS, the patient will therefore not experience the side effects of radical treatment and will enjoy a good quality of life. But regular follow-ups and biopsies are needed that can equally affect the quality of life of these subjects. This strategy can induce important psychological stress for patients, and it is often difficult for doctors to propose this management option to young men with long-term prospects.

For all these reasons and to offer the patient with localized and low-risk tumor therapy that is able to destroy the tumor without causing the unwanted side effects of radical therapies, there is the idea of a so-called focal therapy, a concept borrowed from what is at the base of minimally invasive therapies widely accepted in the therapy of local tumors in many other organs. The challenge of focal therapy is therefore to treat only the localized tumors (indexed lesion relevant in mp-MRI with a PIRADS score ≥4) [64] sparing the rest of the prostate minimizing its potential morbidity (Figs. 13.5 and 13.6). To be effective, focal therapy must be (1) guided by imaging, possibly MRI (to define the exact position of the cancer area and real-time treatment monitoring); (2) able to target only the desired area (dosimetric planning); and (3) followed by the surveillance of the untreated areas.

13.2.3 Focal Treatment

Focal treatments have been developed as treatment options with reduced side effects in case of low-volume localized disease. Several focal treatment techniques with different energy sources have been developed. None of the techniques has been proven to have sufficient efficacy to be a standard treatment according to the guidelines [58]. However, high-intensity focused US (HIFU), cryotherapy, and focal photodynamic therapy are techniques with sufficient data for an initial judgement [58]. Other techniques as irreversible electroporation, radiofrequency abla-

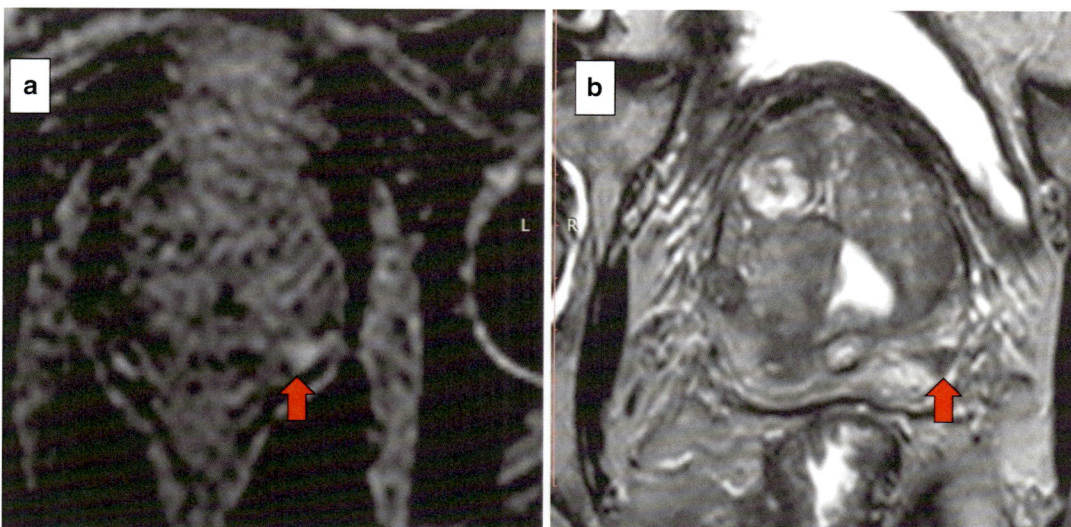

Fig. 13.5 3 T MR images before percutaneous transperineal laser ablation in a 76-year-old man with histopathologically proved prostate cancer (GS 3 + 4). Tumor is located in left peripheral para-basal zone (triangular). (**a**) Axial dynamic contrast-enhanced MR image (36/1.41; FA 14°; temporal resolution, 3.5 s). (**b**) Axial T2-weighted (TR/TE, 5660/104 ms; FA 160°)

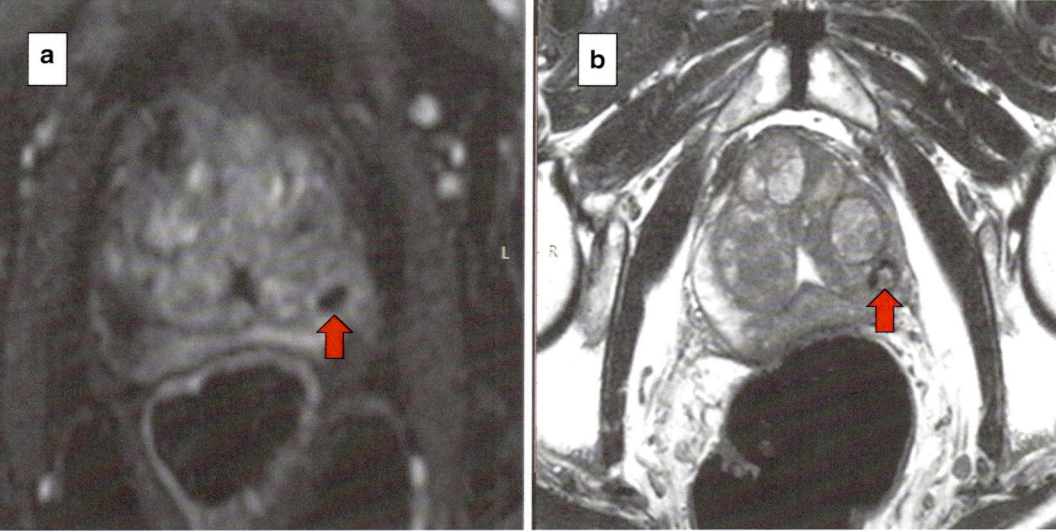

Fig. 13.6 3 T MR images at 1-month follow-up. (**a**) Axial dynamic contrast-enhanced MR image (TR/TE, 36/1.41; FA 14°; temporal resolution, 3.5 s) demonstrates no enhancement in the treated area. (**b**) Axial T2-weighted MR image (TR/TE, 5660/104; FA 160°) ablation cavity

tion, and laser ablation are in earlier development stages. All techniques have in common that they aim to provide equal oncological outcomes with reduced side effects and improved functional outcomes when compared to standard radical therapies [58, 65].

13.2.4 Historical Notes

The first feasibility study was performed on a canine model with a Nd:YAG laser (1064 nm). The author documented an area of well-demarcated coagulative necrosis around the laser fiber that was replaced by a necrotic cavity within a few days due to an enzymatic denaturing process of the tissue [66]. The first clinical application of focal laser ablation (FLA) was performed by Amin for local recurrence of a prostatic carcinoma after external radiotherapy. The procedure was performed under intravenous sedation with 805 nm diode laser. The approach was performed transperineally using 18-gauge needles under US guidance and subsequent CT scan control. The cooling of the bladder and urethra was performed using a continuous perfusion saline solution with triple-lumen urinary catheter. The procedure was well tolerated by the patient with hospital discharge 24 h after treatment. A nonenhancing zone corresponding to the ablated area was visible in the 10-day CT scan. The 3-month biopsy control confirmed the presence of coagulation necrosis in the treated area and tumor cells in the untreated area. A second laser treatment was performed without particular side effects [67]. At that time, the development of the technique was limited by the accuracy to localize the tumor areas in the preoperative evaluation, computer dosimetric planning, and follow-up images.

Numerous preclinical studies followed on canine and rat models *in vivo* and *ex vivo* with laser sources with variable wavelengths from 830 to 980 nm and using different powers and exposure times [68–72]. They all used magnetic resonance imaging to position the fibers in prostate tissue with sufficient accuracy and to assess the extent of necrosis in times varying at 1, 4, 48, and 72 h after treatment. The various studies have verified the correlation rate between planning and histopathologic findings. Thus, a significant difference between the volume of visible necrosis after 1 h and 48 h after FLA could be verified in MRI. The data is explained by the existence of noncoagulated degenerative zone surrounding the coagulative necrosis zone in the acute phase, which develops coagulative necrosis after 48 h. Histopathologic findings were in agreement with cellular damage planning.

Thermometric MR studies described in a phantom prostate have enabled the implementation of FLA under ultrasound, CT, or MRI. The MR thermometry was validated with this model by temperature measure correlation obtained by fluoroptic thermometry [73]. Studies on cadaveric model with MRI thermometry and damage planning have allowed to conclude that MRI real-time thermometry and transperineal fiber guidance through a template are technically feasible [74].

The macroscopic appearance of the FLA coagulation areas corresponds to well-demarcated foci of necrosis surrounded by a small ring of hemorrhage with nonviable glandular tissue after vital staining based on immunoreactivity with cytokeratin [72, 75].

13.2.5 Focal Laser Ablation (FLA)

Focal laser ablation has been investigated with two devices and setups. The Indigo laser system has been developed for treatment of benign prostatic obstruction [76]. Several studies have used the system with a transperineal approach for treatment of PCa [77–80]. Some authors positioned the fiber under 3D MRI reconstruction using a transperineal approach and used the transrectal CEUS immediately after the FLA procedure and treated the vascularized vital residual tissue with another session by placing another fiber [79]. More recently, the system with 17-gauge cooled devices has been used in phase 1 and 2 PCa treatment studies [81, 82]. This system can be applied in-bore with MRI guidance, as it has initially been developed for treatment of brain tumors and works with a wavelength of 980 nm. Therefore, the first PCa studies with the abovementioned system applied FLA in-bore. As the procedure is time consuming, out-of-bore application with MRI-ultrasound fusion has also been investigated [83]. Advantages of FLA focus on localized treatment with reduced side effects as important structures are undamaged [84]. The aim is to spare nearby structures as neurovascular bundles, preserving continence and erectile function. Furthermore, studies show that RP performed after FLA was not more difficult to perform [81]. Thus, radical treatment options are still possible after FLA.

PCa is localized in the peripheral zone, close to the rectum. When FLA is applied and it would extend outside the prostate, the rectal wall could be damaged. Therefore, temperature of vital structures is measured in-bore with MRI sequences or with temperature probes to prevent them from damage [84, 85]. Furthermore, targeting the tumor is a challenge in itself. The system mentioned above uses in-bore tumor localization [85]. The process of correct localization can be time consuming and thus results in a long in-bore time of 2.5–4 h with 4.3 min of treatment time [85]. This makes in-bore treatment expensive, as MRI is an expensive technique. Therefore, the option of MRI-ultrasound fusion has been investigated [78, 83]. This would reduce the costs and improve the ease of application as materials can contain metal (see Appendix).

Also, PCa is visible as a round lesion on MRI most of the time. As FLA produces round lesions this would be ideal. However, studies show that there is still PCa present in follow-up biopsies after treatment [78, 82]. A study that compared MRI imaging and histopathology showed an underestimation of the tumor volume [86]. An ablation volume with a margin of 9 mm around the MRI lesion would achieve complete tumor destruction in their computer-simulated treatment model. In addition, it is suggested that PCa grows in a more dendritic pattern. This could possibly explain the number of positive biopsies at the border of the treatment area in follow-up [84]. In addition to this, a study that performed partial tumor ablation with FLA showed increased mitotic activity (tumor activity) in the border of the ablation zone [81]. This confirms the need for radical tumor ablation. Combining these outcomes, ablation volume increase is needed, shifting towards hemi-ablation [82, 84]. However, the system has only one fiber with the need for fiber replacement to create a larger ablation zone and subsequent longer treatment time (see Appendix).

The EchoLaser system allows the neoplastic tissue to be treated simultaneously with four fibers. This increases the treatment area and allows a more extended treatment area. Furthermore, the laser source settings can be changed per fiber. This makes it possible to model the ablation zone in relation to the site, the shape, and the volume of the lesion. The system uses a 1064 nm wavelength while all recent studies used laser sources with a 980 nm wavelength. Therefore, the first step is the assessment of complete cell death in the ablation zone of a single fiber and in multifiber configurations. Actually ongoing trials are based on three-step protocol. First diagnostic step is based on the use of 3 T multiparametric MRI in order to identify the presence and extension of the index lesion that is biopsied in-bore by using a CAD system. Grade group I and II focal lesion, localized ≥ 1 cm from urethra and bladder neck, undergoes laser ablation with single or double illumination, as reported in the BPH laser ablation protocol. mp-MRI follow-up is at 1, 3, 6, and 12–24 months.

Appendix: Pre- and Postoperative Imaging Diagnostic Techniques

Multiparametric Magnetic Resonance Imaging for Prostate Cancer

Magnetic resonance imaging (MRI) is a scanning method that makes use of a strong magnetic field, radio waves, and dedicated computer software to show detailed images of organs and tissues in the body. The employment of different pulse sequences, or parameters, during the MRI examination helps in highlighting specific differences between healthy and unhealthy tissue. When two or more parameters are used, it goes under the name of multiparametric MRI (mpMRI).

Prostate multiparametric MRI documents gland anatomy and any pathologic process within and around it. Four parameters are routinely used in prostate cancer detection, each highlighting different tissue features. T2-weighted sequence (T2 MRI) yields a multiplanar (3D) map of prostate zone anatomy; a suspicious-looking area is referred to as a region of interest (ROI). Diffusion-weighted imaging (DWI MRI) shows movement of water molecules within a given tissue; cancer cells restrict the motion more than normal cells do, which shows up in DWI MRI.

Dynamic contrast-enhanced imaging (DCE MRI) reveals pathologic blood flow. Prostate cancer develops its own blood vessels, which look abnormal. When injected, the contrast agent is quickly taken up by those aberrant vessels, then washes out, and is later excreted in urine. As well, the pace of the uptake/washout yields additional information about the nature of the neoplasm.

Spectroscopy (MRI-S) may be added as a fourth parameter. When prostate cancer is present, its survival is maintained through certain chemical processes (metabolism) that are distinct from normal cell metabolism. MRI-S gives metabolic information useful in confirming prostate cancer [87, 88].

Multiparametric MRI of the prostate is the imaging of choice for men with rising or abnormally high PSA, a previous negative biopsy with recent increase in prostate-specific antigen (PSA) levels, or the presence of additional findings warranting its use in non-biopsied patients. This exam is also used as active surveillance in patients with proven cancer that do not require therapy at the time.

Prostate mpMRI can rule in or out a biopsy in people already treated for cancer, as mpMRI can confirm therapy success and monitor for disease recurrence outside the treatment area. Malignancy risk assessment of a prostatic lesion detected with magnetic resonance imaging is made using an image-based risk reporting system called Prostate Imaging Reporting and Data System (PI-RADS™v.2) (American college of radiology. MR prostate imaging reporting and data system version 2.0 [internet] Available from: Http://www.Acr.Org/quality-safety/resources/pirads/ [cited 2015 jun 16]). PIRADS v.2 allows for data obtained from the aforementioned MRI parameters to be collected jointly in a unique score; after all imaging sequences are evaluated and a score is given for each, those are combined resulting in a final outcome between 1 and 5 for the suspected lesion.

Prostate Biopsy Techniques

Currently, there are three different MRI-guided biopsy techniques available: MRI-ultrasound fusion, MRI-MRI fusion ("in-bore" biopsy), and cognitive fusion.

The MRI-US fusion biopsy enables the operator to merge the images obtained from the prostatic mpMRI where the index lesion was identified, performed beforehand, and then stored on the device, with real-time US imaging by means of a special 3D software. As the US probe is advanced via a transrectal approach, the fusion software shifts the MRI image accordingly, guiding needle positioning; this allows for better visualization of the lesion and higher procedural accuracy, as many trials have shown [89, 90]. Additionally, needle location in the 3D space can be tracked and recorded for future reference. As a new application of the technique, the MRI-US fusion may gain interest as a guidance tool for selective focal ablation of prostate cancer.

In MRI-MRI fusion ("in-bore" biopsy) the procedure is performed directly in the MRI suite as real-time imaging is obtained during biopsy execution.

The cognitive fusion is an easy-to-use technique simply based on the review, by the biopsy operator, of a previously acquired MRI to help guiding needle positioning under TRUS guidance.

Overall, high-resolution mpMRI of the prostate safely provides all the information needed in order to take the best next step decision in the setting of a neoplastic lesion. Furthermore, it is used to guide precision focal treatments such as focal laser ablation [91].

References

1. Roehrborn CG. Current medical therapies for men with lower urinary tract symptoms and benign prostatic hyperplasia: achievements and limitations. Rev Urol. 2008;10(1):14–25.
2. Roehrborn CG. Combination medical therapy for lower urinary tract symptoms and benign prostatic hyperplasia. Rev Urol. 2005;7(Suppl 8):S43–51.
3. Dindo D, Demartines N, Clavien PA. Classification of surgical complications: a new proposal with evaluation in a cohort of 6336 patients and results of a survey. Ann Surg. 2004;240(2):205–13.
4. Parsons JK. Benign prostatic hyperplasia and male lower urinary tract symptoms: epidemiology and risk factors. Curr Bladder Dysfunct Rep. 2010;5(4):212–8.

5. Rosen RC, Wei JT, Althof SE, Seftel AD, Miner M, Perelman MA, et al. Association of sexual dysfunction with lower urinary tract symptoms of BPH and BPH medical therapies: results from the BPH Registry. Urology. 2009;73(3):562–6.
6. Oelke M, Bachmann A, Descazeaud A, Emberton M, Gravas S, Michel MC, et al. EAU guidelines on the treatment and follow-up of non-neurogenic male lower urinary tract symptoms including benign prostatic obstruction. Eur Urol. 2013;64(1):118–40.
7. Rassweiler J, Teber D, Kuntz R, Hofmann R. Complications of transurethral resection of the prostate (TURP)-incidence, management, and prevention. Eur Urol. 2006;50(5):969–79; discussion 80.
8. Ow D, Papa N, Perera M, Liodakis P, Sengupta S, Clarke S, et al. Trends in the surgical treatment of benign prostatic hyperplasia in a tertiary hospital. ANZ J Surg. 2018;88(1–2):95–9.
9. Cornu JN, Ahyai S, Bachmann A, de la Rosette J, Gilling P, Gratzke C, et al. A Systematic review and meta-analysis of functional outcomes and complications following transurethral procedures for lower urinary tract symptoms resulting from benign prostatic obstruction: an update. Eur Urol. 2015;67(6):1066–96.
10. Robert G, Cornu JN, Fourmarier M, Saussine C, Descazeaud A, Azzouzi AR, et al. Multicentre prospective evaluation of the learning curve of holmium laser enucleation of the prostate (HoLEP). BJU Int. 2016;117(3):495–9.
11. Yu X, Elliott SP, Wilt TJ, McBean AM. Practice patterns in benign prostatic hyperplasia surgical therapy: the dramatic increase in minimally invasive technologies. J Urol. 2008;180(1):241–5; discussion 5.
12. Benoist N, Bigot P, Colombel P, Amie F, Haringanji C, Chautard D, et al. Tuna: clinical retrospective study addressing mid-term outcomes. Prog Urol. 2009;19(1):54–9.
13. Niţă G, Persu C. Radiofrequency ablation in the treatment of benign prostatic hyperplasia (TUNA). In: Handbook E, editor. Endoscopic diagnosis and treatment in prostate pathology. Cambridge, MA: Academic Press; 2016. p. 149–54.
14. Malaeb BS, Yu X, McBean AM, Elliott SP. National trends in surgical therapy for benign prostatic hyperplasia in the United States (2000–2008). Urology. 2012;79(5):1111–6.
15. Perera M, Roberts MJ, Doi SA, Bolton D. Prostatic urethral lift improves urinary symptoms and flow while preserving sexual function for men with benign prostatic hyperplasia: a systematic review and meta-analysis. Eur Urol. 2015;67(4):704–13.
16. Roehrborn CG, Rukstalis DB, Barkin J, Gange SN, Shore ND, Giddens JL, et al. Three year results of the prostatic urethral L.I.F.T. study. Can J Urol. 2015;22(3):7772–82.
17. Yildiz G, Bahouth Z, Halachmi S, Meyer G, Nativ O, Moskovitz B. Allium TPS-a new prostatic stent for the treatment of patients with benign prostatic obstruction: the first report. J Endourol. 2016;30(3):319–22.
18. El-Husseiny T, Buchholz N. Transurethral ethanol ablation of the prostate for symptomatic benign prostatic hyperplasia: long-term follow-up. J Endourol. 2011;25(3):477–80.
19. Shore N, Cowan B. The potential for NX-1207 in benign prostatic hyperplasia: an update for clinicians. Ther Adv Chronic Dis. 2011;2(6):377–83.
20. Elhilali MM, Pommerville P, Yocum RC, Merchant R, Roehrborn CG, Denmeade SR. Prospective, randomized, double-blind, vehicle controlled, multicenter phase IIb clinical trial of the pore forming protein PRX302 for targeted treatment of symptomatic benign prostatic hyperplasia. J Urol. 2013;189(4):1421–6.
21. Marberger M, Chartier-Kastler E, Egerdie B, Lee KS, Grosse J, Bugarin D, et al. A randomized double-blind placebo-controlled phase 2 dose-ranging study of onabotulinumtoxinA in men with benign prostatic hyperplasia. Eur Urol. 2013;63(3):496–503.
22. McVary KT, Roehrborn CG. Three-year outcomes of the prospective, randomized controlled rezum system study: convective radiofrequency thermal therapy for treatment of lower urinary tract symptoms due to benign prostatic hyperplasia. Urology. 2018;111:1–9.
23. Schreuder SM, Scholtens AE, Reekers JA, Bipat S. The role of prostatic arterial embolization in patients with benign prostatic hyperplasia: a systematic review. Cardiovasc Intervent Radiol. 2014;37(5):1198–219.
24. Pisco J, Bilhim T, Costa NV, Ribeiro MP, Fernandes L, Oliveira AG. Safety and efficacy of prostatic artery chemoembolization for prostate cancer-initial experience. J Vasc Interv Radiol. 2018;29(3):298–305.
25. Yassaie O, Silverman JA, Gilling PJ. Aquablation of the prostate for symptomatic benign prostatic hyperplasia: early results. Curr Urol Rep. 2017;18(12):91.
26. Gilling P, Reuther R, Kahokehr A, Fraundorfer M. Aquablation—image-guided robot-assisted water-jet ablation of the prostate: initial clinical experience. BJU Int. 2016;117(6):923–9.
27. Roberts WW. Development and translation of histotripsy: current status and future directions. Curr Opin Urol. 2014;24(1):104–10.
28. Sander S, Beisland HO. Laser in the treatment of localized prostatic carcinoma. J Urol. 1984;132(2):280–1.
29. Shanberg AM, Tansey LA, Baghdassarian R. The use of the neodymium YAG laser in prostatectomy. J Urol. 1985:133.
30. Kandel LB, Harrison LH, McCullogh DL, et al. Transurethral laser prostatectomy: creation of a technique for using the neodymium: yttrium aluminium garnet laser in the canine model. J Urol. 1986:135.
31. Roth RA, Aretz HT. Transurethral ultrasound-guided laser-induced prostatectomy (TULIP procedure): a canine prostate feasibility study. J Urol. 1991;146(4):1128–35.
32. Roth RA, Aretz TH, Lage AL. TULIP Transurethral laser induced prostatectomy under ultrasound guidance. J Urol. 1991:146, 1128–1135.
33. McCullough DL, Roth RA, Babayan RK, Gordon JO, Reese JH, Crawford ED, et al. Transurethral ultrasound-guided laser-induced prostatectomy:

national human cooperative study results. J Urol. 1993;150(5 Pt 2):1607–11.

34. Muschter R, Hofstetter A. Interstitial laser therapy outcome in benign prostatic hyperplasia. J Endourol. 1995;9(2):129–35.

35. Muller-Lisse GU, Schneede P, Heuck AF, Muschter R, Scheidler J, Reiser MF, et al. Magnetic Resonance Imaging in laser induced thermo therapy of the prostate. In: Muller GJ, Roggan A, editors. Laser-induced interstitial thermotherapy. Bellingham, Washington: SPIE—The International Society for Optical Engineering; 1995. p. 340–3.

36. Mueller-Lisse UG, Thoma M, Faber S, Heuck AF, Muschter R, Schneede P, et al. Coagulative interstitial laser-induced thermotherapy of benign prostatic hyperplasia: online imaging with a T2-weighted fast spin-echo MR sequence-experience in six patients. Radiology. 1999;210(2):373–9.

37. Henkel TO, Greschner M, Luppold T, Alken P. Transurethral and transperineal interstitial laser therapy of BPH. In: Mukker G, Roggan A, editors. Laser-induced interstitial thermotherapy. Bellingham, Washington: SPIE—The International Society for Optical Engineering; 1995. p. 416–25.

38. Pacella CM, Mauri G, Achille G, Barbaro D, Bizzarri G, De Feo P, et al. Outcomes and risk factors for complications of laser ablation for thyroid nodules: a multicenter study on 1531 patients. J Clin Endocrinol Metab. 2015;100(10):3903–10.

39. Patelli G, Ranieri A, Paganelli A, Mauri G, Pacella CM. Transperineal laser ablation for percutaneous treatment of benign prostatic hyperplasia: a feasibility study. Cardiovasc Intervent Radiol. 2017;40(9):1440–6.

40. Ahmed M, Solbiati L, Brace CL, Breen DJ, Callstrom MR, Charboneau JW, et al. Image-guided tumor ablation: standardization of terminology and reporting criteria-a 10-year update. J Vasc Interv Radiol. 2014;25(11):1691–705 e4.

41. Sacks D, McClenny TE, Cardella JF, Lewis CA. Society of Interventional Radiology clinical practice guidelines. J Vasc Interv Radiol. 2003;14(9 Pt 2):S199–202.

42. Krambeck AE, Handa SE, Lingeman JE. Experience with more than 1,000 holmium laser prostate enucleations for benign prostatic hyperplasia. J Urol. 2013;189(1 Suppl):S141–5.

43. Tan AHH, Gilling PJ, Kennett KM, Frampton C, Westemberg AM, Fraundorfer MR. A randomized trial comparing holmium laser enucleation of the prostate with transurethral resection of the prostate for the treatment of bladder outlet obstruction secondary to benign prostatic hyperplasia in large glands (40 to 200 grams). J Urol. 2003;170:1270–4.

44. Kim KS, Choi JB, Bae WJ, Kim SJ, Cho HJ, Hong SH, et al. Comparison of photoselective vaporization versus holmium laser enucleation for treatment of benign prostate hyperplasia in a small prostate volume. PLoS One. 2016;11(5):e0156133.

45. Jones P, Rai BP, Somani BK, Aboumarzouk OM. A review of thulium laser vapo-enucleation of the prostate: a novel laser-based strategy for benign prostate enlargement. Arab J Urol. 2015;13(3):209–11.

46. Gilling P, Barber N, Bidair M, Anderson P, Sutton M, Aho T, et al. WATER: a double-blind, randomized, controlled trial of aquablation((R)) vs transurethral resection of the prostate in benign prostatic hyperplasia. J Urol. 2018;199(5):1252–61.

47. Whelan JP, Bowen JM, Burke N, Woods EA, McIssac GP, Hopkins RB, et al. A prospective trial of GreenLight PVP (HPS120) versus transurethral resection of the prostate in the treatment of lower urinary tract symptoms in Ontario, Canada. Can Urol Assoc J. 2013;7(9–10):335–41.

48. Reich O, Gratzke C, Bachmann A, Seitz M, Schlenker B, Hermanek P, et al. Morbidity, mortality and early outcome of transurethral resection of the prostate: a prospective multicenter evaluation of 10,654 patients. J Urol. 2008;180(1):246–9.

49. Ruszat R, Seitz M, Wyler SF, Abe C, Rieken M, Reich O, et al. GreenLight laser vaporization of the prostate: single-center experience and long-term results after 500 procedures. Eur Urol. 2008;54(4):893–901.

50. Gilling P, Anderson P, Tan A. Aquablation of the prostate for symptomatic benign prostatic hyperplasia: 1-year results. J Urol. 2017;197(6):1565–72.

51. Yafi FA, Tallman CT, Seard ML, Jordan ML. Aquablation outcomes for the U.S. cohort of men with LUTS due to BPH in large prostates (80–150 cc). Int J Impot Res. 2018;30(5):209–14.

52. Montorsi F, Naspro R, Salonia A, Suardi N, Briganti A, Zanoni M, et al. Holmium laser enucleation versus transurethral resection of the prostate: results from a 2-center, prospective, randomized trial in patients with obstructive benign prostatic hyperplasia. J Urol. 2004;172(5 Pt 1):1926–9.

53. Ahyai SA, Gilling P, Kaplan SA, Kuntz RM, Madersbacher S, Montorsi F, et al. Meta-analysis of functional outcomes and complications following transurethral procedures for lower urinary tract symptoms resulting from benign prostatic enlargement. Eur Urol. 2010;58(3):384–97.

54. Yu H, Isaacson AJ, Burke CT. Review of current literature for prostatic artery embolization. Semin Intervent Radiol. 2016;33(3):231–5.

55. Gao YA, Huang Y, Zhang R, Yang YD, Zhang Q, Hou M, et al. Benign prostatic hyperplasia: prostatic arterial embolization versus transurethral resection of the prostate-a prospective, randomized, and controlled clinical trial. Radiology. 2014;270(3):920–8.

56. Carnevale FC, Iscaife A, Yoshinaga EM, Moreira AM, Antunes AA, Srougi M. Transurethral Resection of the Prostate (TURP) Versus Original and PErFecTED Prostate Artery Embolization (PAE) Due to Benign Prostatic Hyperplasia (BPH): preliminary results of a single center, prospective, urodynamic-controlled analysis. Cardiovasc Intervent Radiol. 2016;39(1):44–52.

57. Cronin KA, Lake AJ, Scott S, Sherman RL, Noone AM, Howlader N, et al. Annual report to the nation on the status of cancer, part I: national cancer statistics. Cancer. 2018;124(13):2785–800.

58. Mottet N, van den Bergh RCN, Briers E, Bourke L, Cornford P, Santis M, et al. EAU—ESTRO—ESUR—SIOG Guidelines on Prostate Cancer. 2018.

59. Potosky AL, Miller BA, Albertsen PC, Kramer BS. The role of increasing detection in the rising incidence of prostate cancer. JAMA. 1995;273(7):548–52.

60. Epstein JI, Zelefsky MJ, Sjoberg DD, Nelson JB, Egevad L, Magi-Galluzzi C, et al. A contemporary prostate cancer grading system: a validated alternative to the Gleason score. Eur Urol. 2016;69(3):428–35.

61. Heidenreich A, Bastian PJ, Bellmunt J, Bolla M, Joniau S, van der Kwast T, et al. EAU guidelines on prostate cancer. part 1: screening, diagnosis, and local treatment with curative intent-update 2013. Eur Urol. 2014;65(1):124–37.

62. Colin P, Mordon S, Nevoux P, Marqa MF, Ouzzane A, Puech P, et al. Focal laser ablation of prostate cancer: definition, needs, and future. Adv Urol. 2012;2012:589160.

63. Schroder FH, Hugosson J, Roobol MJ, Tammela TL, Ciatto S, Nelen V, et al. Screening and prostate-cancer mortality in a randomized European study. N Engl J Med. 2009;360(13):1320–8.

64. Vargas HA, Hotker AM, Goldman DA, Moskowitz CS, Gondo T, Matsumoto K, et al. Updated prostate imaging reporting and data system (PIRADS v2) recommendations for the detection of clinically significant prostate cancer using multiparametric MRI: critical evaluation using whole-mount pathology as standard of reference. Eur Radiol. 2016;26(6):1606–12.

65. Walser E, Nance A, Ynalvez L, Yong S, Aoughsten JS, Eyzaguirre EJ, et al. Focal laser ablation of prostate cancer: results in 120 patients with low- to intermediate-risk disease. J Vasc Interv Radiol. 2019;30(3):401–9 e2.

66. Johnson DE, Cromeens DM, Price RE. Interstitial laser prostatectomy. Lasers Surg Med. 1994;14(4):299–305.

67. Amin Z, Lees WR, Bown SG. Technical note: interstitial laser photocoagulation for the treatment of prostatic cancer. Br J Radiol. 1993;66(791):1044–7.

68. Peters RD, Chan E, Trachtenberg J, Jothy S, Kapusta L, Kucharczyk W, et al. Magnetic resonance thermometry for predicting thermal damage: an application of interstitial laser coagulation in an in vivo canine prostate model. Magn Reson Med. 2000;44(6):873–83.

69. Fuentes D, Oden JT, Diller KR, Hazle JD, Elliott A, Shetty A, et al. Computational modeling and real-time control of patient-specific laser treatment of cancer. Ann Biomed Eng. 2009;37(4):763–82.

70. van Nimwegen SA, L'Eplattenier HF, Rem AI, van der Lugt JJ, Kirpensteijn J. Nd:YAG surgical laser effects in canine prostate tissue: temperature and damage distribution. Phys Med Biol. 2009;54(1):29–44.

71. Stafford RJ, Fuentes D, Elliott AA, Weinberg JS, Ahrar K. Laser-induced thermal therapy for tumor ablation. Crit Rev Biomed Eng. 2010;38(1):79–100.

72. Colin P, Nevoux P, Marqa M, Auger F, Leroy X, Villers A, et al. Focal laser interstitial thermotherapy (LITT) at 980 nm for prostate cancer: treatment feasibility in Dunning R3327-AT2 rat prostate tumour. BJU Int. 2012;109(3):452–8.

73. Lindner U, Lawrentschuk N, Weersink RA, Raz O, Hlasny E, Sussman MS, et al. Construction and evaluation of an anatomically correct multi-image modality compatible phantom for prostate cancer focal ablation. J Urol. 2010;184(1):352–7.

74. Woodrum DA, Gorny KR, Mynderse LA, Amrami KK, Felmlee JP, Bjarnason H, et al. Feasibility of 3.0T magnetic resonance imaging-guided laser ablation of a cadaveric prostate. Urology. 2010;75(6):1514 e1–6.

75. Evans AJ, Ryan P, Van der Kwast T. Treatment effects in the prostate including those associated with traditional and emerging therapies. Adv Anat Pathol. 2011;18(4):281–93.

76. Martenson AC, De La Rosette JJ. Interstitial laser coagulation in the treatment of benign prostatic hyperplasia using a diode laser system: results of an evolving technology. Prostate Cancer Prostatic Dis. 1999;2(3):148–54.

77. Lindner U, Lawrentschuk N, Weersink RA, Davidson SR, Raz O, Hlasny E, et al. Focal laser ablation for prostate cancer followed by radical prostatectomy: validation of focal therapy and imaging accuracy. Eur Urol. 2010;57(6):1111–4.

78. Lindner U, Weersink RA, Haider MA, Gertner MR, Davidson SR, Atri M, et al. Image guided photothermal focal therapy for localized prostate cancer: phase I trial. J Urol. 2009;182(4):1371–7.

79. Raz O, Haider MA, Davidson SR, Lindner U, Hlasny E, Weersink R, et al. Real-time magnetic resonance imaging-guided focal laser therapy in patients with low-risk prostate cancer. Eur Urol. 2010;58(1):173–7.

80. Atri M, Gertner MR, Haider MA, Weersink RA, Trachtenberg J. Contrast-enhanced ultrasonography for real-time monitoring of interstitial laser thermal therapy in the focal treatment of prostate cancer. Can Urol Assoc J. 2009;3(2):125–30.

81. Bomers JGR, Cornel EB, Futterer JJ, Jenniskens SFM, Schaafsma HE, Barentsz JO, et al. MRI-guided focal laser ablation for prostate cancer followed by radical prostatectomy: correlation of treatment effects with imaging. World J Urol. 2017;35(5):703–11.

82. Eggener SE, Yousuf A, Watson S, Wang S, Oto A. Phase II evaluation of magnetic resonance imaging guided focal laser ablation of prostate cancer. J Urol. 2016;196(6):1670–5.

83. Natarajan S, Jones TA, Priester AM, Geoghegan R, Lieu P, Delfin M, et al. Focal laser ablation of prostate cancer: feasibility of magnetic resonance imaging-ultrasound fusion for guidance. J Urol. 2017;198(4):839–47.

84. Natarajan S, Raman S, Priester AM, Garritano J, Margolis DJ, Lieu P, et al. Focal laser ablation

of prostate cancer: phase I clinical trial. J Urol. 2016;196(1):68–75.

85. Oto A, Sethi I, Karczmar G, McNichols R, Ivancevic MK, Stadler WM, et al. MR imaging-guided focal laser ablation for prostate cancer: phase I trial. Radiology. 2013;267(3):932–40.

86. Le Nobin J, Rosenkrantz AB, Villers A, Orczyk C, Deng FM, Melamed J, et al. Image guided focal therapy for magnetic resonance imaging visible prostate cancer: defining a 3-dimensional treatment margin based on magnetic resonance imaging histology co-registration analysis. J Urol. 2015;194(2):364–70.

87. Barentsz JO, Richenberg J, Clements R, Choyke P, Verma S, Villeirs G, et al. ESUR prostate MR guidelines 2012. Eur Radiol. 2012;22(4):746–57.

88. Yoo S, Kim JK, Jeong IG. Multiparametric magnetic resonance imaging for prostate cancer: a review and update for urologists. Korean J Urol. 2015;56(7):487–97.

89. Yarlagadda VK, Lai WS, Gordetsky JB, Porter KK, Nix JW, Thomas JV, et al. MRI/US fusion-guided prostate biopsy allows for equivalent cancer detection with significantly fewer needle cores in biopsy-naive men. Diagn Interv Radiol. 2018;24(3): 115–20.

90. Kongnyuy M, George AK, Rastinehad AR, Pinto PA. Magnetic resonance imaging-ultrasound fusion-guided prostate biopsy: review of technology, techniques, and outcomes. Curr Urol Rep. 2016; 17(4):32.

91. Westin C, Chatterjee A, Ku E, Yousuf A, Wang S, Thomas S, et al. MRI findings after MRI-guided focal laser ablation of prostate cancer. AJR Am J Roentgenol. 2018;211(3):595–604.

Sergio Sartori, Francesca Di Vece, Paola Tombesi, and Claudio Maurizio Pacella

14.1 Neuroendocrine Neoplasms

Neuroendocrine neoplasms (NEN) encompass a heterogeneous group of tumors that arise from neuroendocrine cells. Neuroendocrine cells are distributed widely throughout the body, and have neurologic and endocrine properties with potential ability to be hormonally active [1–3]. The neuroendocrine system includes neuroendocrine glands such as the pituitary, parathyroids and adrenal glands, endocrine islet tissue incorporated in glandular tissue of thyroid and pancreas, and scattered cells in digestive, respiratory, and genitourinary systems, as well as in the breast skin and central nervous system [4]. NEN include both functioning tumors, which may secrete different peptide hormones (i.e., serotonin, insulin, gastrin, glucagon, and vasoactive intestinal peptide), and nonfunctioning tumors, which are often identified at more advanced stages. From a histologic and prognostic perspective, NEN are usually divided into low-grade indolent tumors and high-grade aggressive carcinomas [5]. However, some histologically low-grade tumors may have aggressive behavior [6].

The bodywide distribution and the heterogeneous behavior of these tumors justify the complexity and confounding classification and nomenclature of NEN, and to date there is no one single system of nomenclature. In brief, gastroenteropancreatic tumors are the most frequent NEN (GEP NEN) and are defined as neuroendocrine tumors (NET) when they are well differentiated, and as neuroendocrine carcinomas if poorly differentiated. Among the non-GEP NEN, lungs are the most common primary site and four types of tumors are defined on the basis of their aggressiveness: typical carcinoid, atypical carcinoid, large cell neuroendocrine carcinoma, and small cell lung cancer [4].

NEN account for about 0.5% of all newly diagnosed malignancies [7]. The incidence has increased over the last decades and to date is approximately 5.86/100000 per year [7]. The most frequent primary sites are gastrointestinal tract (62–67%) and lungs (22–27%), whereas NEN from pancreas are rare with an incidence of less than 1/100000 per year. NEN of unknown origin are relatively uncommon accounting for 10–14% of all NEN [5]. 15 to 20% of NEN are part of inherited genetic syndromes including multiple endocrine neoplasia type 1 and type 2 syndrome, von Hippel-Lindau syndrome, tuberous sclerosis complex, and neurofibromatosis type 1 [7]. The histologic grade does not always

S. Sartori (✉) · F. Di Vece · P. Tombesi
Section of Interventional Ultrasound, St. Anna Hospital, Ferrara, Italy
e-mail: srs@unife.it

C. M. Pacella
Department of Diagnostic Imaging and Interventional Radiology, Regina Apostolorum Hospital, Albano Laziale, Rome, Italy

© Springer Nature Switzerland AG 2020
C. M. Pacella et al. (eds.), *Image-guided Laser Ablation*,
https://doi.org/10.1007/978-3-030-21748-8_14

correlate with clinical behavior [8], and the mitotic count and the Ki-67 index are worldwide considered the most useful tools for prognostic and treatment purposes [9]. 12 to 22% of patients with NEN are metastatic at presentation [7], and the liver is the most frequent site of spreading, followed by lungs and bones [10]. Furthermore, 40% of patients will develop liver metastases (LM) during the course of their disease [11], and LM have a major impact on survival with 5-year survival rates ranging from 24 to 40% [11–14].

14.2 Treatment Strategies

Treatment options depend on several factors such as type of NEN, disease burden, patient's preferences and overall health, symptoms, and possible side effects. The heterogeneity and complexity of NEN make imperative a multidisciplinary approach including medical and radiation oncologists, surgeon, pathologist, endocrinologist, interventional radiologist, and gastroenterologist and pulmonologist when necessary. The goal of primary treatment should be curative, and surgical removal of primary tumor represents the gold standard. However, LM are frequently present at initial diagnosis, or occur in the course of the disease, also in slow-growing tumors [12]. Systemic treatments often obtain disease stabilization, but they rarely achieve objective radiological response [12, 14–16]. Conversely, an aggressive cytoreduction with liver-directed approach can positively impact on both survival and hormonal symptoms control, and is widely recommended [11, 16–20]. Liver resection is worldwide considered the best option to treat LM [11, 13, 16–20], but its feasibility depends on both tumor characteristics such as size, number, and location and patient's characteristics such as age and health status. Therefore, it can usually be offered to a limited number of patients [11, 13, 16]. In prior studies, only 9–25% of patients with LM from NEN underwent hepatic resection [11, 21, 22]. Moreover, most patients undergoing liver surgery experience recurrences within two to 5 years [11, 13, 22], and require further liver-

directed treatments as chemotherapy achieves poor results in the treatment of LM, in particular in well-differentiated tumors [10, 16]. However, other systemic treatments have limited success in obtaining any significant radiological objective response, but they can achieve good symptoms control and, importantly, disease stabilization [10, 16, 18, 19]. They include somatostatin analogues (octreotide and lanreotide), low-dose interferon, peptide receptor radionuclide therapy, and a number of novel targeted agents such as everolimus, an inhibitor of the mammalian target of rapamycin (mTOR, a serine/threonine kinase that plays a crucial role in mediating cell growth), and sunitinib, a tyrosine kinase inhibitor directed against the vascular endothelial growth factor.

In the setting of not infrequently indolent disease progression, or disease stabilized by the above-mentioned systemic treatments, for patients who are not surgical candidates, or have recurrences after surgery, or have multifocal disease requiring a multimodality liver-directed approach, catheter-based treatments like transarterial embolization and chemoembolization, image-guided thermal ablation, and selective internal radiation therapy with yttrium-90 microspheres can be used as a primary approach or as an adjunct to liver resection, in order to obtain complete symptoms control and tumor debulking [11–16]. In the past years, liver debulking interventions were recommended only for patients in whom at least 90% of tumor burden could be removed [23, 24], with 5-year survival rates in excess of 60% [23–25]. However, just fewer than 20% of patients were estimated to be eligible for such an aggressive cytoreduction [17]. Recently, eligibility criteria have been expanded to a 70% debulking threshold, and this approach has been reported to significantly increase the number of eligible patients, while still achieving comparable survival rates [26–28]. Some authors obtained good results adopting a very aggressive and multimodality approach in well-selected patients. In this regard, Gomez et al. reported a 5-year survival rate of 86% in 18 patients with multiple (up to 13) bilobar LM [29], and Elias et al. reported a 3-year survival rate of 84% in 16 patients with a median of 23 LM per patient who were treated with surgical resection combined with intraoperative radiofrequency ablation, in some cases preceded by preoperative selective portal vein embolization; approximately 60% of the LM were surgically excised, and 40% underwent intraoperative radiofrequency ablation [13].

Although surgical resection is still considered the aggressive approach of choice, locoregional liver-directed therapies are gaining increasing importance. Indeed, the percentage of patients undergoing liver surgery remains low, and does not exceed 25% even with the above-mentioned expanded eligibility criteria [11, 26–28]. Moreover, extended resections involving multiple and bilobar LM have to be weighed against the associated morbidity and mortality rates that can be as high as 30% and 1–2%, respectively [11, 16]. Furthermore, 5-year recurrence rates range from 80 to 95% [11, 17, 22, 25] with a median time to recurrence of 21 months [25], requiring repeated treatments. It follows that the achievement of an extended debulking must be balanced with the need of sparing the normal liver parenchyma, as much as possible, to reduce the number of patients who ultimately die of liver failure [11, 17]. In this regard, ablation procedures represent an interesting option when evaluating patients with multiple LM, either as a primary approach or as an adjunct to surgical resection, allowing for both sparing liver parenchyma more than all other liver-directed therapies and repeated treatments [11, 14, 16, 17]. Even though there are no randomized trials comparing thermal ablation with other treatments in patients with LM from NEN, the available data about its efficacy are encouraging. For tumors up to 4 cm in diameter and less than seven to eight in number, 5-year overall survival rates from 54 to 84% have been reported for thermal ablation used alone or in combination with other surgical or nonsurgical treatments [11, 16, 30–33].

Ablation techniques deliver thermal energy, either cooling (cryoablation) or heating the tissues. Radiofrequency ablation (RFA), microwave ablation (MWA), and laser ablation

enable to raise the tissue temperature up to 100 °C, producing coagulative necrosis. RFA has largely become the dominant and most experienced ablation modality, and is extensively used worldwide to ablate both primary and metastatic liver tumors, including LM from NEN [13, 14, 30–39]. MWA systems are gaining increasing interest for the treatment of liver tumors, as they can obtain larger ablation areas and are not affected by the heat sink effect, desiccation, or charring [40–42]. However, the experience with MWA in the treatment of LM from NET is still limited to case reports or very small series [43, 44]. Until last year, laser ablation had also been used quite sporadically in patients with LM from NEN, but thanks to some technical characteristics, it could represent a valid alternative to RFA.

14.3 Laser Ablation

Laser ablation utilizes laser devices that convert electrical energy into light energy, which determines tissue heating and cellular death by coagulative necrosis. Neodymium: Yttrium aluminum garnet (Nd:YAG, wavelength of 1064 nm) and diode (wavelength of 800–980 nm, or 1064 nm) lasers are most commonly used, as penetration of light is optimal in the near infrared spectrum. Laser diodes are replacing the Nd:YAG laser because they are more compact and portable (weighing less than 10 kg), less expensive, and have a tissue penetration compared to Nd:YAG.

Light is delivered via flexible bare-tip fibers with a diameter from 300- to 600-µm. The optical and thermal characteristics of the tissue, as well as the proximity of blood vessels, determine the thermal diffusion of the light energy and define the ablation area. The multifiber technique proposed by Pacella [45] and improved by Di Costanzo [46] uses 300-µm bare-tip fibers that are introduced into the tumor through 21-gauge needles. The diameter of the needles is considerably thinner than that of RFA electrodes or MWA antennas, and for this reason, some authors proposed laser ablation as the technique of choice to ablate lesions in at-risk location or in locations that are difficult to reach [47, 48]. Moreover, each bare-tip fiber provides an almost spherical thermal lesion of 12–15 mm in diameter, and a beam-splitting device or a multisource device allow the use of up to four fibers at once, simultaneously delivering light into each single fiber [49, 50]. By also using, when necessary, the pullback technique [45, 46], these devices enable to achieve ablation areas from 1 to 4–5 cm in diameter, and consequently to treat tumors ranging from 5 mm to 3 cm in diameter obtaining an acceptable safety margin. LM from NEN are frequently multiple and variable in size and often require multiple repeated treatments because, as mentioned above, recurrence rates are very high, making the need of sparing the normal liver parenchyma mandatory. In this setting, the possibility of placing from one to four laser fibers into the tumor makes laser ablation a very flexible technique that enables to tailor the size of each thermal lesion to the size of each nodule, allowing for multiple and repeated treatments over time. In a recent case report, a total of 28 LM from insulin-secreting neuroendocrine tumor of the pancreas underwent successful laser ablation over a period of 3 years; the patient was still alive and disease-free 82 months after the first laser ablation session, and tumoral hormonal secretion was normalized [49].

In a fairly recent preliminary experience from Tombesi et al. [50], 13 patients with a total of 133 LM from NEN (median 7, mean 10.2 ± 7.7, range 3–28) underwent laser ablation in 28 sessions (range 1–5). The diameter of the lesions ranged from 5 to 35 mm, and one to four laser fibers were used according to the tumor size. The outcomes of the treatment were defined according to the recommendations of the International Working Group on the Image-guided Tumor Ablation [51], and complications were classified according to the Cardiovascular and Interventional Society of Europe classification system for complications reporting [52]. Technical success was obtained in all the procedures; contrast-enhanced computed tomography, was performed 1 month after laser ablation, and complete ablation of all the 133 LM was documented, with a technical efficacy of 100%. No procedure-related death occurred, and just one grade 4 complication was observed (0.75%): a bowel perforation that was successfully managed by surgery. Six-month local recurrence was observed in 7/133 LM, with a primary efficacy rate of 94.7%. All local recurrences were successfully retreated by further laser ablation sessions, with a secondary efficacy rate of 100%. After a median follow-up period of 36 months (range 15–54 months), four patients died because of distant hepatic progression or extrahepatic progression, four patients died for causes other than their NEN, three patients were alive and disease-free, and two patients were alive with hepatic distant recurrences [50, 53]. These quite promising preliminary results led the authors to suggest that laser ablation could become not only a valid alternative to RFA, but also the ablative technique of choice for patients with multiple small LM from NEN who are not eligible for surgical resection. Indeed, to date this retrospective study represents the largest series of LM treated with laser ablation, and among the vast literature on RFA of LM from NEN, just three studies involved larger series of LM, with similar or even worse results [14, 32, 37].

Furthermore, in a recent pilot study Pacella et al. [54] reported promising results in the treatment of a small series of large LM from NEN by using laser ablation followed by transarterial chemoembolization (TACE). Complete response was obtained in lesions of 6.4 cm and 7 cm in diameter, and partial response with an estimated volume of ablated tumor tissue of approximately 80% was obtained in a lesion of 12 cm in diameter [54]. Although the number of large lesions treated in this pilot study is quite low, the results suggest that laser ablation combined with catheter-based treatments could be profitably used to significantly reduce the tumor burden in the presence of isolated large LM with diameter also exceeding 5 cm in patients not candidate to surgical resection. Indeed, other authors previously emphasized the role of combined treatment, even though they used TACE as a first procedure to downsizing the initial tumor burden as much as possible, and then treated any residual vital tissue by laser ablation [55].

In both the studies of Tombesi et al. and Pacella et al., laser ablation was performed by using the multifiber technique [45, 46]. In brief, after premedication with short-acting subcutaneous octreotide 1 h before the procedure, and local anesthesia with lignocaine 1% 10 mL and conscious sedation with intravenous midazolam and remifentanil, laser fibers were introduced into the tumor under ultrasonography (US) guidance through 21-gauge Chiba needles. One fiber was used for lesions up to 7 mm in diameter (Fig. 14.1), two laser fibers spaced 12 mm were used for lesions between 7 and 14 mm (Fig. 14.2), three fibers spaced 12–18 mm apart for lesions between 15 and 20 mm (Fig. 14.3), and four fibers spaced 12–18 mm apart arranged in a square configuration for lesions between 21 and 35 mm (Fig. 14.4); the pullback technique [45, 46] was used if the anteroposterior diameter of the nodules exceeded 12 mm. The laser machine was turned on a fixed power of

5 W, and 1800 Joules per fiber were simultaneously delivered in 6 min; further 1800 J were delivered if the pullback technique was used. The completeness of the ablation was assessed by contrast-enhanced US (CEUS) performed about 10 min after the end of the procedure. If no enhancing zone with diameters equal to or greater than those of the treated tumor was depicted by CEUS, the treatment was considered complete. If residual enhancing foci of tumoral tissue were identified, further one or two laser fibers were inserted into the viable foci under CEUS guidance, and further 1800 J per fiber were delivered to complete the treatment.

Although not all the interventional oncology centers routinely perform immediate post-procedural CEUS, in our opinion its implementation is highly recommended to minimize the rate of incomplete ablation with any ablation technique (RFA, MWA, or laser). In a previous experience with RFA of primary and metastatic liver tumors, post-procedural CEUS documented incomplete ablation in 14.4% of the treated lesions, allowing for the retreatment of the residual viable tumoral foci with considerable improvement of the outcome [56].

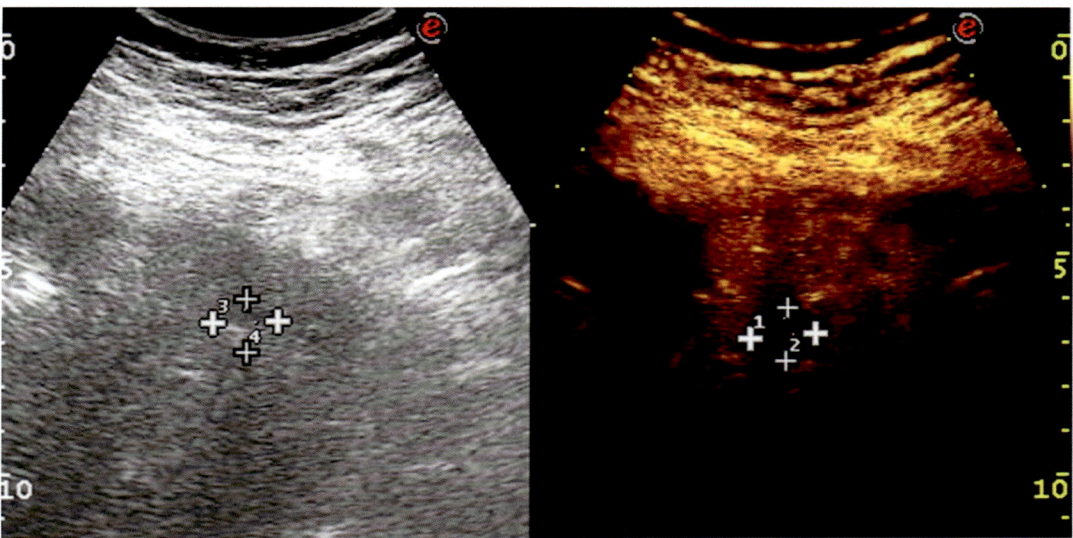

Fig. 14.1 CEUS scan of the left liver lobe showing a 14 × 12 mm thermal lesion obtained with one laser fiber

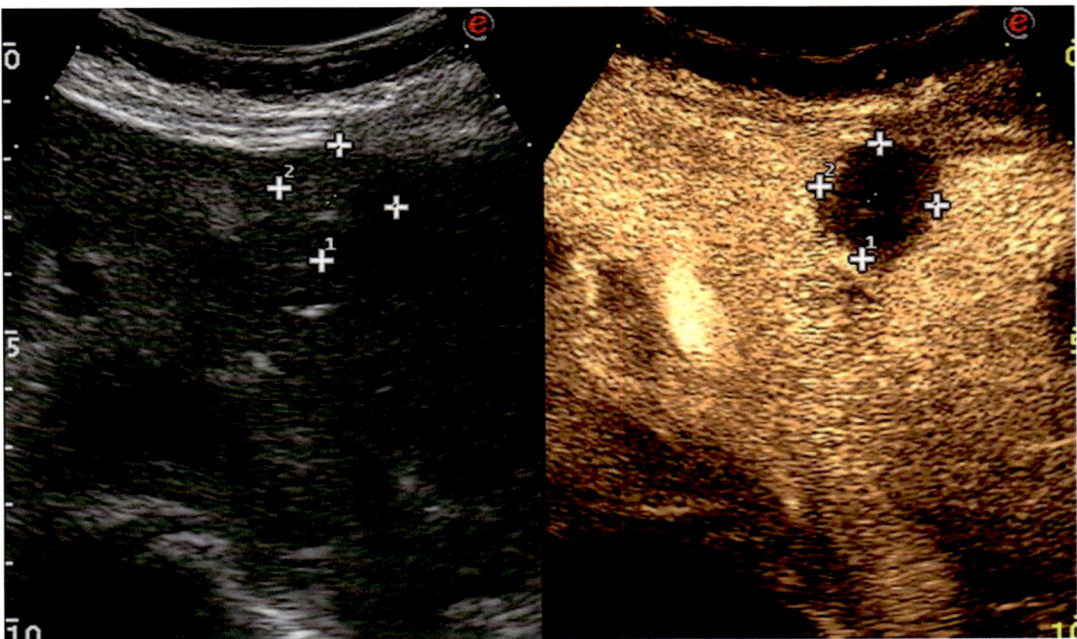

Fig. 14.2 CEUS scan of the right liver lobe showing a 21 × 20 mm thermal lesion obtained with two laser fibers

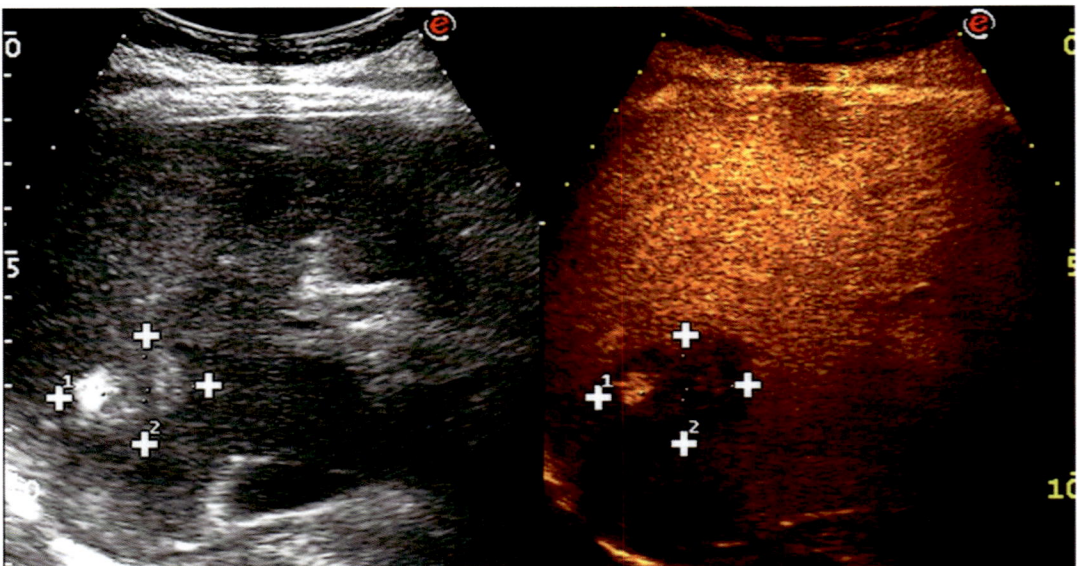

Fig. 14.3 CEUS scan of the right liver lobe showing a 34 × 20 mm thermal lesion obtained with three laser fibers

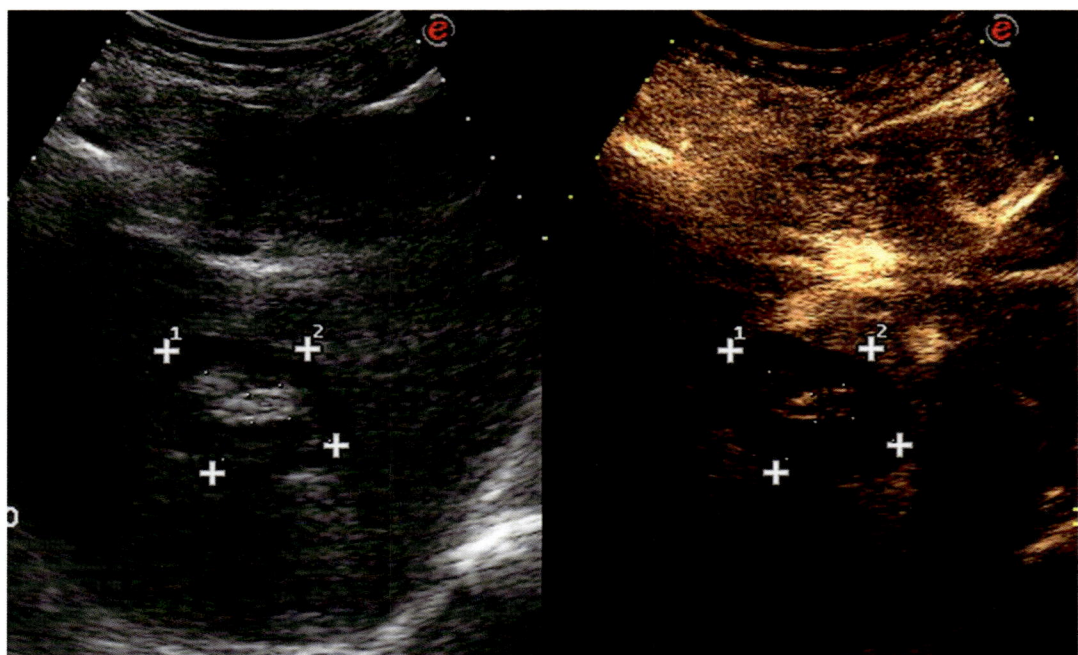

Fig. 14.4 CEUS scan of the right liver lobe showing a 42 × 32 mm thermal lesion obtained with four laser fibers

14.4   Final Considerations

The relative rarity of NEN in the general population, their heterogeneity in either histologic subtype and grade or LM burden, and their variable behavior with wide range of aggressiveness make it nearly impossible to conduct randomized prospective trials to determine the optimal treatment of LM [11, 12, 16]. As a result, the level of evidence of the various approaches is low, and all current recommendations are largely based on retrospective studies. However, there is a large consensus on the fact that an aggressive cytoreduction can achieve significant improvement of survival even in advanced stages of the disease, in particular in patients with indolent disease progression, or disease stabilized by systemic therapies. In this setting, a multimodality approach with liver-directed treatments is strongly recommended, and surgery, transarterial embolization and chemoembolization, selective internal radiation therapy with yttrium-90 microspheres, and image-guided thermal ablation can be profitably used sequentially or in combination with each other, according to tumor and patient characteristics. Among the ablative techniques, at present RFA is the most experienced and used modality to treat LM from NEN, but thanks to its technical characteristics, it is likely that laser ablation could become the ablative approach of choice in the next future.

References

1. Lawrence B, Gustafsson BI, Chan A, et al. The epidemiology of gastroenteropancreatic neuroendocrine tumors. Endocrinol Metab Clin N Am. 2011;40:1–18.
2. Mocellin S, Nitti D. Gastrointestinal carcinoid. Epidemiological and survival evidence from a large population-based study (n 25 531). Ann Oncol. 2013;24:3040–4.
3. Kulke MH, Siu LL, Tepper JE, et al. Future directions in the treatment of neuroendocrine tumors: Consensus report of the National Cancer Institute Neuroendocrine Tumor clinical trials planning meeting. J Clin Oncol. 2011;29:934–43.
4. Bosman FT, Carneiro F, Hruban RH, et al. WHO Classification of Tumours of the Digestive System (ed 4). Lyon, International Agency for Research on Cancer. 2010.
5. Yao JC, Hassan M, Phan A, et al. One hundred years after "carcinoid": Epidemiology of and prognostic factors for neuroendocrine tumors in 35,825 cases in the United States. J Clin Oncol. 2008;26:3063–72.
6. Chandrasekharappa SC, Guru SC, Manickam P, et al. Positional cloning of the gene for multiple endocrine neoplasia-type 1. Science. 1997;276:404–7.
7. American Joint Committee on Cancer (AJCC). AJCC cancer staging handbook: from the ajcc cancer staging manual. 7th ed. New York: Springer; 2010.
8. Moertel CG, Rubin J, Kvols LK. Therapy of metastatic carcinoid tumor and the malignant carcinoid syndrome with recombinant leukocyte A interferon. J Clin Oncol. 1989;7:865–8.
9. Bosman FT, Carneiro F, Hruban RH, et al. World Health Organization classification of tumors. In: Pathology and genetics. Tumors of the digestive system. Lyon: IARC Press; 2010.
10. Pavel M, Baudin E, Couvelard A, et al. ENETS consensus guidelines for the management of patients with liver and other distant metastases from neuroendocrine neoplasms of foregut, midgut, hindgut, and unknown primary. Neuroendocrinology. 2012;95:157–76.
11. Fairweather M, Swanson R, Wang J, et al. Management of neuroendocrine tumor liver metastases: long-term outcomes and prognostic factors from a large prospective database. Ann Surg Oncol. 2017;24:2319–25.
12. Ho AS, Picus J, Darcy MD, et al. Long-term outcome after chemoembolization and embolization of hepatic metastatic lesions from neuroendocrine tumors. Am J Roentgenol. 2007;188:1201–7.
13. Elias D, Goerè D, Leroux G, et al. Combined liver surgery and RFA for patients with gastroenteropancreatic endocrine tumors presenting with more than 15 metastases to the liver. Eur J Surg Oncol. 2009;35:1092–7.
14. Gillams A, Cassoni A, Conway G, Lees W. Radiofrequency ablation of neuroendocrine liver metastases: the Middlesex experience. Abdom Imaging. 2014;30:435–41.
15. Kolbec KJ, Farsad K. Catheter-based treatments for hepatic metastases from neuroendocrine tumors. Am J Roentgenol. 2014;203:717–24.
16. Cavalcoli F, Rausa E, Conte D, et al. Is there still a role for the hepatic locoregional treatment of metastatic neuroendocrine tumors in the era of systemic targeted therapies? World J Gastroenterol. 2017;23(15):2640–50.
17. Howe JR, Cardona K, Fraker DL, et al. The surgical management of small bowel neuroendocrine tumors. Consensus guidelines of the North American Neuroendocrine Tumor Society. Pancreas. 2017;46(6):715–31.
18. Öberg K, Knigge U, Kwekkeboom D, Perren A. ESMO Guidelines Working Group. Neuroendocrine gastro-entero-pancreatic tumors: ESMO Clinical Practice Guidelines for diagnosis, treatment and follow-up. Ann Oncol. 2012;23(Suppl 7):124–30.
19. Kunz PL, Reidy-Lagunes D, Anthony LB, et al. North American Neuroendocrine Tumor Society. Consensus guidelines for the management and treatment of neuroendocrine tumors. Pancreas. 2013;42(4):557–77.
20. Kulke MH, Benson AB, Bergsland E, et al. Neuroendocrine tumors. J Natl Compr Cancer Netw. 2012;10(6):724–64.
21. Sarmiento JM, Heywood G, Rubin J, et al. Surgical treatment of neuroendocrine metastases to the liver: a plea for resection to increase survival. J Am Coll Surg. 2003;197(1):29–37.
22. Mayo SC, de Jong MC, Pulitano C, et al. Surgical management of hepatic neuroendocrine tumor metastasis: results from an international multi-institutional analysis. Ann Surg Oncol. 2010;17(12):3129–36.
23. Oberg K, Astrup L, Eriksson B, Nordic NE Tumour Group. et al. Guidelines for management of gastropancreatic neuroendocrine tumours. Acta Oncol. 2004;43:617–25.
24. Ramage JK, Davies AH, Ardill J. UKNETwork for Neuroendocrine Tumours et al.. Guidelines for the management of gastroenteropancreatic neuroendocrine (including carcinoid) tumours. Gut. 2005;54(suppl 4):iv1–iv16.
25. Maithel SK, Fong Y. Hepatic ablation for neuroendocrine tumor metastases. J Surg Oncology. 2009;100:635–8.
26. Maxwell JE, Sherman SK, O'Dorisio TM, et al. Liver-directed surgery of neuroendocrine metastases: what is the optimal strategy? Surgery. 2016;159:320–33.
27. Chambers AJ, Pasieka JL, Dixon E, et al. The palliative benefit of aggressive surgical intervention for both hepatic and mesenteric metastases from neuroendocrine tumors. Surgery. 2008;144:645–51.
28. Graff-Baker AN, Sauer DA, Pommier SJ, et al. Expanded criteria for carcinoid liver debulking: maintaining survival and increasing the number of eligible patients. Surgery. 2014;156:1369–76.
29. Gomez D, Malik HZ, Al-Muktar KV, et al. Hepatic resection for metastatic gastrointestinal and pancreatic neuroendocrine tumours: outcome and prognostic predictors. HPB. 2007;9:345–51.

30. Amersi FF, McElrath-Garza A, et al. Long-term survival after radiofrequency ablation of complex unresectable liver tumors. Arch Surg. 2016;141:581–7.

31. Taner T, Atwell TD, Zhang L, et al. Adjunctive radiofrequency ablation of metastatic neuroendocrine cancer to the liver complements surgical resection. HPB. 15:190–5.

32. Mazzaglia PJ, Berber E, Milas M, Siperstein AE. Laparoscopic radiofrequency ablation of neuroendocrine liver metastases: a 10-year experience evaluating predictors of survival. Surgery. 2007;142:10–9.

33. Mohan H, Nicholson P, Winter DC, et al. Radiofrequency ablation for neuroendocrine liver metastases: a systematic review. J Vasc Interv Radiol. 2015;26:935–42.

34. Akyildiz HY, Mitchell J, Milas M, et al. Laparoscopic radiofrequency thermal ablation of neuroendocrine hepatic metastases: long-term follow-ups. Surgery. 2010;148:1288–93.

35. Wessels FJ, Schell SR. Radiofrequency ablation treatment of refractory carcinoid hepatic metastases. J Surg Res. 2001;95:8–12.

36. Henn AR, Levine EA, McNulty W, Zagoria RJ. Percutaneous radiofrequency ablation of hepatic metastases for symptomatic relief of neuroendocrine syndromes. Am J Roentgenol. 2003;181:1005–10.

37. Berber E, Flesher N, Siperstein AE. Laparoscopic radiofrequency ablation of neuroendocrine liver metastases. World J Surg. 2002;26:985–90.

38. Hellman P, Ladjevardi S, Skogseid B, et al. Radiofrequency tissue ablation using cooled tip for liver metastases of endocrine tumors. World J Surg. 2002;26:1052–6.

39. Elvin A, Skogseid B, Hellman P. Radiofrequency ablation of neuroendocrine liver metastases. Abdom Imaging. 2005;30:427–34.

40. Qian GJ, Wang N, Shen Q, et al. Efficacy of microwave versus radiofrequency ablation for treatment of small hepatocellular carcinoma: experimental and clinical studies. Eur Radiol. 2012;22:1983–90.

41. Cavagnaro M, Amabile C, Bernardi P, et al. A minimally invasive antenna for microwave ablation therapies: design, performances, and experimental assessment. IEEE Trans Biomed Eng. 2011;58:949–59.

42. Di Vece F, Tombesi P, Ermili F, et al. Coagulation areas produced by cool-tip radiofrequency ablation and microwave ablation using a device to decrease back-heating effects: a prospective pilot study. Cardiovasc Intervent Radiol. 2014;37:723–9.

43. Martin RCG, Scoggins CR, McMasters KM. Safety and efficacy of microwave ablation of hepatic tumors: a prospective review of a 5-year experience. Ann Surg Oncol. 2010;17(1):171–8.

44. Wang W, Seeruttun SR, Fang C, Zhou Z. Comprehensive treatment of a functional pancreatic neuroendocrine tumor with multifocal liver metastases. Chin J Cancer Res. 2014;26(4):501–6.

45. Pacella CM, Bizzarri G, Magnolfi F, Cecconi P, Caspani B, Anelli V, et al. Laser thermal ablation in the treatment of small hepatocellular carcinoma: results in 74 patients. Radiology. 2001;221:712–20.

46. Di Costanzo GG, D'Adamo G, Tortora R, Zanfardino F, Mattera S, Francica G, et al. A novel needle guide system to perform percutaneous laser ablation of liver tumors using the multifiber technique. Acta Radiol. 2013;54:876–81.

47. Tombesi P, Di Vece F, Sartori S. Radiofrequency, microwave, and laser ablation of liver tumors: time to move toward a tailored ablation technique? Hepatoma Res. 2015;1:52–7.

48. Sartori S, Di Vece F, Ermili F, Tombesi P. Laser ablation of liver tumors: An ancillary technique, or an alternative to radiofrequency and microwave? World J Radiol. 2017;9:91–6.

49. Sartori S, Di Vece F, Bianchi L, Tombesi P. Percutaneous laser thermal ablation in a patient with 22 liver metastases from pancreatic neuroendocrine tumor. A case report. EMJ Hepatol. 2018;6(1):95–9.

50. Tombesi P, Di Vece F, Sartori S. Laser ablation for hepatic metastases from neuroendocrine tumors. AJR Am J Roentgenol. 2015;204:W 732.

51. Ahmed M, Solbiati L, Brace CL, Breen DJ, Callstrom MR, Charboneau JW, et al. Image-guided tumor ablation: standardization of terminology and reporting criteria—a 10-year update. J Vasc Intervent Radiol. 2014;25:1691–705.. e4

52. Filippiadis DK, Binkert C, Pellerin O, Hoffmann RT, Krajina A, Pereira PL. CIRSE quality assurance document and standards for classification of complications: the CIRSE classification system. Cardiovasc Intervent Radiol. 2017;40:1141–6.

53. Sartori S, Tombesi P, Di Vece F. Laser thermal ablation in multimodality treatment of liver metastases from neuroendocrine tumors. Echolaser News. 2014;6(Sept):1–3.

54. Pacella CM, Nasoni S, Grimaldi F, et al. Laser ablation with or without chemoembolization for unresectable neuroendocrine liver metastases: a pilot study. Int J Endo Oncol. 2016. doi:https://doi.org/10.2217/ije.15.34.

55. Vogl TJ, Gruber T, Naguib NN, Hammerstingl R, Nour-Eldin NE. Liver metastases of neuroendocrine tumors: treatment with hepatic transarterial chemotherapy using two therapeutic protocols. AJR Am J Roentgenol. 2009;193(4):941–7.

56. Sartori S, Tombesi P, Macario F, Nielsen I, Tassinari D, Catellani M, Abbasciano V. Subcapsular liver tumors treated with percutaneous radiofrequency ablation: a prospective comparison with nonsubcapsular liver tumors for safety and effectiveness. Radiology. 2008;248:670–9.

New Horizons for Laser Ablation: Nanomedicine, Thermometry, and Hyperthermal Treatment Planning Tools

Paola Saccomandi, Emiliano Schena,
and Claudio Maurizio Pacella

15.1 Context

Laser Ablation (LA) technology has proven to be an important tool in the treatment of focal neoplasms. The last two decades have served to study and understand some of the basic principles of this technique. Historically, research on ablative therapies has focused on creating larger or more uniform coagulation areas that are reproducible in the most various clinical situations, improving device engineering and developing new applications. Take into account the characteristics of the tissue such as blood perfusion and thermal and electrical conductivity that are fundamental for the proper engineering of the device, for increasing its performance and optimizing the delivery of energy. In the case of LA technology, differences in the optical properties and refractive index were also taken into due consideration for their crucial role in the penetration of light into different tissues, although research efforts focused primarily on reducing blood flow to the tumor through the technique of arterial or portal embolization [1–3]. Current research seems to be aimed at developing systems able to reduce exposure times, improve predictive abilities, and develop combined therapies to further improve their clinical efficacy. Modern systems use small, compact, high-power laser diode equipment with actively cooled applicators to reduce carbonization during procedures. Moreover, the compatibility with MRI, that enables real-time treatment planning, targeting, monitoring, and evaluation, has helped expand the number of applications in which LA can be safely and effectively applied [4–11]. In addition to advances in imaging and delivery, such as the incorporation of nanotechnologies, next-generation systems incorporate image-guided LA procedures, hyperthermia planning tool, systems for real-time temperature monitoring and thermal dose assessment. Lastly, most of the novel perspectives related to the employment of laser for tumor treatment rely on nanotechnology. Several research groups all over the world are investigating and optimizing the potentialities of nanoparticles as a contrast agent and to enhance the absorption of laser light into the tumor.

P. Saccomandi (✉)
Department of Mechanical Engineering,
Politecnico di Milano, Milan, Italy
e-mail: paola.saccomandi@polimi.it

E. Schena
Department of Measurements and Biomedical
Instrumentation, Università Campus Bio-Medico di
Roma, Rome, Italy

C. M. Pacella
Department of Diagnostic Imaging and Interventional
Radiology, Regina Apostolorum Hospital,
Albano Laziale, Rome, Italy

© Springer Nature Switzerland AG 2020
C. M. Pacella et al. (eds.), *Image-guided Laser Ablation*,
https://doi.org/10.1007/978-3-030-21748-8_15

15.2 Nanoparticle-Enhanced LA for Tumor Treatment

The preferential heating of tumors over the surrounding healthy tissue can be strengthened through light-absorbing nanomaterials. Nanoparticles are nanoscale agents (size ranging from 1 to 100 nm) broadly used in medical field, for drug delivery, imaging contrast, therapy, chemical sensing, and other applications [12]. Several materials are available to synthetize nanoparticles for biomedical uses, as carbon nanotubes, gold nanospheres and nanorods, cadmium selenide quantum dots, and iron oxide, among others. The biodistribution, the potential toxicity, and the clearance are still the main concerns for the use of nanoparticles in the clinical routine, and worldwide research is under development to answer these questions [13].

An important branch of this field is related to the use of nanoparticles to enhance the absorption of laser light by the tissue. The absorption peak of the nanoparticles can be customized by tuning their shape and size, and this feature is particularly relevant in case of gold nanoparticles (GNRs), due to a physical phenomenon known as plasmon surface resonance. They have gained attention due to the intrinsic biocompatibility of the gold, the easy functionalization with other materials (e.g., polyethylene glycol, PEG, to increase blood circulation duration, specific molecular groups for targeting), and the possibility to change the absorption peak within a large spectral range. GNRs available today have absorption peaks ranging in a large portion of the spectrum, including the wavelengths from 520 to 900 nm [14], i.e., the so-called therapeutic window, and suitable for synergy with laser treatment. For instance, gold nanoshells with external diameters of 50–100 nm and gold shell thicknesses of 4–8 nm exhibit strong absorption and low scattering around 800 nm. When shined with a laser wavelength which is low absorbed by the tissue, the nanoparticles induce a strong temperature increase where they are deposited, taking advantage from the bigger absorption coefficient over the normal biological tissue (Fig. 15.1). Gold nanoshells and nanorods are deeply studied because the plasmon surface resonance, and hence their absorption coefficient, can be easily tuned by modifying the core shell diameter over the total diameter in case of nanoshells, and the aspect ratio in case of nanorods. For instance, the absorption coefficient of nanorods can be up to 200 times higher than the one of a normal tissue. When a certain volume (usually <0.01% of volume fraction) of GNRs is administrated into the tumor, the global absorption in the tumor is the function of the absorption characteristic of both the nanomaterials and the tissue. PEGylated nanoparticles are preferentially accumulated into tumor tissues due to the enhanced permeability and retention effect, because the blood vessels of tumors are more leaky, so macromolecules can easily evacuate and get deposited into the tumor cells [14, 15]. A strong research is active in the

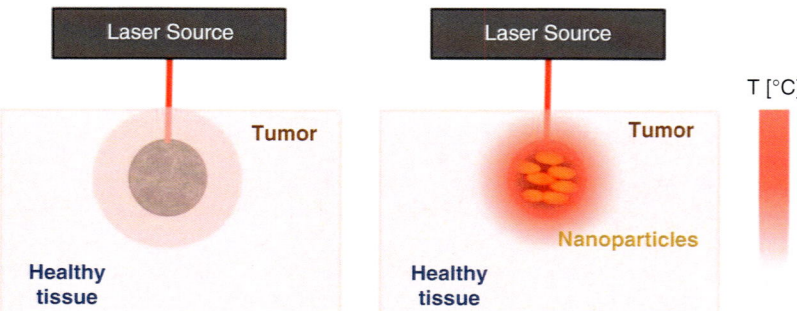

Fig. 15.1 Graphical representation of nanoparticle-mediated LA for tumor treatment. When shined with a laser wavelength which is less absorbed by the tissue, the nanoparticles induce a strong temperature increase where they are deposited, taking advantage from the bigger absorption coefficient over the normal biological tissue

field of functionalization of the gold nanorods. The coating can, indeed, influence the uptake from the tumoral cells, or from the carriers.

The first application of GNR-mediated laser therapy dates back to 2003, when Hirsch and colleagues proposed the use of nanoshells to treat human breast epithelial carcinoma SK-BR-3 cells in mice models, and a 808 nm external laser source was used to irradiate the tumor [16]. The in vivo studies revealed that exposure to low doses of laser light in solid tumors treated with GNRs reached temperature increase of about 40 °C, capable of inducing irreversible tissue damage in less than 10 min; on the other hand, controls treated without GNRs demonstrated significantly lower temperatures on exposure to laser light ($\Delta T < 10$ °C).

Numerous studies regarding the nanoparticle-mediated LA of solid tumors were performed from 2003 till today in this subject, and most of them in in vitro and in vivo settings, within the following kind of tumors: breast [17–19], oral cancer [20], and pancreatic cancer [21, 22], among others. Most of the tests are performed with contactless 808 nm laser source.

A first attempt to bring the mentioned technology on the clinical phase was carried out by Nanospectra Biosciences company, which used PEGylated silica-cored gold nanoshells for the treatment of head and neck, prostate, and lung cancer [23] in the United States. Patients are given a systemic intravenous infusion of nanoparticles and a subsequent escalating dose of near-infrared laser light delivered by optical fiber.

Considering also the need of improving the guidance of the laser therapy, a strong research is active to develop nanoparticles which are visible and quantifiable by diagnostic imaging systems like MRI and computed tomography.

15.3 LA for Tumor Treatment Guided by Temperature Feedback

The irreversible damage of biological tissues during LA is caused by elevated temperature. This damage depends on both temperature value reached within the tissue and exposure time to this hyperthermia. Mathematical models, such as Arrhenius analysis and cumulative equivalent minutes at 43 °C (CEM43) model, provide a relationship between the two mentioned parameters and the cell death [8, 24]. For this reason, the knowledge of temperature trend during the ongoing LA may be useful to help the physician in the optimization of laser settings to remove the whole amount of the tumor while sparing the healthy structures. Since the 1970s, the accurate temperature monitoring has been considered essential in all thermal treatments [25–27].

Two approaches for temperature monitoring are mostly used during LA procedures: contactless methods, relying on the use of diagnostic imaging, and contact ones, based on the use of physical sensors. Among the image-based techniques, there are MRI, CT, ultrasound, and, recently, elastography. Thermometry based on MRI has been assessed on phantom, ex vivo, preclinical, and clinical studies [28–31]. This technique is based on the dependence of a number of magnetic resonance parameters on temperature. The proton density, the proton resonance frequency (PRF), and the relaxation times T1 and T2 have been largely investigated [28, 32, 33]. Among them, the PRF shift of water was particularly appreciated in clinical practice thanks to the linear sensitivity over a wide temperature range suitable for LA purposes (until 100 °C). Valuable features of MR thermometry are related to its noninvasiveness, and the possibility to provide a three-dimensional temperature map with good spatial and temporal resolution [29]; on the other hand it requires the use of MR-compatible systems, in addition bespoke sequences for improving sensitivity and temporal and spatial resolution may be used. Examples of clinical tools based on MR thermometry and approved for intracranial soft-tissue ablation are the Monteris NeuroBlate system (Monteris Medical, Plymouth, MN) and the Medtronic Visualase system (Medtronic Inc., Minneapolis, MN). The NeuroBlate system uses a 1064 nm diode laser, whereas the Visualase system relies on a 980 nm diode laser. They are minimally invasive LA systems, which provide multiple images and the ability to superimpose

MR thermometry and thermal damage estimate maps. The placement of the needle and the surgical approach is performed with stereotactic planning software [34].

Thermometry based on CT images was also proposed to guide thermal treatments [35–37]. In the same way as MRI-based thermometry, CT images allow estimating temperature due to the dependence of physical parameters which influence the formation of the image. The Compton scattering phenomenon and the dependence of the X-ray attenuation coefficient to temperature is the basis of the CT thermometry [38–41]. This technique has not still been investigated on humans, but only on phantoms, and on both ex vivo and in vivo animal models [37, 40, 42, 43]. The main advantage of CT thermometry is the optimal contrast and spatial resolution useful for both the guidance and the monitoring of the ablation treatment. Its image quality is superior if compared to MRI. The main drawbacks of this technique are related to the X-ray dose provided to the patient, the potential concerns related to image artifact due to the presence of metallic parts (which totally confuses the image and impairs CT-based thermometry), and/or movements due to patient respiration.

Ultrasound thermometry is based on the temperature dependence of acoustic properties of biological tissue [44, 45]. As for the MRI, several ultrasound parameters exhibit a dependence with tissue temperature. For instance, changes in sound speed and thermal expansion with temperature cause echo shifts in the backscattered signal. Other ultrasound temperature estimation methods are based on texture features of B-mode ultrasound images, ultrasound contrast agents, tissue shear modulus, and others. Most of the existing ultrasound thermometry methods are applied only within the temperature range of conventional hyperthermia (43–45 °C). When the temperatures are above the mentioned range, the monitoring can become problematic even though the boundaries and size of ablation regions may still be visualized [46].

Recently, the shear-wave elastography technique emerged as a novel tool for real-time and noninvasive monitoring tool for the thermal state of the tissue [47]. This method, applicable with both ultrasound and MRI and known as "virtual palpation," is useful in the diagnosis of some pathologies, where mechanical properties (in particular, elasticity) strongly vary depending on the tissue state. Since a thermal lesion is characterized by higher stiffness with respect to normal tissue, elastography can be an effective tool for the monitoring of thermal effects due to ablation, because of the change of tissue stiffness.

Physical sensors are also known for measuring temperature in this application. They differ from the image-based techniques, because contact between the sensitive element and the tissue is required. Thermocouples consist on metallic wires, quite common also in several fields. They are accurate and affordable; indeed, they are used also to control some commercial ablation systems (RF, MWA). In some advanced models, the clinician can set a temperature threshold, and the energy delivery is adjusted in order to maintain that value for the desired time. Regarding the temperature monitoring during LA, thermocouples are not the best choice. In fact, the self-heating due to the direct absorption of the laser light can entail measurement error higher than 10 °C close to the fiber applicator tip [48]. Another important group of sensors to be employed for LA monitoring is constituted by fiber optic-based sensors like fluoroptic sensors and fiber Bragg gratings. They rely on the change of light reflected due to temperature change, are immune from electromagnetic interferences, and can be used during MR guidance of the treatment. In particular, fiber Bragg gratings are interesting because several sensitive elements can be placed inside one single fiber, hence allowing multipoint temperature measurement [49, 50] with a minimally invasive approach, and in the range of temperature of interest for LA. It is worth highlighting that fiber Bragg gratings are biocompatible, immune from electromagnetic interferences, flexible, and hold the possibility to have long fiber cables to transport the light signal from the measurement site to the processing site. They can be easily embedded inside needles to be inserted inside the ablation target [51], and, in some prototypes, also integrated with the ablation fiber.

15.4 Hyperthermal Treatment Planning (HTP) Tools

Hyperthermal treatment planning (HTP) tools aim at improving the quality of the treatment by means of the definition of the optimal settings [52]. HTP is a computer-aided technology which simulates the interaction between the energy delivered by the laser treatment and the biological tissue. Consequently, HTP can predict the induced tissue temperature distribution, and thus the amount of damaged tissue. The computation can be divided into three main steps: [1] the first step is the generation of the patient model, based on the preoperative images of the patient. This phase is crucial because the geometry and characteristics of the tissue strongly influence the interaction between the tissue and the laser light [2]. The second step focuses on the calculation of the amount of power absorbed by the tissue. The laser light distribution within the tissue is usually calculated using the Monte Carlo simulation and requires information regarding the tissue optical properties at the laser wavelength of choice and the emission modality of the applicator [3]. The third step provides the tissue temperature distribution resulted from the tissue-laser light interaction. This step is crucial because an accurate prediction of temperature distribution inside the target organ can improve the treatment outcomes. The importance of HTP tools in current clinical use is confirmed by the decision of the European Society for Hyperthermic Oncology to include HTP in their quality assurance guidelines for deep hyperthermia [53] and by the recent development of several commercial treatment planning packages (e.g., the Sigma-Hyperplan system, Alba HTPS, VEDO, and Semcad X) [54].

15.5 Conclusions

Basic, applied, and translational research for improving the outcome of the LA witnesses the role of this ablative modality in the clinical pan-orama. In response to clinical needs, the most promising emerging solutions aim at controlling with high accuracy the amount of damaged tissue achieved by LA and at obtaining a more selective tumor treatment that does not injure the healthy tissue and the anatomical structures surrounding the target. Recent efforts are devoted to the development of HTP tools which aid in planning the treatment, to the improvement of new solutions for real-time thermometry, and to the use of tumor-targeted nanoparticles. Some of these solutions are already in use in some advanced clinical centers, whereas the nanoparticles are still a lively research field. Some of these parts are already partially integrated, like computational models and image-based thermometry. The further development of the single solutions will lead to more complex systems able, for instance, to calculate also the amount of nanoparticles to be injected in the tumor, and to give a prediction of the treatment outcome in the postoperative follow-up.

References

1. Ahmed M, Brace CL, Lee FT Jr, Goldberg SN. Principles of and advances in percutaneous ablation. Radiology. 2011;258(2):351–69.
2. Heisterkamp J, van Hillegersberg R, Mulder PG, Sinofsky EL, JN IJ. Importance of eliminating portal flow to produce large intrahepatic lesions with interstitial laser coagulation. Br J Surg. 1997;84(9):1245–8.
3. Vogl TJ, Kreutztrager M, Gruber-Rouh T, Eichler K, Nour-Eldin NE, Zangos S, et al. Neoadjuvant TACE before laser induced thermotherapy (LITT) in the treatment of non-colorectal non-breast cancer liver metastases: feasibility and survival rates. Eur J Radiol. 2014;83(10):1804–10.
4. Fiedler VU, Schwarzmaier HJ, Eickmeyer F, Muller FP, Schoepp C, Verreet PR. Laser-induced interstitial thermotherapy of liver metastases in an interventional 0.5 Tesla MRI system: technique and first clinical experiences. J Magn Reson Imaging. 2001;13(5):729–37.
5. Sequeiros RB, Hyvonen P, Sequeiros AB, Jyrkinen L, Ojala R, Klemola R, et al. MR imaging-guided laser ablation of osteoid osteomas with use of optical instrument guidance at 0.23 T. Eur Radiol. 2003;13(10):2309–14.
6. Lindner U, Lawrentschuk N, Trachtenberg J. Focal laser ablation for localized prostate cancer. J Endourol. 2010;24(5):791–7.

7. Raz O, Haider MA, Davidson SR, Lindner U, Hlasny E, Weersink R, et al. Real-time magnetic resonance imaging-guided focal laser therapy in patients with low-risk prostate cancer. Eur Urol. 2010;58(1):173–7.

8. Stafford RJ, Fuentes D, Elliott AA, Weinberg JS, Ahrar K. Laser-induced thermal therapy for tumor ablation. Crit Rev Biomed Eng. 2010;38(1):79–100.

9. Stafford RJ, Shetty A, Elliott AM, Klumpp SA, McNichols RJ, Gowda A, et al. Magnetic resonance guided, focal laser induced interstitial thermal therapy in a canine prostate model. J Urol. 2010;184(4):1514–20.

10. Sharma M, Balasubramanian S, Silva D, Barnett GH, Mohammadi AM. Laser interstitial thermal therapy in the management of brain metastasis and radiation necrosis after radiosurgery: An overview. Expert Rev Neurother. 2016;16(2):223–32.

11. Natarajan S, Raman S, Priester AM, Garritano J, Margolis DJ, Lieu P, et al. Focal Laser Ablation of Prostate Cancer: Phase I Clinical Trial. J Urol. 2016;196(1):68–75.

12. Zhang L, Gu FX, Chan JM, Wang AZ, Langer RS, Farokhzad OC. Nanoparticles in medicine: therapeutic applications and developments. Clin Pharmacol Ther. 2008;83(5):761–9.

13. Boisselier E, Astruc D. Gold nanoparticles in nanomedicine: preparations, imaging, diagnostics, therapies and toxicity. Chem Soc Rev. 2009;38(6):1759–82.

14. Huang X, Jain PK, El-Sayed IH, El-Sayed MA. Plasmonic photothermal therapy (PPTT) using gold nanoparticles. Lasers Med Sci. 2008;23(3):217–28.

15. Terentyuk GS, Maslyakova GN, Suleymanova LV, Khlebtsov NG, Khlebtsov BN, Akchurin GG, et al. Laser-induced tissue hyperthermia mediated by gold nanoparticles: toward cancer phototherapy. J Biomed Opt. 2009;14(2):021016.

16. Hirsch LR, Stafford RJ, Bankson JA, Sershen SR, Rivera B, Price RE, et al. Nanoshell-mediated near-infrared thermal therapy of tumors under magnetic resonance guidance. Proc Natl Acad Sci U S A. 2003;100(23):13549–54.

17. Lee J, Chatterjee DK, Lee MH, Krishnan S. Gold nanoparticles in breast cancer treatment: promise and potential pitfalls. Cancer Lett. 2014;347(1):46–53.

18. Mooney R, Roma L, Zhao D, Van Haute D, Garcia E, Kim SU, et al. Neural stem cell-mediated intratumoral delivery of gold nanorods improves photothermal therapy. ACS Nano. 2014;8(12):12450–60.

19. Mooney R, Schena E, Saccomandi P, Zhumkhawala A, Aboody K, Berlin JM. Gold nanorod-mediated near-infrared laser ablation: in vivo experiments on mice and theoretical analysis at different settings. Int J Hyperth. 2017;33(2)

20. El-Sayed IH, Huang X, El-Sayed MA. Surface plasmon resonance scattering and absorption of anti-EGFR antibody conjugated gold nanoparticles in cancer diagnostics: applications in oral cancer. Nano Lett. 2005;5(5):829–34.

21. Mocan L, Tabaran FA, Mocan T, Bele C, Orza AI, Lucan C, et al. Selective ex-vivo photothermal ablation of human pancreatic cancer with albumin functionalized multiwalled carbon nanotubes. Int J Nanomedicine. 2011;6:915–28.

22. Guo Y, Zhang Z, Kim DH, Li W, Nicolai J, Procissi D, et al. Photothermal ablation of pancreatic cancer cells with hybrid iron-oxide core gold-shell nanoparticles. Int J Nanomedicine. 2013;8:3437–46.

23. Chen F, Cai W. Nanomedicine for targeted photothermal cancer therapy: where are we now? Nanomedicine (Lond). 2015;10(1):1–3.

24. Dewey WC. Arrhenius relationships from the molecule and cell to the clinic. Int J Hyperth. 2009;25(1):3–20.

25. Christensen DA. Thermal dosimetry and temperature measurements. Cancer Res. 1979;39(6 Pt 2):2325–7.

26. Cetas TC, Connor WG. Thermometry considerations in localized hyperthermia. Med Phys. 1978;5(2):79–91.

27. Cetas TC, Connor WG, Manning MR. Monitoring of tissue temperature during hyperthermia therapy. Ann N Y Acad Sci. 1980;335:281–97.

28. Rieke V, Butts Pauly K. MR thermometry. J Magn Reson Imaging. 2008;27(2):376–90.

29. Todd N, Diakite M, Payne A, Parker DL. In vivo evaluation of multi-echo hybrid PRF/T1 approach for temperature monitoring during breast MR-guided focused ultrasound surgery treatments. Magn Reson Med. 2014;72(3):793–9.

30. Vogl TJ, Straub R, Zangos S, Mack MG, Eichler K. MR-guided laser-induced thermotherapy (LITT) of liver tumours: experimental and clinical data. Int J Hyperth. 2004;20(7):713–24.

31. Saccomandi P, Schena E, Silvestri S. Techniques for temperature monitoring during laser-induced thermotherapy: an overview. Int J Hyperth. 2013;29(7):609–19.

32. de Senneville BD, Mougenot C, Quesson B, Dragonu I, Grenier N, Moonen CT. MR thermometry for monitoring tumor ablation. Eur Radiol. 2007;17(9):2401–10.

33. Allegretti G, Saccomandi P, Giurazza F, Caponero MA, Frauenfelder G, Di Matteo FM, et al. Magnetic resonance-based thermometry during laser ablation on ex-vivo swine pancreas and liver. Med Eng Phys. 2015;37(7):631–41.

34. Munier SM, Hargreaves EL, Patel NV, Danish SF. Effects of variable power on tissue ablation dynamics during magnetic resonance-guided laser-induced thermal therapy with the Visualase system. Int J Hyperth. 2018;34(6):764–72.

35. Fani F, Schena E, Saccomandi P, Silvestri S. CT-based thermometry: an overview. Int J Hyperth. 2014;30(4):219–27.

36. Schena E, Saccomandi P, Giurazza F, Caponero MA, Mortato L, Di Matteo FM, et al. Experimental assessment of CT-based thermometry during laser ablation of porcine pancreas. Phys Med Biol. 2013;58(16):5705–16.

37. Pandeya GD, Klaessens JH, Greuter MJ, Schmidt B, Flohr T, van Hillegersberg R, et al. Feasibility of computed tomography based thermometry during interstitial laser heating in bovine liver. Eur Radiol. 2011;21(8):1733–8.

38. Pandeya GD, Greuter MJ, de Jong KP, Schmidt B, Flohr T, Oudkerk M. Feasibility of noninvasive temperature assessment during radiofrequency liver ablation on computed tomography. J Comput Assist Tomogr. 2011;35(3):356–60.

39. Liguori C, Frauenfelder G, Massaroni C, Saccomandi P, Giurazza F, Pitocco F, et al. Emerging clinical applications of computed tomography. Med Devices. 2015;8:265–78.

40. Homolka P, Gahleitner A, Nowotny R. Temperature dependence of HU values for various water equivalent phantom materials. Phys Med Biol. 2002;47(16):2917–23.

41. Bruners P, Levit E, Penzkofer T, Isfort P, Ocklenburg C, Schmidt B, et al. Multi-slice computed tomography: A tool for non-invasive temperature measurement? Int J Hyperth. 2010;26(4):359–65.

42. Schena E, Saccomandi P, Fong Y. Laser Ablation for Cancer: Past, Present and Future. J Funct Biomater. 2017;8(2)

43. Schena E, Giurazza F, Massaroni C, Fong Y, Park JJ, and Saccomandi P, Thermometry based on computed tomography images during microwave ablation: Trials on ex vivo porcine liver. In: 12MTC 2017 IEEE International Instrumentation and Measurement Technology Conference, Proceedings; 2017.

44. Bowen T, Connor WG, Nasoni RL, Pifer AE, Sholes RR. In: Linzer M, editor. Measurement of the temperature dependence of the velocity of ultrasound in soft tissue: Ultrasonic Tissue Characterization II National Bureau of Standards; 1979. p. 57–61.

45. Martin AR. Temperature dependence of ultrasonic backscattered energy in motion compensated images. IEEE Trans Ultrason Ferr. 2005;52:1644–52.

46. Saccomandi P, Schena E, Diana M, Marescaux J, Costamagna G. Thermal treatments of tumors: principles and methods. In: Sons JW, editor. Biomedical engineering challenges: a chemical engineering insight; 2018. p. 199–228.

47. Zhou Z, Wu W, Sea W. A survey of ultrasound elastography approaches to percutaneous ablation monitoring. Proceedings of the Institution of Mechanical Engineers, Part H. J Eng Med. 2014;22810:1069–82.

48. Schena E, Majocchi L. Assessment of temperature measurement error and its correction during Nd:YAG laser ablation in porcine pancreas. Int J Hyperth. 2014;30(5):328–34.

49. Schena E, Tosi D, Saccomandi P, Lewis E, Kim T. Fiber optic sensors for temperature monitoring during thermal treatments: an overview. Sensors. 2016;(7):16.

50. Saccomandi P, Schena E, Di Matteo FM, Pandolfi M, Martino M, Rea R, et al.. Theoretical assessment of principal factors influencing laser interstitial thermotherapy outcomes on pancreas. In: Proceedings of the Annual International Conference of the IEEE Engineering in Medicine and Biology Society; 2012.

51. Cavaiola C, Saccomandi P, Massaroni C, Tosi D, Schena E. Error of a Temperature Probe for Cancer Ablation Monitoring Caused by Respiratory Movements: Ex Vivo and In Vivo Analysis. IEEE Sensors J. 2016;16(15):5934–41.

52. Paulides MM, Stauffer PR, Neufeld E, Maccarini PF, Kyriakou A, Canters RA, et al. Simulation techniques in hyperthermia treatment planning. Int J Hyperth. 2013;29(4):346–57.

53. Bruggmoser G. Some aspects of quality management in deep regional hyperthermia. Int J Hyperth. 2012;28(6):562–9.

54. Rijnen Z, Bakker JF, Canters RA, Togni P, Verduijn GM, Levendag PC, et al. Clinical integration of software tool VEDO for adaptive and quantitative application of phased array hyperthermia in the head and neck. Int J Hyperth. 2013;29(3):181–93.

Future Perspectives and Clinical Applications

Claudio Maurizio Pacella, Giovanni Mauri, Luca Breschi, and Tian'an Jiang

16.1 Context

Since the last decade of the past century to our days we have witnessed an impetuous flourishing of clinical applications supported by so-called minimally invasive therapies (MIT). These can be thermal and nonthermal. While the latter use chemical agents to kill cells, the former use heat or cold to achieve the same result. Among the thermal ones, using heat as a means of ablation, the technique based on laser light appears fast, precise, and relatively tissue insensitive. The laser ablation technique is currently less widespread than the others probably because while generators are widely available around the world for numerous other clinical procedures [1, 2], applicators for percutaneous ablation are not as common as RF electrodes or MW antennas [3]. With the same results, the laser option appears

more manageable and more versatile than the others and in some specific fields of study the laser methodology can be used more profitably. The use of thin applicators allows to face with greater success and with more safety all the neoplastic lesions difficult to reach and close to vital structures in the various organs candidates for focal ablation [3–7]. In all cases where the clinical condition of the subject to be treated is compromised, the technique is more useful and more reliable as in cirrhotic patients with evident coagulopathy or in patients with renal tumors at risk of bleeding or still in pulmonary nodules in patients with ventilation disorders [4, 8–10].

Laser ablation technology has proven to be an important tool in the treatment of focal neoplasms. The last two decades have served to study and understand some of the basic principles of this technique [11]. Historically, research on ablative therapies has focused on creating larger or more uniform coagulation areas that are reproducible in the most various clinical situations, improving device engineering, and developing new applications [3, 12–14]. Take into account the characteristics of the tissue such as tissue perfusion and thermal and electrical conductivity that are fundamental for the proper engineering of the device, for increasing its performance and optimizing the delivery of energy. In the case of laser ablation technology, differences in the optical properties and refractive index were also taken into due consideration for their crucial role in the penetration of

C. M. Pacella (✉)
Department of Diagnostic Imaging and Interventional Radiology, Regina Apostolorum Hospital, Albano Laziale, Rome, Italy

G. Mauri
Division of Interventional Radiology, European Institute of Oncology, IRCCS, Milan, Italy

L. Breschi
Elesta Srl, Florence, Italy

T. Jiang
Department of Ultrasound, First Affiliated Hospital, College of Medicine, Zhejiang University, Hangzhou, China

© Springer Nature Switzerland AG 2020
C. M. Pacella et al. (eds.), *Image-guided Laser Ablation*,
https://doi.org/10.1007/978-3-030-21748-8_16

light into different tissues, although research efforts focused primarily on reducing blood flow to the tumor through the technique of arterial or portal embolization [3, 13, 15]. Current research seems to be aimed at developing systems able to reduce exposure times, improve predictive abilities, and develop combined therapies to further improve their clinical efficacy. Modern systems use small, compact, high-power laser diode equipment with actively cooled applicators to reduce carbonization during procedures. Moreover, the compatibility with MRI, that enables real-time treatment planning, targeting, monitoring, and evaluation, has helped expand the number of applications in which LA can be safely and effectively applied [16–23]. In addition to advances in imaging and delivery, such as the incorporation of nanotechnologies, next-generation systems incorporate models of MR-gLA procedures for human-assisted computational tools for planning, MR model-assisted temperature monitoring, thermal dose assessment, and optimal control [20].

16.2 Future Perspectives and Clinical Applications

This book presents an overview of the various laser light methodologies that have occurred over time and technological changes to improve their clinical success. In light of the experience accumulated over the years and the results obtained so far in the various fields of application, we can suggest in which field of study this option is appropriate and where it should be used most. Here we list the applications where, in our opinion, it is possible to make the most of the characteristics of this methodology.

An important field is the treatment of hepatocellular carcinomas in cirrhotic patients. The European Association for the Study of the Liver (EASL) [24] writes in the paragraph on locoregional treatments that "laser ablation in patients with hepatocellular carcinoma within the Milan criteria […] gave results […] not inferior to RFA in complete tumor ablation, time to local progression and OS. However, laser ablation requires more operator skills than RFA or MWA due to the need to place more fibers within the same

tumor, with adequate spatial distribution, although it may be safer in difficult places" [5, 6].

Although more experience and special attention are needed to correctly position several fibers within the target lesion, this option offers the double benefit of safely treating nodules at risk sites and at the same time achieving a high rate of complete ablation. With only two thin sources it is possible to obtain an area of 4–5 cm of max diameter [25–27] (Figs. 16.1 and 16.2). Worthy of note is the fact that the percutaneous placement of two thin needles for proper targeting of the neoplastic nodule requires the same skill needed to place an RF electrode or a MW antenna, particularly as laser is generally provided with advanced guidance systems for multiple-fiber insertion [26]. In this scenario, improvement in image guidance, with larger application of advanced techniques such as fusion imaging or augmented reality, can make easier the application of this technique even for less experienced operators.

We believe that laser technology in the treatment of liver metastases will be more and more applied in the future, for particularly good results in terms of high rate of local control of the disease, with few local relapses and good effects on survival, as shown by the data published by the Frankfurt group [28]. Particularly, the use of advanced imaging modalities, such as real-time MR monitoring of the ablation maneuver, might allow the operator to conclude the ablative treatment only after obtaining a sufficient safety margin at the periphery of the metastasis [29]. The safety margin plays a major role in the local control of metastatic disease with clear positive effects on patient survival [30, 31] (Chap. 4).

Given its characteristics, the laser technique may be ideal also in the treatment of hepatic metastases from neuroendocrine tumors, due to the high degree of safety, flexibility, and repeatability of the method in the treatment of patients with numerous lesions disseminated in the liver parenchyma not susceptible to surgery and/or treatment embolizing [32, 33] (Chap. 14).

Due to the very small size of applicators and fibers, laser ablation can be regarded as the technique of choice for the percutaneous treatment of small pathological lymph nodes, both in the abdomen and in the neck [7, 34–37] (Chaps. 5 and 8).

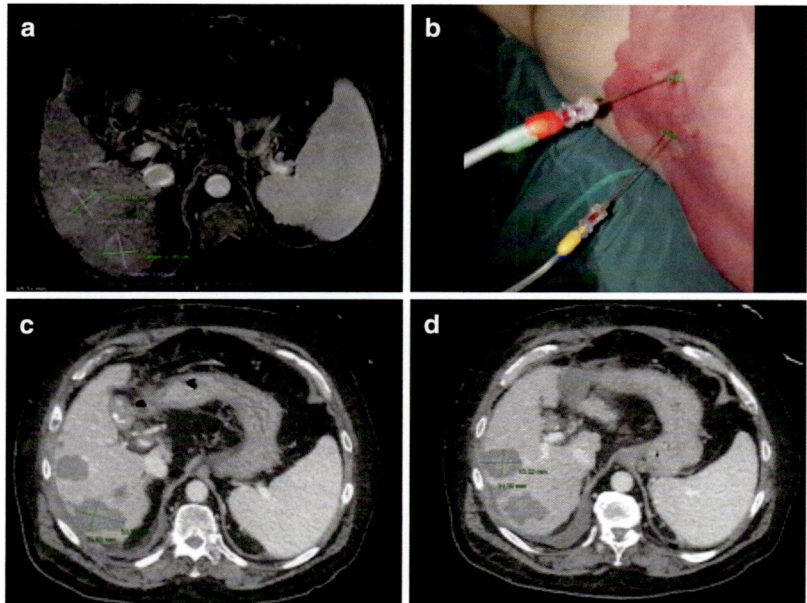

Fig. 16.1 Representative cases of HCC of 3 cm in maximum diameter completely ablated using novel guidance system and two heat sources. (**a**) MRI imaging showing two recurrent HCC in the sixth segment 32 and 34 mm in size in a patient with low platelet count (35,000/mm³). (**b**) Due to coagulopathy only two needles in each nodule were inserted. (**c, d**) CT imaging showing complete necrosis of nodules. Ablation area was 53 × 34 mm and 43 × 31 mm, respectively, after delivering of 10,800 J per lesion. It is noteworthy that the two lesions were treated simultaneously in the same session of LA (courtesy of Dr. Giovan Guseppe Di Costanzo, A. Cardarelli Hospital, Naples, Italy)

Fig. 16.2 Representative US images of the 43 × 31 mm coagulation zone of the sixth segment appreciable in Fig. 12.1c, d obtained after the ablation maneuver. **e-1**. US axial image after LA treatment and **e-2**. US axial image during the administration of ecocontrast shows large non-vascularized coagulation zone (courtesy of Dr. Giovan Giuseppe Di Costanzo, A. Cardarelli Hospital, Naples, Italy)

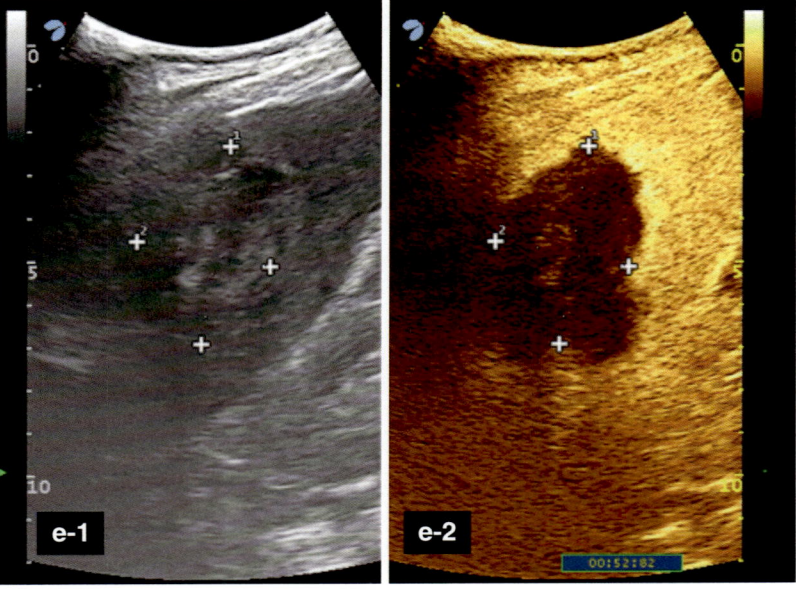

An interesting role could have the laser methodology in the percutaneous treatment of renal cell carcinoma in stage T1a, to date prevalent prerogative of RFA and cryotherapy, especially in cases at risk of bleeding [10] (Chap. 6).

An interesting chapter should be opened in the treatment of early-stage breast cancer (T1a and T1b according to TNM). Furthermore, a much more interesting field of investigation could be the treatment of small (≤2 cm) breast lesions classified as lesions of uncertain malignant potential (B3) that are a heterogeneous group of abnormalities with a borderline histological spectrum, and a variable but low risk of associated neoplasia [38, 39] (Chap. 10).

The trans-gastric endoscopic treatment of the endocrine and neoplastic focal lesions of the pancreas with curative and palliative intent is undoubtedly an interesting application certainly anticipating future developments with relevant clinical results. The thinness of the fibers facilitates the endoscopic approach compared to other ablative techniques [40–43]. However, this particular approach should be considered in particular cases because the percutaneous route is very useful and handy, especially when it is necessary to place several applicators for lesions larger than 2–3 cm (Chap. 11).

As we have already succinctly reported in the 3rd and more extensively in the 12th chapter of this book, the ablation of the primary and secondary nodular pathology of the lung is, in our opinion, much easier and profitable with laser light because this methodology is not conditioned by electrical conductivity of the lung, as it happens with the radiofrequency and with its dielectric properties as the relative capacity of storage of energy (permittivity—how much a material will be able to store the charge) and the mass conductivity (the loss of energy inside the material) which influences the heating of tissue induced by microwaves [44]. In other words, due to the reduced influence of the pulmonary electrical conductivity in the deposition of heat, there is a greater diffusion of energy in the tissue and therefore it is possible to obtain larger areas of coagulation of predictable volume [45]. Not to mention the advantage of having very thin and manageable introducers with far fewer complications [4, 46–48] (Chap. 12).

The pioneering approach to percutaneous treatment of benign thyroid lesions has long been known. Since the early 1990s the group of Rome has hypothesized and developed the debulking of benign cold thyroid nodules with well-established and validated results such as to propose this treatment as an alternative to the surgical approach [49, 50]. The rationale behind this proposal is the finding that "the occurrence of thyroid nodular disease in the general population is definitely high and the number of benign lesions that grow or become symptomatic accordingly increasing. In these cases, a timely and appropriate use of thermal ablation is followed by the modification of the natural history of the growing benign nodules. Therefore, non-surgical treatment of nodules that are cause of concern avoids the unfavorable influence of thyroidectomy on quality of life (due to aesthetic damage and long-term replacement therapy), decreases direct and indirect costs of treatment and allows more appropriate use of surgical facilities" (Chap. 7).

For pre-toxic and toxic nodules, interesting studies have recently been conducted to reduce the administration of radioiodine in large nodules above 13 mL—combined treatment—and to completely eliminate the use of radioiodine therapy in nodules of less than 13 mL [51, 52] (Chap. 7).

The percutaneous approach is proving very useful in the treatment of a few thyroid carcinomas such as papillary microcarcinoma (PTM) or anaplastic carcinoma and more generally in the disease of the neck and secondary malignant lymph nodes [7, 53–55] (Chap. 8).

Finally, we must emphasize the interesting chapter on opening in the percutaneous treatment of benign prostatic hyperplasia (BPH). There are numerous surgical and minimally invasive therapies in BPH treatment and urologists are always looking for new solutions. Starting from some long-standing studies published at the dawn of laser technology in the 1990s [56] in which the percutaneous treatment of BPH was performed with an extra-urethral transperineal approach, we again proposed this option using thin needles. It is easy to think that this solution makes this approach easier and more manageable compared to the old solutions with larger devices and more complex systems [57]. There are now results in the medium-long term (average follow-up period of 16 months—data not yet published) that attest to the validity of the method and the durability over time of the improvements. Additionally, the thin needle is easy to use in the ablation of localized non-advanced prostate cancer. Even in this specific field of research, this option could be very useful and gives us interesting results, helping to reduce the excessive number of patients subjected to surgical and radiotherapy overtreatments [58–61] (Chap. 13).

Preliminary experimental studies in vitro and ex vivo with different types of nanoparticles have described the various mechanisms with which the nanosystem induces the death of cells such as pancreatic cancer by apoptosis for depolarization of the mitochondrial membrane or decreasing cell proliferation thanks to the progressive increase of nanoparticles in the tissue with consequent increase of power density applied [62–64]. The presence of nanoparticles in tumor tissue reinforces the specificity of focal laser ablation for tumor tissue and reduces the morbidity of adjacent healthy tissue as demonstrated, albeit not specifically, in prostatic adenocarcinoma [58, 60, 61]. All these experimental experiences will, in the close future, lead to clinical applications at least in particular types of tumors. The mechanism of action of nanoparticles can be used effectively for example in the multimodal selective treatment of a very aggressive tumor such as pancreatic cancer or in localized and non-advanced tumors such as those of the prostate. In both cases, the preferential accumulation of nanoparticles in the target area selectively confines heat into the tumor leading to complete ablation without damaging adjacent vital structures such as those surrounding the pancreas or prostate gland [65, 66]. The simultaneous measurement of tissue temperature can also provide crucial information about the status of the ongoing treatment and can support the clinician in the real-time optimization of the procedure. The laser-nanoparticle combination or drug-aided photocoagulation methods can represent a very interesting frontier of research for the future, but to date commercially available systems do not yet seem to add value to the laser alone, in terms of neither efficacy nor safety.

Furthermore, although we have not devoted a chapter to the discussion of laser applications in brain pathology in this book, we cannot close this last chapter without mentioning the use of the laser technology with cooled devices in the management of radiosurgery-resistant metastases,

radiation necrosis, surgically inaccessible malignant gliomas, and ablation of epileptogenic foci [22]. It is noteworthy that neurosurgical operators use the same devices that have been used in phase 1 studies in the focal treatment of non-advanced prostate cancer [67].

16.3 Conclusion

It is our strong belief that laser represents one of the most vivid and most versatile minimally invasive techniques for percutaneous ablation [68, 69]. The very small caliber of the applicators, together with the high precision of energy delivery and the high predictability of the ablated zone, makes this technique still extremely fascinating. Several new clinical applications have been recently reported, with a potentially relevant impact on the medicine of tomorrow. Clinical studies on larger series and in novel application will provide more robust results on the potential clinical role of laser, and technological advancements, such as the application of nanoparticles, will easily open new scenarios in the next future.

References

1. Niemz MH. Laser-Tissue Interactions -Fundamental and Applications. New York: Springer-Verlag; 2004.
2. Jordan DJ, Mafi P, Mafi R, Malahias M, Gawad AE. The Use of LASER and its Further Development in Varying Aspects of Surgery. Open Med J. 2016;3(3):288–99.
3. Ahmed M, Brace CL, Lee FT Jr, Goldberg SN. Principles of and advances in percutaneous ablation. Radiology. 2011;258(2):351–69.
4. Weigel C, Rosenberg C, Langner S, Frohlich CP, Hosten N. Laser ablation of lung metastases: results according to diameter and location. Eur Radiol. 2006;16(8):1769–78.
5. Francica G, Petrolati A, Di Stasio E, Pacella S, Stasi R, Pacella CM. Effectiveness, safety, and local progression after percutaneous laser ablation for hepatocellular carcinoma nodules up to 4 cm are not affected by tumor location. AJR Am J Roentgenol. 2012;199(6):1393–401.
6. Di Costanzo GG, Tortora R, D'Adamo G, De Luca M, Lampasi F, Addario L, et al. Radiofrequency ablation versus laser ablation for the treatment of small hepatocellular carcinoma in cirrhosis: a randomized trial. J Gastroenterol Hepatol. 2015;30(3):559–65.

7. Mauri G, Cova L, Ierace T, Baroli A, Di Mauro E, Pacella CM, et al. Treatment of metastatic lymph nodes in the neck from papillary thyroid carcinoma with percutaneous laser ablation. Cardiovasc Intervent Radiol. 2016;39(7):1023–30.

8. Arienti V, Pretolani S, Pacella CM, Magnolfi F, Caspani B, Francica G, et al. Complications of laser ablation for hepatocellular carcinoma: a multicenter study. Radiology. 2008;246(3):947–55.

9. Pacella CM, Francica G, Di Lascio FM, Arienti V, Antico E, Caspani B, et al. Long-term outcome of cirrhotic patients with early hepatocellular carcinoma treated with ultrasound-guided percutaneous laser ablation: a retrospective analysis. J Clin Oncol. 2009;27(16):2615–21.

10. Sartori S, Mauri G, Tombesi P, Di Vece F, Bianchi L, Pacella CM. Ultrasound-guided percutaneous laser ablation is safe and effective in the treatment of small renal tumors in patients at increased bleeding risk. Int J Hyperth. 2018;35(1):19–25.

11. Muller GJ, Roggan A. Laser-induced interstitial thermotherapy. Washington SPIE-The International Society for Optical Engineering: Bellingham; 1995.

12. Heisterkamp J, van Hillegersberg R, Sinofsky E, JN IJ. Heat-resistant cylindrical diffuser for interstitial laser coagulation: comparison with the baretip fiber in a porcine liver model. Lasers Surg Med. 1997;20(3):304–9.

13. Heisterkamp J, van Hillegersberg R, Mulder PG, Sinofsky EL, JN IJ. Importance of eliminating portal flow to produce large intrahepatic lesions with interstitial laser coagulation. Br J Surg. 1997;84(9): 1245–8.

14. Pacella CM, Bizzarri G, Francica G, Bianchini A, De Nuntis S, Pacella S, et al. Percutaneous laser ablation in the treatment of hepatocellular carcinoma with small tumors: analysis of factors affecting the achievement of tumor necrosis. J Vasc Interv Radiol. 2005;16(11):1447–57.

15. Vogl TJ, Kreutztrager M, Gruber-Rouh T, Eichler K, Nour-Eldin NE, Zangos S, et al. Neoadjuvant TACE before laser induced thermotherapy (LITT) in the treatment of non-colorectal non-breast cancer liver metastases: feasibility and survival rates. Eur J Radiol. 2014;83(10):1804–10.

16. Fiedler VU, Schwarzmaier HJ, Eickmeyer F, Muller FP, Schoepp C, Verreet PR. Laser-induced interstitial thermotherapy of liver metastases in an interventional 0.5 Tesla MRI system: technique and first clinical experiences. J Magn Reson Imaging. 2001;13(5):729–37.

17. Sequeiros RB, Hyvonen P, Sequeiros AB, Jyrkinen L, Ojala R, Klemola R, et al. MR imaging-guided laser ablation of osteoid osteomas with use of optical instrument guidance at 0.23 T. Eur Radiol. 2003;13(10):2309–14.

18. Lindner U, Lawrentschuk N, Trachtenberg J. Focal laser ablation for localized prostate cancer. J Endourol. 2010;24(5):791–7.

19. Raz O, Haider MA, Davidson SR, Lindner U, Hlasny E, Weersink R, et al. Real-time magnetic resonance imaging-guided focal laser therapy in patients with low-risk prostate cancer. Eur Urol. 2010;58(1):173–7.

20. Stafford RJ, Fuentes D, Elliott AA, Weinberg JS, Ahrar K. Laser-induced thermal therapy for tumor ablation. Crit Rev Biomed Eng. 2010;38(1): 79–100.

21. Stafford RJ, Shetty A, Elliott AM, Klumpp SA, McNichols RJ, Gowda A, et al. Magnetic resonance guided, focal laser induced interstitial thermal therapy in a canine prostate model. J Urol. 2010;184(4):1514–20.

22. Sharma M, Balasubramanian S, Silva D, Barnett GH, Mohammadi AM. Laser interstitial thermal therapy in the management of brain metastasis and radiation necrosis after radiosurgery: An overview. Expert Rev Neurother. 2016;16(2):223–32.

23. Natarajan S, Raman S, Priester AM, Garritano J, Margolis DJ, Lieu P, et al. Focal Laser Ablation of Prostate Cancer: Phase I Clinical Trial. J Urol. 2016;196(1):68–75.

24. Galle PR, Forner A, Llovet JM, Mazzaferro V, Piscaglia F, Raoul J-L, et al. EASL Clinical Practice Guidelines: Management of hepatocellular carcinoma. J Hepatol. 2018;69:182–236.

25. Pacella CM, Francica G, Di Costanzo GG. Laser ablation: an alternative to radiofrequency ablation for hepatocellular carcinoma in cirrhotic patients? Hepat Oncol. 2015;2(2):111–5.

26. Di Costanzo GG, D'Adamo G, Tortora R, Zanfardino F, Mattera S, Francica G, et al. A novel needle guide system to perform percutaneous laser ablation of liver tumors using the multifiber technique. Acta Radiol. 2013;54(8):876–81.

27. Di Costanzo GG, Francica G, Pacella CM. Laser ablation for small hepatocellular carcinoma: State of the art and future perspectives. World J Hepatol. 2014;6(10):704–15.

28. Vogl TJ, Straub R, Eichler K, Woitaschek D, Mack MG. Malignant liver tumors treated with MR imaging-guided laser-induced thermotherapy: experience with complications in 899 patients (2,520 lesions). Radiology. 2002;225(2):367–77.

29. Vogl TJ, Dommermuth A, Heinle B, Nour-Eldin NE, Lehnert T, Eichler K, et al. Colorectal cancer liver metastases: long-term survival and progression-free survival after thermal ablation using magnetic resonance-guided laser-induced interstitial thermotherapy in 594 patients: analysis of prognostic factors. Investig Radiol. 2014;49(1):48–56.

30. Francica G, Petrolati A, Di Stasio E, Pacella S, Stasi R, Pacella CM. Influence of ablative margin on local tumor progression and survival in patients with HCC </=4 cm after laser ablation. Acta Radiol. 2012;53(4):394–400.

31. Shyn PB, Mauri G, Alencar RO, Tatli S, Shah SH, Morrison PR, et al. Percutaneous imaging-guided cryoablation of liver tumors: predicting local

progression on 24-hour MRI. AJR Am J Roentgenol. 2014;203(2):W181–91.

32. Tombesi P, Di Vece F, Sartori S. Laser ablation for hepatic metastases from neuroendocrine tumors. AJR Am J Roentgenol. 2015;204(6):W732.

33. Pacella C, Nasoni S, Grimaldi F, Di Stasio E, Misischi I, Bianchetti S, et al. Laser ablation with or without chemoembolization for unresectable neuroendocrine liver metastases: a pilot study. Int J Endo Oncol. 2016;3(2):97–107.

34. Pacella CM, Stasi R, Bizzarri G, Pacella S, Graziano FM, Guglielmi R, et al. Percutaneous laser ablation of unresectable primary and metastatic adrenocortical carcinoma. Eur J Radiol. 2008;66(1):88–94.

35. Jiang T, Deng Z, Tian G, Chen F, Bao H, Li J, et al. Percutaneous laser ablation: a new contribution to unresectable high-risk metastatic retroperitoneal lesions? Oncotarget. 2017;8(2):2413–22.

36. Jiang T, Chai W. Endoscopic ultrasonography (EUS)-guided laser ablation (LA) of adrenal metastasis from pancreatic adenocarcinoma. Lasers Med Sci. 2018;33(7):1613–6.

37. Yun M, Zhao Q, Zhong L, Chen F, Jiang T. Preliminary results of ultrasound-guided laser ablation for unresectable metastases to retroperitoneal and hepatic portal lymph nodes. World J Surg Oncol. 2016; 14:165.

38. Nori J, Gill MK, Meattini I, Delli Paoli C, Abdulcadir D, Vanzi E, et al. The evolving role of ultrasound guided percutaneous laser ablation in elderly unresectable breast cancer patients: a feasibility pilot study. Biomed Res Int. 2018;2018:9141746.

39. Mauri G, Sconfienza LM, Sardanelli F. Imaging-guided Percutaneous Ablation: A Step Forward to Minimize the Invasiveness of Breast Cancer Treatment. Radiology. 2019;290(3):849–50.

40. Di Matteo F, Picconi F, Martino M, Pandolfi M, Pacella CM, Schena E, et al. Endoscopic ultrasound-guided Nd:YAG laser ablation of recurrent pancreatic neuroendocrine tumor: a promising revolution? Endoscopy. 2014;46(Suppl 1):UCTN:E380-1.

41. Di Matteo F, Grasso R, Pacella CM, Martino M, Pandolfi M, Rea R, et al. EUS-guided Nd:YAG laser ablation of a hepatocellular carcinoma in the caudate lobe. Gastrointest Endosc. 2011;73(3): 632–6.

42. Di Matteo FM, Saccomandi P, Martino M, Pandolfi M, Pizzicannella M, Balassone V, et al. Feasibility of EUS-guided Nd:YAG laser ablation of unresectable pancreatic adenocarcinoma. Gastrointest Endosc. 2018;88(1):168–74 e1.

43. Jiang T, Guo Tian G, Bao H, Chen F, Deng Z, Ba JL, et al. EUS dating with laser ablation against the caudate lobe or left liver tumors: a win–win proposition? Cancer Biol Ther. 2018;19(3):145–52.

44. Schepps JL, Foster KR. The UHF and microwave dielectric properties of normal and tumour tissues: variation in dielectric properties with tissue water content. Phys Med Biol. 1980;25(6):1149–59.

45. Knappe V, Mols A. Laser therapy of the lung: biophysical background. Radiologe. 2004;44(7):677–83.

46. Zhao Q, Tian G, Chen F, Zhong L, Jiang T. CT-guided percutaneous laser ablation of metastatic lung cancer: three cases report and literature review. Oncotarget. 2017;8(2):2187–96.

47. Regine R, Stavolo C, Maglione F. Laser thermoablation of small pulmonary tumors: immediate and long-term follow-up CT features. In: C 23; First World Congress of Thoracic Imaging and Diagnosis in Chest Disease. Naples: Pozzuoli; 2005.

48. Sponza M, Aprile G, Gasparini D, Iaiza E, De Pauli F, Giovannoni M, et al. Percutaneous laser-induced thermoablation (LIT) of non-resectable lung metastases and primary lung tumors: A preliminary evaluation of technical aspects and local efficiency. ASCO Annual Meeting Proceedings (Post-Meeting Edition). J Clin Oncol. 2006;24:18S.

49. Papini E, Rago T, Gambelunghe G, Valcavi R, Bizzarri G, Vitti P, et al. Long-term efficacy of ultrasound-guided laser ablation for benign solid thyroid nodules. Results of a three-year multicenter prospective randomized trial. J Clin Endocrinol Metab. 2014;99(10):3653–9.

50. Pacella CM, Mauri G, Achille G, Barbaro D, Bizzarri G, De Feo P, et al. Outcomes and Risk Factors for Complications of Laser Ablation for Thyroid Nodules: A Multicenter Study on 1531 Patients. J Clin Endocrinol Metab. 2015;100(10):3903–10.

51. Chianelli M, Bizzarri G, Todino V, Misischi I, Bianchini A, Graziano F, et al. Laser ablation and 131-iodine: a 24-month pilot study of combined treatment for large toxic nodular goiter. J Clin Endocrinol Metab. 2014;99(7):E1283–6.

52. Pacella CM, Mauri G. Is there a role for minimally invasive thermal ablations in the treatment of autonomously functioning thyroid nodules? Int J Hyperth. 2018;34(5):636–8.

53. Pacella CM, Bizzarri G, Spiezia S, Bianchini A, Guglielmi R, Crescenzi A, et al. Thyroid tissue: US-guided percutaneous laser thermal ablation. Radiology. 2004;232(1):272–80.

54. Papini E, Guglielmi R, Gharib H, Misischi I, Graziano F, Chianelli M, et al. Ultrasound-guided laser ablation of incidental papillary thyroid microcarcinoma: a potential therapeutic approach in patients at surgical risk. Thyroid. 2011;21(8):917–20.

55. Valcavi R, Piana S, Bortolan GS, Lai R, Barbieri V, Negro R. Ultrasound-guided percutaneous laser ablation of papillary thyroid microcarcinoma: a feasibility study on three cases with pathological and immunohistochemical evaluation. Thyroid. 2013;23(12):1578–82.

56. Mueller-Lisse UG, Thoma M, Faber S, Heuck AF, Muschter R, Schneede P, et al. Coagulative interstitial laser-induced thermotherapy of benign prostatic hyperplasia: online imaging with a T2-weighted fast spin-echo MR sequence--experience in six patients. Radiology. 1999;210(2):373–9.

57. Patelli G, Ranieri A, Paganelli A, Mauri G, Pacella CM. Transperineal laser ablation for percutaneous treatment of benign prostatic hyperplasia: a feasibility study. Cardiovasc Intervent Radiol. 2017;40(9):1440–6.

58. Feng Y, Fuentes D, Hawkins A, Bass J, Rylander MN, Elliott A, et al. Nanoshell-mediated laser surgery simulation for prostate cancer treatment. Eng Comput. 2009;25(1):3–13.

59. Stern JM, Cadeddu JA. Emerging use of nanoparticles for the therapeutic ablation of urologic malignancies. Urol Oncol. 2008;26(1):93–6.

60. Stern JM, Stanfield J, Kabbani W, Hsieh JT, Cadeddu JA. Selective prostate cancer thermal ablation with laser activated gold nanoshells. J Urol. 2008;179(2):748–53.

61. Schwartz JA, Price RE, Gill-Sharp KL, Sang KL, Khorchani J, Goodwin BS, et al. Selective nanoparticle-directed ablation of the canine prostate. Lasers Surg Med. 2011;43(3):213–20.

62. Mocan L, Tabaran FA, Mocan T, Bele C, Orza AI, Lucan C, et al. Selective ex-vivo photothermal ablation of human pancreatic cancer with albumin functionalized multiwalled carbon nanotubes. Int J Nanomedicine. 2011;6:915–28.

63. Mocan T, Matea CT, Cojocaru I, Ilie I, Tabaran FA, Zaharie F, et al. Photothermal treatment of human pancreatic cancer using pegylated multi-walled carbon nanotubes induces apoptosis by triggering mitochondrial membrane depolarization mechanism. J Cancer. 2014;5(8):679–88.

64. Guo Y, Zhang Z, Kim DH, Li W, Nicolai J, Procissi D, et al. Photothermal ablation of pancreatic cancer cells with hybrid iron-oxide core gold-shell nanoparticles. Int J Nanomedicine. 2013;8:3437–46.

65. Saccomandi P, Lapergola A, Longo F, Schena E, Quero G. Thermal ablation of pancreatic cancer: A systematic literature review of clinical practice and pre-clinical studies. Int J Hyperth. 2018: 1–21.

66. Colin P, Mordon S, Nevoux P, Marqa MF, Ouzzane A, Puech P, et al. Focal laser ablation of prostate cancer: definition, needs, and future. Adv Urol. 2012;2012:589160.

67. Lindner U, Weersink RA, Haider MA, Gertner MR, Davidson SR, Atri M, et al. Image guided photothermal focal therapy for localized prostate cancer: phase I trial. J Urol. 2009;182(4):1371–7.

68. Sartori S, Di Vece F, Ermili F, Tombesi P. Laser ablation of liver tumors: An ancillary technique, or an alternative to radiofrequency and microwave? World J Radiol. 2017;9(3):91–6.

69. Schena E, Saccomandi P, Fong Y. Laser Ablation for Cancer: Past, Present and Future. J Funct Biomater. 2017;8:2.

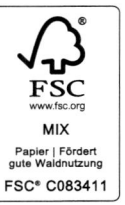

Zeitfracht Medien GmbH
Ferdinand-Jühlke-Straße 7
99095 Erfurt, Deutschland
produktsicherheit@kolibri360.de